PCAT *

Pharmacy College Admission Test

6TH EDITION

Marie A. Chisholm-Burns, Pharm.D., MPH, MBA, FCCP, FASHP
Dean and Professor
University of Tennessee College of Pharmacy
Memphis, Knoxville, and Nashville, Tennessee

Contributing Authors:

Alan Wolfgang, Ph.D.
Assistant Dean for Student Affairs
The University of Georgia College of Pharmacy
Athens, Georgia

Mark A. McCombs, M.S.
Senior Lecturer, Department of Mathematics
University of North Carolina at Chapel Hill
Chapel Hill, North Carolina

Suzanne Carpenter, M.S.
Associate Professor of Chemistry
Armstrong Atlantic State University
College of Science and Technology
Savannah, Georgia

Christina Spivey, Ph.D.
Assistant Professor
Department of Clinical Pharmacy
University of Tennessee College of Pharmacy
Memphis, Tennessee

Sara Gremillion, Ph.D.
Assistant Professor, Department of Biology
Armstrong Atlantic State University
College of Science and Technology
Savannah, Georgia

BARRON'S

*PCAT is a registered trademark of Pearson, which does not endorse this book.

ISBN: 978-1-4380-0381-8

Library of Congress Catalog Card No.: 2014931004

10%
POST-CONSUMER
WASTE
Paper contains a minimum
of 10% post-consumer
waste (PCW). Paper used
in this book was derived
from certified, sustainable
forestlands.

PRINTED IN THE UNITED STATES OF AMERICA
9 8 7 6 5 4 3 2 1

Contents

Introduction

For many colleges and schools of pharmacy, grades achieved in college pre-pharmacy courses and Pharmacy College Admission Test (PCAT) scores are the most important criteria used to evaluate students for admission. Therefore, it is very important for you to perform your very best on the PCAT. The PCAT was developed to provide college admission committees with comparable information about the academic abilities of applicants in designated areas.

This study guide can be very useful in preparing you for the PCAT, and for pharmacy education in general. When used properly and in combination with other materials, this guide will enhance your chances in the applicant pool of a college or school of pharmacy. All chapters are written by practicing pharmacists and/or educators (professors or instructors) with extensive experience in the admission procedures of U.S. pharmacy schools. In addition, each of the chapter authors has special expertise in the designated subject; this will further help you do your best on the PCAT.

This guide should help focus your review by outlining and reviewing subjects that are currently included on the PCAT. In addition, this guide can be very useful in the early stages of your pre-pharmacy education by pointing out the areas that will be covered on the PCAT. Thus, you will be able to prioritize topics for studying, a step that will aid you in achieving your desired score.

Remember, your pre-pharmacy courses are designed to serve as the foundation for your pharmacy education, and the PCAT is intended to determine your grasp of this material and your ability to apply it during your continued education. To be successful on the PCAT, it is important that you not only understand the material in a particular course, but that you can also apply it in your future program of higher education. If you take your pre-pharmacy courses with this in mind, the PCAT should be less difficult.

Use this and any other study guide as just that—a guide to what and how to study. The chance that the same exact questions contained in this text will be on the exam you take is remote; however, the likelihood that the same material will be covered is great. When reviewing a particular question, do not just look for the sentence or phrase that "answers the question"; study the topic and refresh your understanding of the material. Pay particular attention to facts that are related but differ in a "testable" way. For example, do you remember the terms *mitosis* and *meiosis*? You may remember these words and perhaps know that they have something to do with cell propagation, but that is not enough. If the multiple-choice answers to a question on the PCAT include descriptions of both mitosis and meiosis, you must be able to distinguish between the terms to select the correct answer, or risk receiving no more credit than someone who never took a biology course.

This book reviews all sections of the PCAT (as of 2014) and therefore serves as a good focal point to begin studying for the exam. Please keep in mind, however, that this is a guide; its purpose is not to review all required pre-pharmacy courses, but rather to aid you in studying for the PCAT. For optimal performance, it is strongly suggested that you use this guide along with your pre-pharmacy coursework to prepare for the PCAT.

FORMAT AND USE OF THIS BOOK

The format of this book is user-friendly. Chapter 1 covers general information about the pharmacy profession, pharmacy school admissions, and pharmacy education. In Chapters 2 and 3, general information on the PCAT and specific test-taking strategies and tactics are presented, respectively. Six chapters addressing verbal ability, biology, chemistry, quantitative ability, reading comprehension, and essay writing follow. Also, each chapter (with the exception of the essay chapter) has a set of questions with full explanatory answers to test, review, and enhance your knowledge of the various subjects. The chapter on writing your PCAT essay contains helpful tips on writing effectively. Finally, so you can practice taking the exam and evaluate your skills, two sample PCATs with full explanatory answers are provided in Chapters 10 and 11.

Planning for a Career in Pharmacy

A CAREER IN PHARMACY

Over the last few decades, pharmacy practice has undergone significant changes. Since the 1960s, the pharmacy profession has branched out in many directions other than traditional pharmacy settings (community and hospital). Once you have graduated from pharmacy school and have successfully passed a pharmacy state board licensure examination, career opportunities in pharmacy are great. These opportunities include, but are not limited to, community pharmacy (chain and independent), hospital pharmacy, pharmaceutical industry, government agencies, geriatric pharmacy, clinical pharmacy, pharmacy services, managed-care pharmacy, pharmaceutical research, pharmacy and medical education, nuclear pharmacy, and other specialty areas.

Job opportunities are diverse for a person who earns a degree in pharmacy. In addition, postgraduate training or graduate education provides an excellent opportunity for continuing your pharmacy education, thereby enhancing your career opportunities in this field. Although career counseling is best done in a pharmacy program, the purpose of this section is to familiarize you with several pharmacy careers (see the list that follows). Once accepted into a pharmacy school, you should inquire further about career opportunities in pharmacy.

Examples of Career Opportunities in Pharmacy

Academia
  Administration
  Biological Science
  Clinical Pharmacy
  Continuing Education
  Experiential Education
  Medicinal Chemistry
  Pharmaceutics
  Pharmacy Administration
  Pharmacy Practice

Administration
  Continuing Education
  Professional Relations
Business
  Administration
  Management
  Marketing
  Sales
Chain (Community)
  Apothecary
  Franchise
  Home Health Care
  Long-term Care
  Specialty Pharmacy

Clinical
Adult Medicine
Ambulatory Care
Clinical Coordinator
Clinical Manager
Critical Care
Drug Information
Family Medicine
Geriatrics
Infectious Disease
Internal Medicine
Nutrition
Oncology
Pain Management
Pediatrics
Pharmacokinetics
Poison Control
Psychiatry
Surgery
Transplantation
Computer Technology
Consultant
Clinical Pharmacy
Home Health Care
Long-term Care
Drug Information
Federal
Alcohol, Drug Abuse, and
Mental Health
Armed Services
Clinical Pharmacy
Drug Enforcement Administration
Food and Drug Administration
Health Administration
Health Care Financing
Indian Health Services
Hospital
Administration
Clinical Pharmacy
Inventory Control
Staff

Independent
Clinical Pharmacy
Franchise
Home Health Care
Long-term Care
Specialty Pharmacy
Industry
Regulatory Affairs
Medical Communication
Medication Safety
Mail-Order Pharmacy
Managed Care Pharmacy
Nuclear Pharmacy
Pharmacy Associations
Research and Development
Biological Sciences
Clinical Outcomes
Informatics
Medicinal Chemistry
Pharmaceutical Research
Pharmaceutics
Pharmacogenomics
Pharmacognosy
Pharmacology
Pharmacy Administration
Pharmacy Practice
State
Board of Pharmacy
Clinical Outcomes
Department of Consumer
Affairs
Department of Health
Technical/Scientific
Drug Information
Manufacturing
Postmarketing Surveillance
Product Control
Veterans Administration Facilities

IMPORTANT CONSIDERATIONS IN PLANNING YOUR PHARMACY EDUCATION

On the following page is a flowchart that displays some general guidelines to help you in planning your pharmacy education and completing the admission process at a U.S. college/school of pharmacy. For additional information, refer to the pre-pharmacy advisor at the institution where you are taking your pre-pharmacy required courses and the college/school of pharmacy you wish to attend. The information given in this chapter should not replace or supersede information obtained from your pre-pharmacy advisor or the college/school of pharmacy in which you would like to continue your education.

Pre-Pharmacy Curricula

You should be familiar with the requirements of each of the institutions to which you plan to apply. Many students who apply to pharmacy school have more than the minimum pre-pharmacy course requirements and/or have attended college for more than two years. The pre-pharmacy required coursework may be able to be completed within two years (of course, this depends on the individual requirements of the pharmacy school); however, there are some schools that require more than two years of coursework. Obviously, the pre-pharmacy curricula at each school may vary, but there are typically some similarities that will give you an idea of the type of courses required. Below is an outline detailing the subject areas covered by many pre-pharmacy curricula. Please note: additional coursework may be required and the courses listed below may or may not be required at many schools of pharmacy; therefore, it is imperative to check with the school of pharmacy for its exact pre-pharmacy requirements.

Remember

The information provided in this book regarding the PCAT is current at the time of the book's writing; for the most recent PCAT updates and information, please refer to the official PCAT website at *www.pcatweb.info.*

PRE-PHARMACY CURRICULUM OUTLINE

- Humanities and Fine Arts Courses
  - English—two courses or one year.
  - Literature—one course.
  - Communication/Speech—one course.
- Social Science Courses
  - History—one or more courses.
  - Political Science—one course. This may be covered with an additional History course.
  - Economics—one course.
  - Other Social Science elective—one course (e.g., Sociology, Psychology, Anthropology, or additional History courses).
- Math and Science Courses
  - Pre-Calculus—one course. Some programs may only require Calculus courses, but prerequisites may be required of some post-secondary applicants.
  - Calculus/Analytical Geometry—one or two courses.
  - Statistics—one course.

PHARMACY SCHOOL APPLICANT GUIDELINES

Identify pharmacy school(s) of interest.
Important considerations that may help you
in the identification process include:
- school's geographical location;
- your program preference;
- cost and scholarship availability;
- school's reputation; and
- academic requirements for admission.

Identify what pre-pharmacy courses are required.
- This information will vary between different
  pharmacy schools.
- Since many pre-pharmacy courses are sequential,
  it is important to focus on the scheduling of courses.
- As soon as possible, make an appointment
  to consult with the pre-pharmacy advisor
  at your school.

Take pre-pharmacy courses.
- It is important to make the best grades and
  get the best background possible in these
  courses. Keep materials from courses as they
  may be helpful to study for the PCAT.

**Apply to pharmacy school(s) and/or
PharmCAS (*www.pharmcas.org*).**
Check with your pre-pharmacy advisor
concerning the most appropriate
time to apply.
- Apply as early as possible and when
  appropriate, considering when you will
  be finished with pre-pharmacy requirements.
- If faculty or personal references are
  required, select professors and others who
  know you well, will provide a good
  reference, and will send it in *on time*.
- If the school utilizes PharmCAS, check to
  see if supplemental forms are required.

Register to take the PCAT.
Allow yourself the opportunity to take
the PCAT more than once; check with
your pre-pharmacy advisor and the
PCAT website (*www.pcatweb.info*)
for scheduling and registration.
Check with the pharmacy school(s)
concerning policy on taking the PCAT
more than once and how multiple
PCAT scores are considered in the
admission process.

**Complete the application
process and await status letter.**
Make sure you follow up if you
are offered admission. You will
need to confirm and may have
to provide a tuition deposit and/or
complete a background check.

**Check with each pharmacy
school/college about interview.**

**Is the PCAT required by
the pharmacy school(s)
to which you are applying?**

YES

NO

- Biological Sciences—two courses or one year with labs. Some programs may require Anatomy and Physiology and/or Microbiology as pre-pharmacy courses.
- Chemistry—four courses or two years. These courses include General Chemistry and Organic Chemistry with labs. Some programs may require Biochemistry.
- Physics—up to two courses or one year. Physics is not required by some programs.

Each institution's program will have its own pre-pharmacy course requirements; you should obtain this information directly from the desired school. Many colleges and universities offer pre-professional advising programs to assist students in course selection. Utilize these advisors and the recruitment and admission staff of your desired pharmacy program as important resources. Since many programs only accept students once a year, if you do not complete the pre-pharmacy curriculum by the designated time, it may delay acceptance by an entire academic year. If you have previously completed coursework for which you expect to receive credit, in lieu of some specific pre-pharmacy prerequisites, verify whether the course will satisfy requirements early in your application process.

Doctorate of Pharmacy Degree Curricula

DOCTORATE OF PHARMACY DEGREE ("2+4," "3+4," AND "4+4" PROGRAMS)

Each school or college of pharmacy has a list of courses that are considered prerequisites to the pharmacy professional program. For many schools, the pre-pharmacy prerequisites can take two years or longer to complete. A two-year pre-pharmacy curriculum, along with the four-year professional curriculum, comprises what is called a "2+4" professional doctor of pharmacy degree program. There are a few pharmacy programs in which students take courses year round (i.e., they attend classes in the summer), and thereby complete the equivalent of a standard four-year curriculum in three calendar years. Some programs require three years of pre-pharmacy coursework ("3+4" program). Some programs require eighty or more hours of pre-pharmacy coursework, and may even require applicants to have earned a bachelor's degree (such programs are referred to as "4+4" programs); thus, it could take considerably longer than two years to complete the pre-pharmacy requirements for many schools.

DOCTORATE OF PHARMACY DEGREE ("0+6" PROGRAM)

Another variation of the "2+4" program is the "0+6" program. This program allows students to be accepted directly into the school or college of pharmacy where they will complete the pre-pharmacy core as part of a six-year academic program. Most of these programs also consider applicants to the professional program; however, if the student is accepted, he or she will enter at the beginning of the third year of the program.

PharmCAS

The Pharmacy College Application Service (PharmCAS) is a centralized application service designed to assemble, process, and distribute applicants' information. Some

TIP

Familiarize yourself with PharmCAS by obtaining information from their online site, *www.PharmCAS.org.*

pharmacy programs utilize this service to gather admission data from applicants, advisors, and other sources. The system is similar to those used by other professional programs such as medical schools, law schools, and veterinary medicine programs. The PharmCAS system has been used by some schools since the early 2000s application cycle, but is not used by all pharmacy programs. The information presented here is current as of the preparation of this edition of the book.

PharmCAS is designed to be a comprehensive application system providing a mechanism to distribute information about an applicant to one or more participating pharmacy schools. According to the information detailed on the PharmCAS website, the system operates to benefit applicants, participating pharmacy schools, and advisors of pre-pharmacy students. Information for each participating school is provided on the PharmCAS site. Listed below are some examples of the information that is provided:

1. application deadlines
2. transcript submission requirements
3. pre-pharmacy requirements
4. recommendation submission procedures
5. any special or additional requirements for specific schools

Non-participating schools—those NOT participating in PharmCAS—are listed and links to various school websites are provided. Be aware that PharmCAS participating schools may still require that supplemental application data be submitted directly to the school to which the student is applying.

As of 2013, the application fee for an individual to submit an application to a single participating school is $150. There is a graduated fee scale to apply for more than one school. For example, to apply for a second school, an additional $55 is required. The PharmCAS website contains the most current information.

The PharmCAS website lists several sources of instructions. Applicants are encouraged to familiarize themselves with the "Step-by-Step" checklist, PharmCAS Application Instructions, and Applicant Code of Conduct. Visit the PharmCAS website at *www.PharmCAS.org.*

In addition to various supplemental materials that may be required by schools participating in PharmCAS, applicants must submit transcript request forms to the registrar of each U.S. and Canadian college or university they have attended. A requirement as of 2014 is the provision for Letters of Reference to be submitted via PharmCAS. There are currently three categories of Letter of Reference procedures for participating schools: (1) No letters of reference; (2) Letters submitted directly to the school (and not to PharmCAS); and (3) Letters submitted electronically to PharmCAS, which are then distributed to the applicant's specified schools. Again, the applicant should consult the PharmCAS website for specific instructions for the program or programs in which he or she is interested.

Some participating pharmacy programs offer an "Early Decision" process via the PharmCAS system. As of the 2013–2014 application cycle, the early decision application deadline is September 3. The PharmCAS website indicates that an applicant must contact the schools offering early decision to obtain information regarding early decision guidelines. Additionally, if you are offered admission as an early decision application participant, you are obligated to accept that offer AND you will not be permitted to apply to another PharmCAS institution. PharmCAS institutions that participate in the early decision process will announce those choices by a date selected annually.

Part of the application process for PharmCAS requires that the applicant enter all coursework and grades using personal transcripts or grade reports. These entries are verified by PharmCAS upon receipt of official copies of your transcripts. Additional copies of your official transcripts may be required by the institution(s).

Students who have completed college-level work at foreign institutions must contact the schools to which they are applying, or get specific information from the school's website. Usually, foreign transcripts must be submitted to a service that specializes in this type of evaluation. Individual schools vary in their procedures for accepting credit toward the completion of pre-pharmacy coursework from non-U.S. accredited programs.

Applicants who submitted and paid for an application to PharmCAS in the pervious cycle are eligible to have their application information carried over to the new cycle. Please refer to the application instructions on the PharmCAS website for further details.

The PharmCAS system offers a mechanism for an applicant to pursue a number of pharmacy programs while possibly reducing the amount of repeated materials that must be submitted. Currently, more than one-half of all pharmacy programs utilize PharmCAS. Applicants should contact each pharmacy school of interest to obtain admission requirements.

For current information on PharmCAS, please visit *www.pharmCAS.org*, as information in this section may change.

TIP

Make sure that you check to see if any additional materials are required, even if a school uses PharmCAS.

U.S. Colleges and Schools of Pharmacy Admission Requirements

Applications for admission to schools and colleges of pharmacy have increased significantly in the twenty-first century. For example, the American Association of Colleges of Pharmacy (AACP) reported an average application-to-enrollment ratio of approximately 3:1 for U.S. schools of pharmacy in 1990; however, in 2012 the average applicant-to-enrollment ratio was about 6.4:1. The increased number of applicants can be interpreted in many ways in terms of pharmacy practice and education. You should prepare yourself to be the most competitive.

As of 2014, there were approximately 130 schools of pharmacy with accreditation status in the U.S. The listing of schools can be found through the Accreditation Council of Pharmacy Education website (*www.acpe-accredit.org*) or through the AACP website (*www.aacp.org*). All schools of pharmacy utilize the college pre-pharmacy grade point average (GPA) in evaluating candidates for admission. In addition to the GPA, the PCAT is utilized by most pharmacy schools in selecting students. Therefore, the two main academic performance selection criteria for admission are the PCAT scores and the pre-pharmacy GPA. Schools also conduct interviews to evaluate students for acceptance; however, whether a candidate is selected for an interview is often dependent on his or her GPA and PCAT performance.

Since acceptance into pharmacy school is very competitive, it is extremely important for you to do your best in both.

U.S. Colleges and Schools of Pharmacy

The following information represents the U.S. colleges and schools of pharmacy as reported by the Accreditation Council for Pharmacy Education (ACPE). Greater than 95% of the schools listed here have been accredited by ACPE. To obtain the most current information and accreditation status, contact the specific college or school of pharmacy in which you are interested.

Albany College of Pharmacy
Appalachian College of Pharmacy
Auburn University
Belmont University
Butler University
California Health Sciences University
California Northstate University
Campbell University
Cedarville University
Chicago State University
Concordia University
Creighton University
Drake University
Duquesne University
D'Youville College
East Tennessee State University
Farleigh Dickinson University
Ferris State University
Florida A&M University
Hampton University
Harding University
Howard University
Husson University
Idaho State University
Lake Erie College of Osteopathic Medicine
Lipscomb University
Loma Linda University
Long Island University
Manchester University
Marshall University
Massachusetts College of Pharmacy and Health Sciences (MCPHS) University—Boston
MCPHS University—Manchester
MCPHS University—Worcester
Mercer University
Midwestern University—Chicago

Midwestern University—Glendale
North Dakota State University
Northeastern Ohio Medical University
Northeastern University
Notre Dame of Maryland University
Nova Southeastern University
Ohio Northern University
Ohio State University
Oregon State University
Pacific University
Palm Beach Atlantic University
Philadelphia College
Presbyterian College
Purdue University
Regis University
Roosevelt University
Rosalind Franklin University
Roseman University of Health Sciences
Rutgers University
Samford University
Shenandoah University
South Carolina College of Pharmacy
South College
South Dakota State University
South University
Southern Illinois University—Edwardsville
Southwestern Oklahoma State University
St. John Fisher College
St. John's University
St. Louis College of Pharmacy
Sullivan University
Temple University
Texas A&M University—Kingsville
Texas Southern University
Texas Tech University
Thomas Jefferson University

Touro College
Touro University
Union University
University of Arizona
University of Arkansas
University at Buffalo—State University
of New York
University of California—
San Diego
University of California—
San Francisco
University of Charleston
University of Cincinnati
University of Colorado
University of Connecticut
University of Findlay
University of Florida
University of Georgia
University of Hawaii
University of Houston
University of Illinois
University of the Incarnate Word
University of Iowa
University of Kansas
University of Kentucky
University of Louisiana
University of Maryland
Univeristy of Maryland Eastern Shore
University of Michigan
University of Minnesota
University of Minnesota—Duluth
University of Mississippi
University of Missouri

University of Montana
University of Nebraska
University of New England
University of New Mexico
University of North Carolina
University of North Texas
University of Oklahoma
University of the Pacific
University of Pittsburgh
University of Puerto Rico
University of Rhode Island
University of Saint Joseph
University of the Sciences in
Philadelphia
University of Southern California
University of South Florida
University of Tennessee
University of Texas
University of Toledo
University of Utah
University of Washington
University of Wisconsin
University of Wyoming
Virginia Commonwealth University
Washington State University
Wayne State University
West Virginia University
Western New England University
Western University of Health Sciences
Wilkes University
Wingate University
Xavier University of Louisiana

Directory of U.S. Colleges and Schools of Pharmacy (by State)

ALABAMA

Harrison School of Pharmacy
Auburn University
2316 Walker Building
Auburn University, Alabama 36849-5501
(334) 844-8348
pharmacy.auburn.edu/
Professional Degree Offered: Doctor of Pharmacy

McWhorter School of Pharmacy
Samford University
800 Lakeshore Drive
Birmingham, Alabama 35229
(205) 726-2982
pharmacy.samford.edu
Professional Degree Offered: Doctor of Pharmacy

ARIZONA

College of Pharmacy—Glendale
Midwestern University
19555 North 59th Avenue
Glendale, Arizona 85308
(623) 572-3215
www.midwestern.edu/programs-and-admission/
    az-pharmacy.html
Professional Degree Offered: Doctor of Pharmacy

College of Pharmacy
University of Arizona
1295 N. Martin Avenue
P.O. Box 210202
Tucson, Arizona 85721
(520) 626-1427
www.pharmacy.arizona.edu/
Professional Degree Offered: Doctor of Pharmacy

ARKANSAS

College of Pharmacy
Harding University
915 East Market Avenue
Searcy, Arkansas 72149
(501) 279-5528
www.harding.edu/pharmacy
Professional Degree Offered: Doctor of Pharmacy

College of Pharmacy
University of Arkansas for Medical Sciences
4301 West Markham Street, Slot 522
Little Rock, Arkansas 72205
(501) 686-5557
www.uams.edu/cop/
Professional Degree Offered: Doctor of Pharmacy

CALIFORNIA

College of Pharmacy
California Health Sciences University
120 N. Clovis Avenue
Clovis, California 93612
(559) 325-3600
chsn.org
Professional Degree Offered: Doctor of Pharmacy

College of Pharmacy
California Northstate University
10811 International Drive
Rancho Cordova, California 95670
(916) 631-8108
pharmacy.cnsu.edu/home
Professional Degree Offered: Doctor of Pharmacy

School of Pharmacy
Loma Linda University
West Hall 1316
11262 Campus Street
Loma Linda, California 92350
(909) 558-1300
www.llu.edu/pharmacy/index.page
Professional Degree Offered: Doctor of Pharmacy

College of Pharmacy
Touro University—California
1310 Club Drive, Mare Island
Vallejo, California 94592
(707) 638-5200
cop.tu.edu/index.html
Professional Degree Offered: Doctor of Pharmacy

Skaggs School of Pharmacy and Pharmaceutical
   Sciences
University of California—San Diego
9500 Gilman Drive, MC 0657
La Jolla, California 92093-0657
(858) 822-4900
www.pharmacy.ucsd.edu/
Professional Degree Offered: Doctor of Pharmacy

School of Pharmacy
University of California at San Francisco
513 Parnassus Avenue
UCSF Box 0150, Room S-960
San Francisco, California 94143
(415) 476-2732
pharmacy.ucsf.edu/
Professional Degree Offered: Doctor of Pharmacy

Thomas J. Long School of Pharmacy
   and Health Sciences
University of the Pacific
3601 Pacific Avenue
Stockton, California 95211
(209) 946-2211
www.pacific.edu/Academics/Schools-and-Colleges/
   Thomas-J-Long-School-of-Pharmacy-and-
   Health-Sciences.html
Professional Degree Offered: Doctor of Pharmacy

School of Pharmacy
University of Southern California
1985 Zonal Avenue
Los Angeles, California 90089-9121
(323) 442-1369
pharmacyschool.usc.edu
Professional Degree Offered: Doctor of Pharmacy

College of Pharmacy
Western University of Health Sciences
309 E. Second Street
Pomona, California 91766-1854
(909) 469-5335
www.westernu.edu/pharmacy
Professional Degree Offered: Doctor of Pharmacy

COLORADO

School of Pharmacy
Regis University
3333 Regis Boulevard
Denver, Colorado 80221-1099
(303) 458-4344
www.regis.edu/RHCHP/Schools/School-of-
   Pharmacy.aspx#.Uh0GVGSDQXw
Professional Degree Offered: Doctor of Pharmacy

Skaggs School of Pharmacy and Pharmaceutical
   Sciences
University of Colorado Anschutz Medical
   Campus
Mail Stop C238
Pharmacy and Pharmaceutical Sciences Building
12850 East Montview Boulevard
Aurora, Colorado 80045
(303) 724-2882
www.ucdenver.edu/pharmacy
Professional Degree Offered: Doctor of Pharmacy

CONNECTICUT

School of Pharmacy
The University of Connecticut
69 North Eagleville Road, Unit 3092
Storrs, Connecticut 06269-3092
(860) 486-2216
pharmacy.uconn.edu/
Professional Degree Offered: Doctor of Pharmacy

School of Pharmacy
University of St. Joseph
229 Trumbull Street
Hartford, Connecticut 06103-0501
(860) 231-5858
www.usj.edu/academics/schools/school-of-pharmacy
Professional Degree Offered: Doctor of Pharmacy

DISTRICT OF COLUMBIA

College of Pharmacy
Howard University
2300 Fourth Street, Northwest
Washington, DC 20059
(202) 806-6530
www.pharmacy.howard.edu/
Professional Degree Offered: Doctor of Pharmacy

FLORIDA

College of Pharmacy and Pharmaceutical Sciences
Florida Agricultural and Mechanical University
1415 South Martin Luthur King, Jr. Boulevard
Tallahassee, Florida 32307
(850) 599-3301
pharmacy.famu.edu/
Professional Degree Offered: Doctor of Pharmacy

College of Pharmacy
Nova Southeastern University
3200 South University Drive
Fort Lauderdale, Florida 33328
(954) 262-1300
pharmacy.nova.edu
Professional Degree Offered: Doctor of Pharmacy

Lloyd L. Gregory School of Pharmacy
Palm Beach Atlantic University
901 South Flagler Drive
West Palm Beach, Florida 33416-4708
(561) 803-2000
www.pba.edu/school-of-pharmacy
Professional Degree Offered: Doctor of Pharmacy

College of Pharmacy
University of Florida
101 S. Newell Drive
Gainesville, Florida 32610
(352) 273-6312
pharmacy.ufl.edu/
Professional Degree Offered: Doctor of Pharmacy

College of Pharmacy
University of South Florida
12901 Bruce B. Downs Boulevard
Tampa, Florida 33612
(813) 974-5699
health.usf.edu/nocms/pharmacy/
Professional Degree Offered: Doctor of Pharmacy

GEORGIA

College of Pharmacy and Health Sciences
Mercer University
3001 Mercer University Drive
Atlanta, Georgia 30341-4415
(678) 547-6232
cophs.mercer.edu
Professional Degree Offered: Doctor of Pharmacy

School of Pharmacy
Philadelphia College of Osteopathic Medicine
625 Old Peachtree Road, NW
Suwanee, Georgia 30024
(678) 225-7500
*www.pcom.edu/Academic_Programs/aca_pharmd/
pharmacy.php*
Professional Degree Offered: Doctor of Pharmacy

School of Pharmacy
South University
709 Mall Boulevard
Savannah, Georgia 31406
(912) 201-8120
www.southuniversity.edu/
Professional Degree Offered: Doctor of Pharmacy

College of Pharmacy
The University of Georgia
250 W. Green Street
Athens, Georgia 30602-2351
(706) 542-1911
www.rx.uga.edu/
Professional Degree Offered: Doctor of Pharmacy

HAWAII

College of Pharmacy
The University of Hawaii at Hilo
200 West Kawili Street
Hilo, Hawaii 96720-4091
(808) 933-2909
pharmacy.uhh.hawaii.edu
Professional Degree Offered: Doctor of Pharmacy

IDAHO

College of Pharmacy
Idaho State University
970 South 5th Street, Stop 8288
Pocatello, Idaho 83209-8288
(208) 282-3475
pharmacy.isu.edu/live/
Professional Degree Offered: Doctor of Pharmacy

ILLINOIS

College of Pharmacy
Chicago State University
9501 South King Drive
206 Douglas Hall
Chicago, Illinois 60628-1598
(773) 821-2500
www.csu.edu/collegeofpharmacy/
Professional Degree Offered: Doctor of Pharmacy

Chicago College of Pharmacy
Midwestern University
555 31st Street
Downers Grove, Illinois 60515
(630) 515-6171
www.midwestern.edu/programs-and-admission/
il-pharmacy.html
Professional Degree Offered: Doctor of Pharmacy

College of Pharmacy
Roosevelt University
1400 N. Roosevelt Boulevard
Schaumburg, Illinois 60173
(847) 619-7300
www.roosevelt.edu/Pharmacy.aspx
Professional Degree Offered: Doctor of Pharmacy

College of Pharmacy
Rosalind Franklin University of Medicine and
    Science
3333 Green Bay Road
North Chicago, Illinois 60064
(847) 578-8831
www.rosalindfranklin.edu/cop/Home.aspx
Professional Degree Offered: Doctor of Pharmacy

School of Pharmacy
Southern Illinois University, Edwardsville
Campus Box 2000
Edwardsville, Illinois 62026-2000
(618) 650-5150
www.siue.edu/pharmacy/
Professional Degree Offered: Doctor of Pharmacy

College of Pharmacy
University of Illinois at Chicago
833 South Wood Street, m/c 874
Chicago, Illinois 60612
(312) 996-7242
www.uic.edu/pharmacy/
Professional Degree Offered: Doctor of Pharmacy

INDIANA

College of Pharmacy and Health Sciences
Butler University
Pharmacy Building 107
4600 Sunset Avenue
Indianapolis, Indiana 46208
(317) 940-9969
www.butler.edu/cophs/
Professional Degree Offered: Doctor of Pharmacy

College of Pharmacy
Manchester University
10627 Diebold Road
Fort Wayne, Indiana 46845
(260) 470-2700
pharmacy.manchester.edu/
Professional Degree Offered: Doctor of Pharmacy

School of Pharmacy and Pharmaceutical Sciences
Purdue University
575 Stadium Mall Drive
West Lafayette, Indiana 47907
(765) 494-1361
www.pharmacy.purdue.edu/
Professional Degree Offered: Doctor of Pharmacy

IOWA

College of Pharmacy and Health Sciences
Drake University
Cline 106
2507 University Avenue
Des Moines, Iowa 50311-4505
(515) 271-3018 or 1-800-44-DRAKE (ext. 3018)
www.drake.edu/cphs
Professional Degree Offered: Doctor of Pharmacy

College of Pharmacy
The University of Iowa
115 South Grand Avenue
Iowa City, Iowa 52242
(319) 335-8794
www.pharmacy.uiowa.edu/
Professional Degree Offered: Doctor of Pharmacy

KANSAS

School of Pharmacy
University of Kansas
2010 Becker Drive
Lawrence, Kansas 66047-1620
(785) 864-3591
pharmacy.ku.edu/
Professional Degree Offered: Doctor of Pharmacy

KENTUCKY

College of Pharamcy
Sullivan University
2100 Gardiner Lane
Louisville, Kentucky 40205
(502) 413-8640
www.sullivan.edu/pharmacy
Professional Degree Offered: Doctor of Pharmacy

College of Pharmacy
University of Kentucky
789 South Limestone
Lexington, Kentucky 40536-0596
(859) 323-2755
pharmacy.mc.uky.edu
Professional Degree Offered: Doctor of Pharmacy

LOUISIANA

School of Pharmacy
The University of Louisiana at Monroe
1800 Bienville Drive
Monroe, Louisiana 71201
(318) 342-1600
rxweb.ulm.edu/pharmacy/
Professional Degree Offered: Doctor of Pharmacy

College of Pharmacy
Xavier University of Louisiana
1 Drexel Drive
New Orleans, Louisiana 70125
(504) 520-7580
www.xula.edu/cop/index.php
Professional Degree Offered: Doctor of Pharmacy

MAINE

School of Pharmacy
Husson University
One College Circle
Bangor, Maine 04401
(207) 404-5660
www.husson.edu/pharmacy
Professional Degree Offered: Doctor of Pharmacy

College of Pharmacy
University of New England
716 Stevens Avenue
Portland, Maine 04103
(207) 221-4225
www.une.edu/pharmacy
Professional Degree Offered: Doctor of Pharmacy

MARYLAND

School of Pharmacy
Notre Dame of Maryland University
4701 North Charles Street
Baltimore, Maryland 21210
(410) 532-5551
www.ndm.edu/academics/school-of-pharmacy
Professional Degree Offered: Doctor of Pharmacy

School of Pharmacy
University of Maryland
20 North Pine Street
Baltimore, Maryland 21201
(410) 706-7650
www.pharmacy.umaryland.edu/
Professional Degree Offered: Doctor of Pharmacy

School of Pharmacy
University of Maryland Eastern Shore
117 Somerset Hall
Princess Anne, Maryland 21853
(410) 651-2200
www.umes.edu/pharmacy
Professional Degree Offered: Doctor of Pharmacy

MASSACHUSETTS

School of Pharmacy—Boston
MCPHS University
179 Longwood Avenue
Boston, Massachusetts 02115
(617) 732-2781
www.mcphs.edu/campuses/boston
Professional Degree Offered: Doctor of Pharmacy

School of Pharmacy—Worcester
MCPHS University
19 Foster Street
Worcester, Massachusetts 01608
(508) 890-8855
www.mcphs.edu/campuses/worcester
Professional Degree Offered: Doctor of Pharmacy

Bouvé College of Health Sciences—School of
  Pharmacy
Northeastern University
140 The Fenway
360 Huntington Avenue
Mailstop R218TF
Boston, Massachusetts 02115
(617) 373-3380
www.northeastern.edu/bouve/pharmacy
Professional Degree Offered: Doctor of Pharmacy

School of Pharmacy
Western New England College
1215 Wilbraham Road
Springfield, Massachusetts 01119
(413) 796-2300
www.wne.edu/pharmacy/home.cfm
Professional Degree Offered: Doctor of Pharmacy

MICHIGAN

College of Pharmacy
Ferris State University
220 Ferris Drive, PHR 105
Big Rapids, Michigan 49307
(231) 591-3780
www.ferris.edu/colleges/pharmacy/homepage.htm
Professional Degree Offered: Doctor of Pharmacy

College of Pharmacy
The University of Michigan
428 Church Street
Ann Arbor, Michigan 48109-1065
(734) 764-7312
pharmacy.umich.edu
Professional Degree Offered: Doctor of Pharmacy

Eugene Applebaum College of Pharmacy
  and Health Sciences
Wayne State University
259 Mack Avenue
Detroit, Michigan 48201
(313) 577-1716
www.cphs.wayne.edu
Professional Degree Offered: Doctor of Pharmacy

MINNESOTA

College of Pharmacy
University of Minnesota
5-130 Weaver-Densford Hall
308 Harvard Street, SE
Minneapolis, Minnesota 55455
(612) 624-1900
www.pharmacy.umn.edu
Professional Degree Offered: Doctor of Pharmacy

College of Pharmacy, Duluth
University of Minnesota
232 Life Science
1110 Kirby Drive
Duluth, Minnesota 55812
(218) 726-6000
www.pharmacy.umn.edu/duluth
Professional Degree Offered: Doctor of Pharmacy

MISSISSIPPI

School of Pharmacy
The University of Mississippi
P.O. Box 1848
University, Mississippi 38677-1848
(662) 915-7265
www.pharmacy.olemiss.edu/
Professional Degree Offered: Doctor of Pharmacy

MISSOURI

St. Louis College of Pharmacy
4588 Parkview Place
St. Louis, Missouri 63110-1088
(314) 367-8700
www.stlcop.edu
Professional Degree Offered: Doctor of Pharmacy

School of Pharmacy
University of Missouri—Kansas City
UMKC Health Sciences Building
2464 Charlotte Street
Kansas City, Missouri 64108
(816) 235-2833
pharmacy.umkc.edu
Professional Degree Offered: Doctor of Pharmacy

MONTANA

Skaggs School of Pharmacy
The University of Montana
32 Campus Drive, 340 Skaggs Building
Missoula, Montana 59812-1512
(406) 243-4621
pharmacy.health.umt.edu/
Professional Degree Offered: Doctor of Pharmacy

NEBRASKA

School of Pharmacy and Health Professions
Creighton University
2500 California Plaza
Criss III, Room 151
Omaha, Nebraska 68178
(402) 280-2662
spahp.creighton.edu/node/3487
Professional Degree Offered: Doctor of Pharmacy

College of Pharmacy
University of Nebraska Medical Center
986000 Nebraska Medical Center
Omaha, Nebraska 68198-6000
(402) 559-4333
www.unmc.edu/pharmacy/
Professional Degree Offered: Doctor of Pharmacy

NEVADA

College of Pharmacy
Roseman University of Health Sciences
11 Sunset Way
Henderson, Nevada 89014
(702) 940-4433
*www.roseman.edu/explore-our-colleges/college-of-
    pharmacy*
Professional Degree Offered: Doctor of Pharmacy

NEW HAMPSHIRE

School of Pharmacy—Manchester
MCPHS University
1260 Elm Street
Manchester, New Hampshire 03101
(603) 314-0210
www.mcphs.edu/campuses/manchester
Professional Degree Offered: Doctor of Pharmacy

NEW JERSEY

School of Pharmacy
Farleigh Dickinson University
Becton College
Mailstop M-SP1-01
230 Park Avenue
Florham Park, New Jersey 07932
(973) 443-8401
www.fdu.edu/academic/pharmacy
Professional Degree Offered: Doctor of Pharmacy

Ernest Mario School of Pharmacy
Rutgers, the State University of New Jersey
160 Frelinghuysen Road
Piscataway, New Jersey 08854
(848) 445-2675
pharmacy.rutgers.edu/
Professional Degree Offered: Doctor of Pharmacy

NEW MEXICO

College of Pharmacy
University of New Mexico
MSC 09 5360
1 University of New Mexico
Albuquerque, New Mexico 87131-0001
(505) 272-3241
hsc.unm.edu/pharmacy/
Professional Degree Offered: Doctor of Pharmacy

NEW YORK

Albany College of Pharmacy and Health Sciences
106 New Scotland Avenue
Albany, New York 12208
(888) 203-8010
www.acphs.edu
Professional Degree Offered: Doctor of Pharmacy

School of Pharmacy
D'Youville College
320 Porter Avenue
Buffalo, New York 14201
(716) 829-7846
www.dyc.edu/academics/pharmacy
Professional Degree Offered: Doctor of Pharmacy

Arnold and Marie Schwartz College of Pharmacy
and Health Sciences
Long Island University
75 Dekalb Avenue
Brooklyn, New York 11201
(718) 488-1004
www.liu.edu/pharmacy/
Professional Degree Offered: Doctor of Pharmacy

Wegmans School of Pharmacy
St. John Fisher College
3690 East Avenue
Rochester, New York 14618
(585) 385-8430
www.sjfc.edu/pharmacy
Professional Degree Offered: Doctor of Pharmacy

College of Pharmacy and Health Sciences
St. John's University
8000 Utopia Parkway
Queens, New York 11439
(718) 990-6275
*www.stjohns.edu/academics/schools-and-colleges/
college-of-pharmacy-and-health-sciences*
Professional Degree Offered: Doctor of Pharmacy

Touro College of Pharmacy—New York
230 West 125th Street
New York, New York 10027
(646) 981-4700
www.pharmacy.touro.edu
Professional Degree Offered: Doctor of Pharmacy

School of Pharmacy and Pharmaceutical Sciences
University at Buffalo—State University
of New York
John and Editha Kapoor Hall
South Campus, 285 Kapoor Hall
Buffalo, New York 14214-8033
(716) 645-2825
www.pharmacy.buffalo.edu/
Professional Degree Offered: Doctor of Pharmacy

NORTH CAROLINA

College of Pharmacy and Health Sciences
Campbell University
P.O. Box 1090
Buies Creek, North Carolina 27506
(800) 760-9734, ext. 1690
www.campbell.edu/cphs
Professional Degree Offered: Doctor of Pharmacy

Eshelman School of Pharmacy
University of North Carolina at Chapel Hill
CB #7355
Chapel Hill, North Carolina 27599-7355
(919) 966-9429
www.pharmacy.unc.edu/
Professional Degree Offered: Doctor of Pharmacy

School of Pharmacy
Wingate University
515 N. Main Street
Levine College of Health Sciences
Wingate, North Carolina 28174
(704) 233-8633
pharmacy.wingate.edu/
Professional Degree Offered: Doctor of Pharmacy

NORTH DAKOTA

College of Pharmacy, Nursing, and
   Allied Sciences
North Dakota State University
NDSU Dept. 2650
123 Sudro Hall
PO Box 6050
Fargo, North Dakota 58108-6050
(701) 231-7456
www.ndsu.nodak.edu/pharmacy/
Professional Degree Offered: Doctor of Pharmacy

OHIO

School of Pharmacy
Cedarville University
251 N. Main Street
Cedarville, Ohio 45314
(937) 766-7480
www.cedarville.edu/Academics/Pharmacy.aspx
Professional Degree Offered: Doctor of Pharmacy

College of Pharmacy
Northeastern Ohio Medical University
4209 State Route 44
P.O. Box 95
Rootstown, Ohio 44272
(800) 686-2511
www.neomed.edu/academics/pharmacy
Professional Degree Offered: Doctor of Pharmacy

Rudolph H. Raabe College of Pharmacy
Ohio Northern University
525 S. Main Street
Roberston-Evans Pharmacy 132
Ada, Ohio 45810
(419) 772-2275
www.onu.edu/academics/pharmacy
Professional Degree Offered: Doctor of Pharmacy

College of Pharmacy
The Ohio State University
217 Lloyd M. Parks Hall
500 West 12th Avenue
Columbus, Ohio 43210
(614) 292-2266
www.pharmacy.ohio-state.edu
Professional Degree Offered: Doctor of Pharmacy

James L. Winkle College of Pharmacy
University of Cincinnati
3225 Eden Avenue
136 Health Professions Building
Cincinnati, Ohio 45267-0004
(513) 558-3784
www.pharmacy.uc.edu/
Professional Degree Offered: Doctor of Pharmacy

College of Pharmacy
University of Findlay
300 Davis Street
Findlay, Ohio 45840
(419) 434-5327
www.findlay.edu/pharmacy
Professional Degree Offered: Doctor of Pharmacy

College of Pharmacy
The University of Toledo
300 Arlington Avenue, MS 1014
Toledo, Ohio 43614
(419) 383-1904
www.utoldeo.edu/pharmacy
Professional Degree Offered: Doctor of Pharmacy

OKLAHOMA

College of Pharmacy
Southwestern Oklahoma State University
100 Campus Drive
Weatherford, Oklahoma 73096
(580) 774-3105
www.swosu.edu/pharmacy/
Professional Degree Offered: Doctor of Pharmacy

College of Pharmacy
University of Oklahoma
P.O. Box 26901
Oklahoma City, Oklahoma 73126-0901
(405) 271-6484
pharmacy.ouhsc.edu
Professional Degree Offered: Doctor of Pharmacy

OREGON

College of Pharmacy
Oregon State University
203 Pharmacy Building
Corvallis, Oregon 97331
(541) 737-3424
pharmacy.oregonstate.edu/
Professional Degree Offered: Doctor of Pharmacy

School of Pharmacy
Pacific University
222 Southeast 8th Avenue
Hillsboro, Oregon 97123
(503) 352-2218
www.pacificu.edu/pharmd/
Professional Degree Offered: Doctor of Pharmacy

PENNSYLVANIA

Mylan School of Pharmacy
Duquesne University
600 Forbes Avenue
Pittsburgh, Pennsylvania 15282
(412) 396-6000
www.pharmacy.duq.edu
Professional Degree Offered: Doctor of Pharmacy

School of Pharmacy
Lake Erie College of Osteopathic Medicine
1858 West Grandview Boulevard
Erie, Pennsylvania 16509-1025
(814) 866-6641
www.lecom.edu
Professional Degree Offered: Doctor of Pharmacy

School of Pharmacy
Temple University
3307 North Broad Street
Philadelphia, Pennsylvania 19140
(215) 707-4900
www.temple.edu/pharmacy/
Professional Degree Offered: Doctor of Pharmacy

Jefferson School of Pharmacy
Thomas Jefferson University
901 Walnut Street
Health Professions Academic Building
Philadelphia, Pennsylvania 19107 .
(877) 533-3247 or (215) 503-8890
www.jefferson.edu/pharmacy.html
Professional Degree Offered: Doctor of Pharmacy

School of Pharmacy
University of Pittsburgh
Student Services
1104 Salk Hall
3501 Terrace Street
Pittsburgh, Pennsylvania 15261
(412) 383-9000
www.pharmacy.pitt.edu/
Professional Degree Offered: Doctor of Pharmacy

Philadelphia College of Pharmacy
University of the Sciences in Philadelphia
600 South 43rd Street
Philadelphia, Pennsylvania 19104
(215) 596-8800
www.usip.edu/pcp/
Professional Degree Offered: Doctor of Pharmacy

Nesbitt College of Pharmacy and Nursing
Wilkes University
Stark Learning Center
84 West South Street
Wilkes-Barre, Pennsylvania 18766
(570) 408-4298
www.wilkes.edu/pages/373.asp
Professional Degree Offered: Doctor of Pharmacy

PUERTO RICO

School of Pharmacy
University of Puerto Rico
Medical Sciences Campus
P.O. Box 365067
San Juan, Puerto Rico 00936-5067
(787) 758-2525 ext. 5400
farmacia.rcm.upr.edu/
Professional Degree Offered: Doctor of Pharmacy

RHODE ISLAND

College of Pharmacy
University of Rhode Island
Pharmacy Building
7 Greenhouse Road
Kingston, Rhode Island 02881
(401) 874-2761
www.uri.edu/pharmacy/
Professional Degree Offered: Doctor of Pharmacy

SOUTH CAROLINA

School of Pharmacy
Presbyterian College
307 North Broad Street
Clinton, South Carolina 29325
(864) 938-3900
pharmacy.presby.edu
Professional Degree Offered: Doctor of Pharmacy

South Carolina College of Pharmacy
MUSC Campus
280 Calhoun Street
MSC 141
Charleston, South Carolina 29425
(843) 792-3740
www.sccp.sc.edu
Professional Degree Offered: Doctor of Pharmacy

South Carolina College of Pharmacy
USC Campus
715 Sumter Street
Coker Life Science Building
Columbia, South Carolina 29208
(803) 777-4151
www.sccp.sc.edu
Professional Degree Offered: Doctor of Pharmacy

SOUTH DAKOTA

College of Pharmacy
South Dakota State University
Avera Health and Science Center 133
Box 2202C
Brookings, South Dakota 57007
(605) 688-6197
www.sdstate.edu/pha/index.cfm
Professional Degree Offered: Doctor of Pharmacy

TENNESSEE

School of Pharmacy
Belmont University
1900 Belmont Boulevard
Nashville, Tennessee 37212-3757
(615) 460-8122
www.belmont.edu/pharmacy
Professional Degree Offered: Doctor of Pharmacy

Bill Gatton College of Pharmacy
East Tennessee State University
P.O. Box 70414
Johnson City, Tennessee 37614-1704
(423) 439-6338
www.etsu.edu/pharmacy
Professional Degree Offered: Doctor of Pharmacy

College of Pharmacy
Lipscomb University
One University Park Drive
Nashville, Tennessee 37204
(615) 966-6656
www.lipscomb.edu/pharmacy
Professional Degree Offered: Doctor of Pharmacy

School of Pharmacy
South College
3904 Lonas Drive
Knoxville, Tennessee 37909
(865) 251-1800
www.southcollegetn.edu/pharmacy
Professional Degree Offered: Doctor of Pharmacy

School of Pharmacy
Union University
1050 Union University Drive
Jackson, Tennessee 38305
(731) 661-5910
www.uu.edu/academics/sop
Professional Degree Offered: Doctor of Pharmacy

College of Pharmacy
University of Tennessee
Health Science Center
881 Monroe Avenue, Suite 226
Memphis, Tennessee 38163
(901) 448-6036
www.uthsc.edu/pharmacy
Professional Degree Offered: Doctor of Pharmacy

TEXAS

Irma Lerma Rangel College of Pharmacy
Texas A&M University Health Science Center
MSC 131, 1010 West Avenue B
Kingsville, Texas 78363
(361) 221-0604
pharmacy.tamhsc.edu
Professional Degree Offered: Doctor of Pharmacy

College of Pharmacy and Health Sciences
Texas Southern University
3100 Cleburne Street
Houston, Texas 77004
(713) 313-6700
*www.tsu.edu/academics/colleges__schools/
College_of_Pharmacy_and_Health_Sciences/
pharm_main.php*
Professional Degree Offered: Doctor of Pharmacy

School of Pharmacy
Texas Tech University Health Sciences Center
1300 Coutler, Suite 2210
Amarillo, Texas 79106
(806) 354-5418
www.ttuhsc.edu/sop/
Professional Degree Offered: Doctor of Pharmacy

College of Pharmacy
University of Houston
141 Science & Research Building 2
Houston, Texas 77204-5000
(713) 743-1239
www.uh.edu/pharmacy
Professional Degree Offered: Doctor of Pharmacy

Feik School of Pharmacy
University of the Incarnate Word
4301 Broadway, CPO #99
San Antonio, Texas 78209-6397
(210) 883-1000
www.uiw.edu/pharmacy/
Professional Degree Offered: Doctor of Pharmacy

College of Pharmacy
University of North Texas System
3500 Camp Bowie Boulevard
Fort Worth, Texas 76107
(717) 735-2000
web.unthsc.edu/education/scp
Professional Degree Offered: Doctor of Pharmacy

College of Pharmacy
The University of Texas at Austin
2409 University Avenue
Stop: A1900
Austin, Texas 78712-0120
(512) 471-1737
www.utexas.edu/pharmacy/
Professional Degree Offered: Doctor of Pharmacy

UTAH

College of Pharmacy
University of Utah
30 South 2000 East
Salt Lake City, Utah 84112-5820
(801) 581-6731
www.pharmacy.utah.edu/
Professional Degree Offered: Doctor of Pharmacy

VIRGINIA

Appalachian College of Pharmacy
1060 Dragon Road
Oakwood, Virginia 24631
(276) 498-4190 ext. 5233
www.acp.edu
Professional Degree Offered: Doctor of Pharmacy

School of Pharmacy
Hampton University
Kittrell Hall
Hampton, Virginia 23668
(757) 727-5071
pharm.hamptonu.edu
Professional Degree Offered: Doctor of Pharmacy

Bernard J. Dunn School of Pharmacy
Shenandoah University
1775 N. Sector Court
Winchester, Virginia 22601
(540) 665-1282 or (888) 420-7877
pharmacy.su.edu
Professional Degree Offered: Doctor of Pharmacy

School of Pharmacy
Virginia Commonwealth University
P.O. Box 980581
410 North 12th Street, Room 500
Richmond, Virginia 23298-0581
(804) 828-3000
www.pharmacy.vcu.edu/
Professional Degree Offered: Doctor of Pharmacy

WASHINGTON

School of Pharmacy
University of Washington
H362 Health Sciences Building, Box 357631
Seattle, Washington 98195-7631
(206) 543-6100
sop.washington.edu/
Professional Degree Offered: Doctor of Pharmacy

College of Pharmacy
Washington State University
P.O. Box 646510
Pullman, Washington 99164-6510
(509) 368-6605
www.pharmacy.wsu.edu/
Professional Degree Offered: Doctor of Pharmacy

WEST VIRGINIA

School of Pharmacy
Marshall University
One John Marshall Drive
Huntington, WV 25755-2950
(304) 696-7302
www.marshall.edu.wpmu/pharmacy
Professional Degree Offered: Doctor of Pharmacy

School of Pharmacy
University of Charleston
2300 MacCorkle Avenue, Southeast
Charleston, West Virginia 25304
(304) 357-4889
pharmacy.ucwv.edu/pharmacy
Professional Degree Offered: Doctor of Pharmacy

School of Pharmacy
West Virginia University
P.O. Box 9500
Morgantown, West Virginia 26506-9500
(304) 293-1894
www.hsc.wvu.edu/sop/
Professional Degree Offered: Doctor of Pharmacy

WISCONSIN

School of Pharmacy
Concordia University
12800 North Lake Shore Drive
Mequon, Wisconsin 53097
(262) 243-5700
www.cuw.edu/programs/pharmacy
Professional Degree Offered: Doctor of Pharmacy

School of Pharmacy
University of Wisconsin—Madison
777 Highland Avenue
Madison, Wisconsin 53705-2222
(608) 262-6234
www.pharmacy.wisc.edu/
Professional Degree Offered: Doctor of Pharmacy

WYOMING

School of Pharmacy
University of Wyoming
Health Sciences Center, Room 292
Department 3375
1000 East University Avenue
Laramie, Wyoming 82071
(307) 766-6120
uww.uwyo.edu/Pharmacy/
Professional Degree Offered: Doctor of Pharmacy

TIP

Provide additional information that you think is important for the committee to understand your interest in pharmacy and their program in particular.

Admission Committees

The individuals who wrote the "Admission Committees" and the "Interview Process" sections of this book have served on pharmacy school admission committees for several years. Based on their experiences, they have summarized their observations of students who were successful in being accepted into a college/school of pharmacy. The following describes the purpose of the admission committee and provides tips to successfully guide you through the admission process.

The purpose of the admission committee for a pharmacy school is to select the most qualified students to enter the program. The phrase "most qualified student" will have a slightly different interpretation by each committee and may vary slightly within an institution from year to year. As soon as possible, contact the institutions in which you are interested and request materials regarding application requirements. Much of this data may be available on the school's website, and therefore it is important to review materials most schools make available on the Internet. By reviewing these materials you should be able to determine not only the requirements for the institution, but which factors are utilized to select students for admission.

The committees will use various sources of information and mechanisms to compare students to make selection decisions. You should make sure that the information requested is provided for the committee. If you have a special interest, ability, or experience that you think would be helpful in your application, include a letter or other supporting documentation in the materials you submit to the institution(s) for the committee to consider.

As important as it is for you to do well academically and to take the required courses, the practice of pharmacy requires various skills and talents that you may develop and enhance prior to attending a pharmacy school. Some of these areas include:

- Work Experience
- Verbal and Written Communication Skills
- Community Involvement/Leadership
- Entrepreneurial Ability

Some institutions will request information regarding the activities listed above as part of the application, others may rely on recommendations to provide this information. Schools utilize a personal interview as part of the application process to give the student a chance to present information regarding his or her personal and academic background. You should determine how to best develop and exhibit your skills in these areas, and also how to communicate this information to the pharmacy college(s)/school(s). If your current school has a career center that offers practice interviews, take advantage of that opportunity to optimize your interview skills.

Work experience provides the student with a background about the workplace in general. It also gives students a chance to develop good work habits and communication skills. Work experience in the profession of pharmacy will be an excellent way for you to understand what pharmacy is about and whether your interests and skills are compatible. Also, you will be able to find out more information about the variety of career opportunities that exist in the practice of pharmacy. Work experience in pharmacy is great, but other jobs can also be supportive and provide information about a student's interests and abilities. Work in a doctor's office, a health clinic, or hospital setting should provide the student with a background in health care issues, contact with patients, and a chance to see various health care professionals in action. Additionally, seemingly unrelated jobs in retail or food services still provide a medium for the student to develop good work skills, communication skills, and the ability to work with people. No matter what work experience you have, try to see what aspects of that job might apply to your activities as a pharmacist or pharmacy student. Make sure to communicate this effectively to the admission committee.

Communication skills are important in all aspects of pharmacy. Students and pharmacists must be able to communicate effectively with a wide range of people. Also, they must be able to communicate about potentially complex subject matter in a manner that is effective for their audience, whether it be a patient, another student, a professor or other health care professional. Additionally, the ability to listen effectively is just as important as the ability to communicate.

Community involvement is a way for the admission committee to determine more about the character of an applicant. The practice of pharmacy requires that a person be empathetic to the needs of the patient or other professional contact. This means that a pharmacist can be most effective when he or she can "put him- or herself in the other's shoes." By showing a history of participation in organizations that show compassion by assisting others, you may be more likely to have the desired character to practice effectively and ethically. It is suggested that you show a history of participation in these types of activities, not just recent participation in one or two events to have something to place on an application or state in an interview. Make sure that you can talk about the type of activities or events you have been involved in, not just list organizations or events.

Entrepreneurship is the interest in new opportunities—not only business ventures, but also professional development and new ways of doing things. Pharmacy, like most professions, will go through various changes throughout one's career, and the ability and interest to pursue new avenues of practice assures that one will continue to be competent and competitive in practice. A committee might assess an applicant's entrepreneurial abilities through questions in the interview such as "tell me about a project you instituted or carried out with others." By asking such a question, the committee might be looking for creativity, leadership skills, and motivation.

It is important to consider the composition of the admission committee. Committees may consist of any combination of faculty members, pharmacists, non-pharmacists, alumni members, students, and administrative members. Be sure to think in terms of what that type of individual would want to know about you that will help them realize you will be a good pharmacy student and practitioner.

Not all students will have experience or strong backgrounds in each of the areas mentioned; however, you want to have a good mixture of skills and talents. Do not go out and try to "check-off all the boxes" just to satisfy the committee. It is important that you represent yourself completely and honestly to the committee so that your interest can best be served and the committee can assess not only what you bring to the program, but how the program will benefit your development as a pharmacist.

The Interview Process

Schools require an interview as part of the admission process. The structure and goals of this process will vary between programs. This general information regarding interviews is meant to help you have a better idea of what to expect, and therefore be more effective in communicating your abilities and desires to the interviewers. One of the most positive benefits of preparing yourself for an interview is that it gives you a structured assessment of your strengths, weaknesses, and professional goals. By quantifying these at this critical time in your career, you will be sure of your goals and motivation for your chosen career path.

There are many texts providing copious information on how interviews are structured and can prepare you for this event. Most of these address the pursuit of a job in your chosen field. This fact makes their recommendations a bit more structured than might be appropriate for an academic interview for a position in a professional program. Overall, the committee or interviewer is not looking for one right person for the job. They look for a wide range of backgrounds and interests that will not only assure student success in a rigorous academic program, but will also provide support for a variety of practice settings. Not everyone will work in a direct patient care environment for his or her whole career. As important as patient empathy is to a health care professional, some are going to be better than others and some will work in an area where this skill is not the most important one required on a case-by-case basis. There is room for diversity in pharmacy programs in every sense of the word. Thus, interviewers may evaluate candidates on a range of criteria including communication skills, critical thinking, maturity, and motivation. Just as interviewees will vary, so will the interviewers. Some will be more skilled than others and some may look at the applicant in terms of their own career choices. It is important for you to try and listen to the interviewer, and determine what is meant by the question being asked and how you should best relate your own feelings while being sensitive to the setting and the audience. One thing that comes through in the interview texts reviewed is that honesty is the best policy. If you feel that you have to compromise your interests to say what the interviewer wants to hear, you should review your choice of this institution or career pursuit.

Overall, the greatest benefit to be gained by the interview is for the committee to see the sincerity of the interest you have in the program and a career in pharmacy. Also, it is important that you receive positive reinforcement of your goals and helpful information from the institution administering the interview.

TIP

Get as much information as possible about the program and have some good questions ready (for example, a question about points that were brought up by committee members). This shows that you are "thinking on your feet."

Based on our experience, here are three of the most common topics discussed during a pharmacy application interview:

- Professional Background
- Academic Background
- Personal Background

The following table lists questions you may want to consider as you prepare for the interview process.

- What qualities do you possess that you believe are complementary to the pharmacy profession?

- What have you done to increase the likelihood of your acceptance into pharmacy school? What sets you apart from other applicants?

- What are your plans if you do not gain entry to pharmacy school this year?

- Describe a project you worked on that required problem-solving and critical thinking skills.

- What skills and abilities have facilitated your academic success thus far and which will promote your success in pharmacy school?

- Describe an obstacle you have faced in the past and what you learned about yourself as a result.

- Name five things you are most proud of.

- What are the advantages and disadvantages of working with a team on a project?

- Describe your best friend. How would your best friend describe you?

- What are the most important attributes of a good pharmacist?

- Describe an ethical dilemma you have faced in the past and how you resolved the dilemma.

- Do you have any hobbies? What do you do to have fun and relax?

PROFESSIONAL BACKGROUND

Basically, you have been preparing all of your life for the interview. However, you should spend some significant time before the interview making an "inventory" of your answer to the question "why pharmacy?" Here are some self-assessment questions to help prepare you for this type of discussion.

- Why have you chosen pharmacy as a career path? When did you first consider pharmacy as a career?
- Do you know anyone who is a pharmacist?
- What other careers did you consider?
- What steps have you taken to learn more about pharmacy as a profession?
- Who influenced your choice of career, and how (actively or through example)?
- Who would you consider to be your mentor? Why?
- What type of jobs have you held? What have been your likes and dislikes about those jobs? Have these jobs influenced your decision to pursue pharmacy as a career?
- What other careers or academic pursuits interest you?
- What jobs are available to pharmacists? What type of career in pharmacy interests you most?
- What will you do if you are not admitted into a school or college of pharmacy?
- Have you held any leadership positions such as in an organization or on a sports team?
- What hobbies or extracurricular activities are you involved in?
- What are your opinions on professional and community service?
- How would you describe yourself? What are your strengths and weaknesses?
- What is the most challenging personal situation you have faced? How did you cope?
- Can you provide an example of a situation in which you faced a moral or ethical dilemma? How did you confront or resolve this situation?

Pointer

Avoid yes or no answers to questions posed to you, as well as one-line answers.

Any student can come up with answers to these types of questions. Ideally, there is no right or wrong answer. What the committee should be looking for is the background information that you relate to support your answers. Understand that any answer to the questions, such as the ones above, should include an implicit explanation of why or how you arrived at that decision. This is the best way to relate to the committee the maturity of your decision-making process and career interest. It also helps minimize the problem with a difficult interviewer who may be looking for your answer to match his or her choices. If you have a good explanation of how you arrived at that decision, it validates your answer.

Be aware of the professional questions being posed to you as an applicant. The interviewers have been in their profession a long time and often can only relate to subject matter that they have come to accept as common knowledge. An example of a question being asked about a professional setting scenario is—"What would you do if a patient comes in and needs a prescription refill and there are no refills indicated on the prescription?" The possible answers are myriad, and often the question is asked of a student who has retail pharmacy experience and has observed a pharmacist handle this situation many times. If you do not have any experience or any idea of how to answer this question, consider explaining your lack of experience in that area and that this is the type of thing you know training in the professional program will provide. Then, try to relate the question to something you are more familiar with. For example, you might respond, "It sounds like this is a question that deals with utilizing appropriate people skills and ethical behavior on the part of the pharmacist; let me tell you about a situation that I dealt with in a job where we had an employee who was involved in stealing. . . ." This allows you to put the question on your own terms and to talk about something with which you are familiar. Follow-up your description with a question as to whether that scenario related sufficiently to the professional question posed by the interviewer(s).

Ideally, you will have some pharmacy or related experiences to utilize in the interview. This not only shows your competency in areas that you have been trained, but also, that you are making your decision regarding a career choice based on personal experience. Pharmacy jobs for pre-pharmacy students can be difficult to obtain, particularly if you are in an area with a high concentration of pharmacy students. Often, students first think of retail or community pharmacy because this practice option is so visible, but do not neglect opportunities in hospitals, clinics, long-term care facilities and many other areas where pharmacists or other healthcare professionals have the opportunity to work with interested students. Hopefully you started working in a related area as early as high school. In doing this, you may have had the opportunity to advance to a position which provides direct contact with the operation of a pharmacy. If you are unable to obtain a job in a pharmacy, you may be able to obtain relevant experience by shadowing pharmacists or volunteering in health care settings that provide pharmacy services.

ACADEMIC BACKGROUND

The nature of academic performance reported to the institution you are applying to is very quantitative. All require that transcripts be provided and often calculate a single grade point average (GPA) for ranking the applicant pool. Some interviews may be conducted "blind" in that the interviewers do not have access to the student's credentials prior to the interview. In this case, you may still bring this information into the process if they refer to your performance or discuss this as part of the interview. If academic success is a strong point in your background, by all means, include it in your discussions. Most interviewers will have had the chance to review a student's admission file before and during the interview. It is important that all available materials, transcripts, and other required information have been provided and that your application is as complete as possible. Also, the committee may ask specific questions regarding courses in which you did especially well or faced challenges. Do not try to ignore bad academic events or specific grades. Address them honestly to the committee and explain any extenuating circumstances which may have adversely affected performance in the short term. In most circumstances, you should avoid blaming the instructor in a course; it is important to take responsibility for your own performance. Point out improvements or trends which show improved effort or understanding of vital material. Talk about additional courses that you may have taken which, even though not required, might provide a benefit during the pharmacy program or in professional practice. Even courses in business, psychology, writing or education can be very applicable and helpful in one's career pursuit. Usually, high school grades or performance are not an issue, but if you had a particularly good experience in a class or with a teacher who was pivotal in your career choice or academic performance, it would be good to include this in your discussion.

Be aware of the pre-pharmacy requirements for the program and discuss how you plan to complete any remaining courses in time to begin the professional program in the desired term. If you have courses for which you hope to receive credit toward pharmacy prerequisites, check that out with the admission office before the interview. Often the interviewers are faculty who, though familiar with the requirements of the program, are not the ones to make transfer credit decisions. Thus, questions concerning transfer credit should be addressed to the admissions office.

Often you will be asked if you have applied to other pharmacy or academic programs. Again, be honest and discuss other plans you have or pursuits you have considered. Considering other programs or even other academic pursuits, which are based on the interests you have stated in the interview, should be a positive factor and show that you are a serious and mature student. However, if you detect that the interviewers feel some competitiveness toward another pharmacy program which you are considering, tell them that this shows how serious you are about your pursuit of a career in pharmacy. We believe it is a good idea to consider and apply to any program you feel you could attend and get the education that will allow you to pursue your career goals.

TIP ✏️

Don't just state that you were a member of a particular organization. Discuss what you did in it to show your leadership abilities or interest in providing service to the community.

PERSONAL BACKGROUND

The interview is a chance to put some "personality" into your application. The process prior to the time of the interview is very quantitative, with GPAs and PCAT scores often being the primary consideration that allowed you an interview. It is your responsibility to make the impression on the interviewers that you will do well in their institution and will be the type of pharmacist they want to represent their institution. Talk not only about the experiences in your background that led you to pharmacy, but also talk about the experiences that helped you to develop a personality that will support you through the academic program and as a pharmacist. Include information about outside activities, sports, and hobbies. Include involvement in organizations in addition to academic pursuits, such as membership in service groups. Membership in honor societies should be mentioned; discuss activities or opportunities that were provided during your membership, not just that you were a member because of your grades or other academic qualities.

The various background areas overlap, each one providing important information in how you got to where you are and what type of student and person you are. Therefore, it is natural that the relationship between academics, professional pursuits, and personality will be extensions of each other.

ON-SITE ESSAY

Some schools may require that you complete an essay during your interview at the school/college. Examples of possible essay topics include:

- You just learned your patient has been nonadherent to his medication. Describe how you would convince this patient to take his medication as prescribed, and the importance of medication adherence.
- What are two (2) messages or themes about responsibility for personal health care and well being that you feel are important to advance to American teenagers today?
- What one or two areas of health maintenance and disease treatment should U.S. scientific research efforts and resources be directed toward during the next 10 years?
- What are some knowledge or skill requirements essential for practitioners in today's community and environment? Why?

The length of the essay and the time allotted for completion of the essay will vary by school/college. Essay evaluation criteria may include use of language, grammar, punctuation, clarity, and cohesiveness. We recommend that you take a few minutes at the beginning of the essay-writing session to prepare an outline to help guide your writing process. We also recommend that you save a few minutes at the end of the essay-writing session to review and edit your essay as necessary. Other general essay-writing tips can be found in Chapter 9.

CONCLUSION OF THE INTERVIEW

At the end of the interview make sure you summarize your interest in the program and "wrap-up" any issues regarding remaining coursework. State your plans for future academic terms, and make sure you know what the next step will be and when you can expect to hear from the committee regarding the results of your application.

> ## TIPS FOR SUCCESSFUL INTERVIEWING
>
> - Arrive on time for the interview. Arriving late may send the message that the interview is not a priority to you.
> - Try not to appear nervous. Arriving to the interview early will give you the opportunity to adjust to the environment and may decrease your anxiety.
> - Dress professionally.
> - Be courteous.
> - Be positive, friendly, and smile.
> - Answer all questions as completely as possible.
> - Speak clearly.
> - Make eye contact with the interviewers.
> - Don't exhibit unnecessary movements.
> - Educate yourself on the institution.
> - If you have questions, ask if there is enough time to ask your questions. If so, ask questions.
> - If you have any additional materials that you want the committee to review, bring them with you to the interview.
> - Listen attentively and learn from the interview. The information exchange should be a two-way process.
> - Bring a pen and notebook to the interview. Have a list of questions that you may want to ask and make notes as appropriate.
> - Don't limit yourself to one or two word answers.

Graduate Degrees in Pharmacy

Master of Science (M.S.) and Doctor of Philosophy (Ph.D.) degrees are available for pharmacy disciplines including, but not limited to, medicinal chemistry, pharmaceutics, pharmacology, pharmacy care administration, and toxicology. For more information regarding graduate programs, you should contact the specific college or school of pharmacy in which you are interested.

Postgraduate Training: Residencies and Fellowships

A graduate of a college or school of pharmacy may decide to pursue postgraduate training in a specific area of pharmacy practice or pharmacy research (see the later section, entitled "Residency and Fellowship Programs: Areas of Pharmacy Practice and Research"). Residencies and fellowships are two distinct types of postgraduate training programs. General requirements for an applicant seeking a residency or fellowship include graduating from an accredited college or school of pharmacy and an interest in and aptitude for advanced training in pharmacy. A resident or fellow receives a stipend plus benefits (insurance, vacation, etc.). The amount of the stipend and the specific benefits vary according to the individual program.

RESIDENCIES

A residency is an organized, directed postgraduate training program in a defined area of pharmacy practice. Residencies are typically one year in duration; however, some may be longer. The primary goal of a residency is to train pharmacists in a specific area of pharmacy practice. The objective of a residency is to develop competent practitioners who are able to provide pharmacy services such as clinical, drug information, pharmacotherapeutic dosing and monitoring, and administration.

A pharmacy practice residency is a general residency in pharmacy practice. In addition to pharmacy practice residencies, a host of specialized residencies exists. A specialized residency focuses on a particular niche of pharmacy practice; pediatric pharmacy, psychiatric pharmacy, and nuclear pharmacy are all examples of specialized residencies. Whether the residency is a pharmacy practice residency or a specialty residency, training typically involves structured rotations within the pharmacy department as well as medical rotations with physicians and other health care professionals. The practice experiences of residents are closely directed and evaluated by qualified practitioner-preceptors who are trained in particular areas of pharmacy practice.

The American Society of Health-System Pharmacists is the accrediting body for residencies. To obtain a list of postgraduate pharmacy practice residency programs, write to or visit:

American Society of Health-System Pharmacists
7272 Wisconsin Avenue
Bethesda, MD 20814
www.ashp.org/menu/residents.asp

FELLOWSHIPS

A fellowship is a directed, highly individualized postgraduate program, typically two years in duration, that is designed to prepare the participant to become an independent researcher. The primary goal of a fellowship is to develop competency in scientific pharmacy research. A fellow works under the close direction and instruction of a qualified researcher-preceptor. Many fellowships are affiliated with a college or school of pharmacy. To obtain a list of postgraduate fellowship programs, you can write to or visit:

American College of Clinical Pharmacy
13000 W. 87th St. Parkway
Lenexa, Kansas 66215-4530
www.accp.com

RESIDENCY AND FELLOWSHIP PROGRAMS: AREAS OF PHARMACY PRACTICE AND RESEARCH

Administration
Ambulatory Care
Cardiology
Clinical Informatics
Clinical Pharmaceutical Sciences
Clinical Pharmacology
Community Pharmacy
Critical Care
Drug Development
Drug Information
Emergency Medicine
Endocrinology
Family Medicine
Geriatrics
HIV Pharmacy
Hospice
Immunology
Infectious Disease
Internal Medicine
Managed Care
Nephrology
Neurology
Nuclear Pharmacy

Nutrition
Obstetrics-Gynecology
Oncology
Outcomes Research
Pain Management
Patient Safety
Pediatrics
Pharmacoeconomics
Pharmacoepidemiology
Pharmacogenomics
Pharmacokinetics
Pharmacometrics
Pharmacotherapy
Pharmacy Practice
Primary Care
Psychiatric Pharmacy
Pulmonary
Rheumatology
Toxicology
Translational Research
Transplantation
Women's Health

The PCAT

CHAPTER 2

WHAT IS THE PCAT?

The Pharmacy College Admission Test (PCAT) is a national examination developed by Pearson Education, Inc. The PCAT was developed to provide admission committees of pharmacy schools with comparable information about the academic abilities of applicants in six topic areas: verbal ability, reading comprehension, chemistry, biology, quantitative ability (math), and writing.

The computer-based exam consists of 232 multiple-choice questions and one essay topic. The stem portion of each multiple-choice question may be presented as a question, partial statement, or problem scenario followed by four possible answers. Only one answer is correct. Often the other choices are distractors, may contain errors, do not apply to the question, or may not be the best answer to the question. Often the distractors are taken from the same content area of study as the correct answer, so it is important to recognize specific facts, not just be familiar with topics. The PCAT score is calculated from the number of correct answers. There is NO penalty for guessing, so candidates should not leave any answers blank.

PCAT Contents

As of April 2014, the following is a description of the PCAT's six scoring sections:

- **Verbal Ability.** This section consists of 40 word-pairing analogies and sentence completion questions. Twenty-five minutes are given to complete this section.
- **Biology.** This section consists of 48 general biology, microbiology, and anatomy and physiology questions. Thirty-five minutes are given to complete this section.
- **Reading Comprehension.** This section consists of six reading passages and 48 questions that test candidates' evaluation, comprehension, and analytical skills. Fifty minutes are given to complete this section.
- **Quantitative Ability.** This section consists of 48 basic math, algebra, precalculus, calculus, probability, and statistics questions. No calculators are allowed during the exam. Forty-five minutes are given to complete this section.
- **Chemistry.** This section consists of 48 general and organic chemistry and basic biochemistry processes questions. Some may involve calculations; remember, no calculators are allowed. Thirty-five minutes are given to complete this section.
- **Writing.** The candidate will be requested to compose one problem-solving essay. Thirty minutes will be given to write the essay.

Usually the PCAT exam includes multiple-choice experimental questions being tested for possible use in future exams. There is no way to know which items are experimental, so candidates will want to do their best to answer each question correctly.

The Exam

PCAT Sections	2014–2015 PCAT Section Subtests/% of Item Types	Number of Items in Section	Number of Minutes to Complete PCAT Section
1. Verbal Ability	Analogies—62% Sentence Completion—38%	40 Items	25 Minutes
2. Biology	General Biology—50% Microbiology—20% Anatomy & Physiology—30%	48 Items	35 Minutes
3. Reading Comprehension	Comprehension—30% Evaluation—30% Analysis—40%	6 Reading Passages & 48 Items	50 Minutes
4. Quantitative Ability	Basic Math—15% Algebra—20% Probability & Statistics—20% Precalculus—22% Calculus—22%	48 Items	45 Minutes
5. Chemistry	General Chemistry—50% Organic Chemistry—30% Basic Biochemistry Processes—20%	48 Items	35 Minutes
6. Writing	Problem Solving Conventions of Language	1 Topic	30 Minutes

PCAT Scoring

Your score report will include separate scaled scores and percentile scores for each of the five multiple-choice content areas. It will also include a composite scaled score and percentile score for the overall multiple-choice exam. Scaled scores are computed from raw scores for each individual test offering so that results can be compared from one test offering to the next. The scaled scores will range from 200 to 600.

Additionally, a percentile score is computed by distributing your performance in a norm group or pool of candidates. The percentile reported for individual sections and the composite score indicate the percentage of students who scored below you. For example, a 75th percentile score on the biology section indicates that you did better than 75% of the students in the norm group. Immediately after taking the PCAT, students receive preliminary scores for each of the five content areas and the overall composite score; these preliminary scores will very closely approximate the official PCAT scores received several weeks after taking the test. Students can use these preliminary scores to assess how well they performed on the PCAT and whether they may need to take the test again to improve their scores.

You will receive a single writing score that is based both on mechanics and on the development and presentation of the composition. The writing score is reported on a scale of 1.0 to 6.0, and a mean score for all individuals taking that administration of the PCAT is also shown.

TIP ✏️

Check with the school to ensure that your score is as competitive as possible.

The scores used by numerous pharmacy programs in evaluating candidates vary. Some use scaled scores; others use percentiles. Some have minimum scores required in each of the PCAT sections; some use composite scores. Many will use a candidate's highest score on a single attempt if the candidate has taken the test more than once; however, this might not always be the case.

After a candidate has taken the PCAT five times, submission of a written request is required for a sixth test. Candidates registering for more than the fifth time still register online, but they must be prepared to provide documentation explaining the circumstances that require taking the PCAT again. If the requested documentation is not provided, a candidate's registration will be cancelled. Further details on this policy and the type of documentation that may be required can be found on the PCAT website.

When Is the PCAT Offered?

The PCAT is administered at Pearson VUE Test Centers on multiple dates. To obtain exact dates, visit the PCAT website at *www.pcatweb.info*. Accommodations may be made for individuals with disabilities. Deadlines for registration for the PCAT are generally approximately eight weeks prior to the testing date—onsite, same-day registration is not available.

Fees

For the most current information visit the PCAT website at *www.pcatweb.info*. The following is the PCAT fee as of 2014.

Online Registration Fee $199.00

For more information concerning special fees, visit the PCAT website.

PCAT Information

For more information concerning the PCAT, contact Pearson at the address or phone number or visit the website below.

NCS Pearson, Inc.
PCAT Customer Relations—PCAT
19500 Bulverde Road
San Antonio, Texas 78259
1-800-622-3231
www.pcatweb.info

The authors strongly recommend reviewing the PCAT candidate information booklet available at *www.pcatweb.info*.

When Should You Take the PCAT?

Many considerations are involved in the decision of when and how often to take the PCAT. Many colleges/schools of pharmacy do not penalize applicants for taking the test more than once and often use the highest scores. This practice differs from institution to institution, so you will need to check with the college/school that you are interested in attending. In addition, it is strongly recommended that you take the PCAT no later than the fall of the year prior to the semester that you want to begin pharmacy school. This strategy will allow you to retake the PCAT in the winter if desired or necessary.

The ultimate decision of when and how often to take the PCAT is an individualized one and depends on many circumstances, such as when you feel most comfortable taking the test (this may depend on the number of pre-pharmacy courses you have taken). Other factors that may affect your decision are the admissions policy of the pharmacy college or school you wish to attend and your previous PCAT scores.

Strategies to Increase Your Score

CHAPTER 3

PCAT STRATEGIES

When taking the PCAT, work at a comfortable pace but keep in mind that there is a time limit for each section. Be sure to answer every question. Your total PCAT score and the score you receive on each section of the test (excluding the PCAT essay) reflect the number of correct answers only. Some tests penalize for guessing by subtracting the number of wrong answers from the number of correct answers; with the PCAT, however, this is not the case. Although guesses are not likely to make much difference in your scores, you should not ignore this chance to avoid the total loss of points from unanswered questions.

The PCAT is divided into six sections. Three sections are specifically related to coursework covered in the pre-pharmacy curriculum: chemistry, biology, and mathematics. Two sections are more comprehensive in nature and measure skills acquired through lifelong learning: verbal ability and reading comprehension. Because the verbal ability and reading comprehension sections assess skills acquired over a long period of time, they tend to be more difficult to study for in advance. The essay is a combination of comprehensive learning, life experiences, and skills potentially obtained during your pre-pharmacy work.

When you take the practice PCAT tests in this book and the actual PCAT test, make sure to keep track of the time allotted for each test section. Pace yourself and work quickly but calmly through all the questions. Although you may be forced to guess on some questions, there is a chance that some of your guesses will be correct.

FIFTEEN PRESCRIPTIONS TO INCREASE YOUR SCORE

The first section of this chapter discussed general PCAT strategies. In this section you are given fifteen "prescriptions" to improve your PCAT test scores. Students who have taken the PCAT and employed these test-taking tactics have found them quite useful:

Remember

On the PCAT, your score is computed from the number of correct answers only. You are NOT penalized for guessing.

- **Rx 1.** Get an adequate amount of sleep the night before the test.
- **Rx 2.** Allow yourself plenty of time to get to the testing site.
- **Rx 3.** Bring an accurate watch.
- **Rx 4.** Bring two forms of proper identification (e.g., driver's license, passport).
- **Rx 5.** Wear comfortable clothes.
- **Rx 6.** Know what to expect. After studying this preparation manual, you will be familiar with the types of questions that may appear on the PCAT.
- **Rx 7.** Read and memorize the directions for each question type or section.
- **Rx 8.** Pace yourself. Work within the time restriction.
- **Rx 9.** Look at all the possible answers before making your final choice.
- **Rx 10.** Eliminate as many wrong answers as possible.
- **Rx 11.** Answer every question.
- **Rx 12.** In preparing for the verbal ability section, consider reviewing a vocabulary study manual.
- **Rx 13.** In the reading comprehension section, when asked to find the main idea, be sure to check the opening and summary sentences of the passage.
- **Rx 14.** You cannot use a calculator on the PCAT; therefore, rounding numbers to do the math problems accurately and quickly may be beneficial.
- **Rx 15.** Do not bring cell phones and other electronic devices to the PCAT as they are not allowed in the testing area. Your PCAT score will be cancelled if you break this rule.

Verbal Ability Review and Practice

CHAPTER 4

TIPS FOR THE VERBAL ABILITY SECTION

The verbal ability section of the PCAT is designed to test your knowledge of words (vocabulary) and the relationships between them by using sentence completion and analogy-type questions. This section consists of approximately 40 questions, with about 62% involving analogies and 38% involving sentence completion. You will have 25 minutes to complete the verbal ability section. To study for the verbal ability section, you can use texts designed to help you increase your "word power" or vocabulary. Studying material on the roots of words and on prefixes and suffixes may also help you prepare for this section of the PCAT.

Analogy questions test your understanding of how paired vocabulary words and ideas relate to each other. They are expressed as A : B :: C : D. In words, A is to B as C is to D; for example, meow is to cat as bark is to dog. The notion of a proportion should be familiar to you from mathematics. In an analogy, however, the proportion is a logical or verbal one.

There are a number of different kinds of analogy relationships including association (e.g., cause and effect, affiliation, sequence, function, purpose or use), part to whole, whole to part, synonyms, antonyms, classification (e.g., members of a class or category), and characteristic (e.g., location, having or lacking an attribute). It is not necessary for you to memorize all the types of analogies, but becoming familiar with some of the main types can help you identify them and answer the questions on the analogy section more quickly. You should first identify the part of speech represented by the words in the analogy; then look for that part of speech among the answer selections.

TIP

Be sure to familiarize yourself with the different kinds of analogy relationships.

Other strategies include:

> - Eliminating answer choices that do not have a clear and reasonable relationship to the word in question
>
> - Consider whether both words in the first set of words are concrete items (e.g., painting is to wall . . .), abstract concepts (e.g., valor is to chivalry . . .), or a combination of both (e.g., knight is to chivalry . . .); then, look for the answer choice that might best complete the pattern with the word in question
>
> - Remember that many words have more than one meaning, and an answer choice may be correct due to a lesser-known definition
>
> - Consider the pattern of the first word set (e.g., a noun followed by a verb) and apply this pattern when selecting an answer choice

The practice questions and answers in this chapter will demonstrate and explain the different types of analogies and provide insight into formulating a correct answer. For a complete survey of analogies, you may wish to consult *Barron's Miller Analogies Test*.

Once you have spent some time preparing yourself by studying vocabulary reviews and "word power" exercises and are ready to test your ability in this area, complete the verbal ability questions in this book. The explanatory answers for the analogy questions are designed to help you become familiar with the various types of analogies; therefore, you should read them carefully.

Sentence completion questions are also included in the verbal section of the PCAT. You will be given a sentence in which either one word or two words will be omitted. You will be asked to choose which of the four answer choices provided best completes the sentence based on sentence context and reading comprehension. There will be only one correct response. The correct utilization of vocabulary skills, logic, grammar, and sentence tone and style will help you to eliminate the incorrect responses, allowing you to choose the answer that makes the most sense and best completes the sentence. In sentences that have two, or double, blanks, the correct answer will provide the best word choices for BOTH blanks. Even if you are unfamiliar with one or more of the words listed in the answer choices or the subject base of the sentence, by using clues embedded in the sentence you should still be able to choose the word or words that correctly complete the sentence. Thus, the sentence fragment may contain clues to help you eliminate unfamiliar words in the answers listed so that you may choose the correct answer.

Answer Sheet
VERBAL ABILITY

1	Ⓐ Ⓑ Ⓒ Ⓓ				26	Ⓐ Ⓑ Ⓒ Ⓓ			
2	Ⓐ Ⓑ Ⓒ Ⓓ				27	Ⓐ Ⓑ Ⓒ Ⓓ			
3	Ⓐ Ⓑ Ⓒ Ⓓ				28	Ⓐ Ⓑ Ⓒ Ⓓ			
4	Ⓐ Ⓑ Ⓒ Ⓓ				29	Ⓐ Ⓑ Ⓒ Ⓓ			
5	Ⓐ Ⓑ Ⓒ Ⓓ				30	Ⓐ Ⓑ Ⓒ Ⓓ			
6	Ⓐ Ⓑ Ⓒ Ⓓ				31	Ⓐ Ⓑ Ⓒ Ⓓ			
7	Ⓐ Ⓑ Ⓒ Ⓓ				32	Ⓐ Ⓑ Ⓒ Ⓓ			
8	Ⓐ Ⓑ Ⓒ Ⓓ				33	Ⓐ Ⓑ Ⓒ Ⓓ			
9	Ⓐ Ⓑ Ⓒ Ⓓ				34	Ⓐ Ⓑ Ⓒ Ⓓ			
10	Ⓐ Ⓑ Ⓒ Ⓓ				35	Ⓐ Ⓑ Ⓒ Ⓓ			
11	Ⓐ Ⓑ Ⓒ Ⓓ				36	Ⓐ Ⓑ Ⓒ Ⓓ			
12	Ⓐ Ⓑ Ⓒ Ⓓ				37	Ⓐ Ⓑ Ⓒ Ⓓ			
13	Ⓐ Ⓑ Ⓒ Ⓓ				38	Ⓐ Ⓑ Ⓒ Ⓓ			
14	Ⓐ Ⓑ Ⓒ Ⓓ				39	Ⓐ Ⓑ Ⓒ Ⓓ			
15	Ⓐ Ⓑ Ⓒ Ⓓ				40	Ⓐ Ⓑ Ⓒ Ⓓ			
16	Ⓐ Ⓑ Ⓒ Ⓓ				41	Ⓐ Ⓑ Ⓒ Ⓓ			
17	Ⓐ Ⓑ Ⓒ Ⓓ				42	Ⓐ Ⓑ Ⓒ Ⓓ			
18	Ⓐ Ⓑ Ⓒ Ⓓ				43	Ⓐ Ⓑ Ⓒ Ⓓ			
19	Ⓐ Ⓑ Ⓒ Ⓓ				44	Ⓐ Ⓑ Ⓒ Ⓓ			
20	Ⓐ Ⓑ Ⓒ Ⓓ				45	Ⓐ Ⓑ Ⓒ Ⓓ			
21	Ⓐ Ⓑ Ⓒ Ⓓ				46	Ⓐ Ⓑ Ⓒ Ⓓ			
22	Ⓐ Ⓑ Ⓒ Ⓓ				47	Ⓐ Ⓑ Ⓒ Ⓓ			
23	Ⓐ Ⓑ Ⓒ Ⓓ				48	Ⓐ Ⓑ Ⓒ Ⓓ			
24	Ⓐ Ⓑ Ⓒ Ⓓ				49	Ⓐ Ⓑ Ⓒ Ⓓ			
25	Ⓐ Ⓑ Ⓒ Ⓓ				50	Ⓐ Ⓑ Ⓒ Ⓓ			

Practice Questions

50 Questions

ANALOGIES (25 QUESTIONS)

Directions: Choose the word that **best** completes the analogy.

1. HUMIDITY : SWAMP :: ARIDITY :

   (A) Ocean
   (B) Air conditioning
   (C) Sea level
   (D) Desert

2. HYPNOSIS : TRANCE :: STROKE :

   (A) Embolism
   (B) Paralysis
   (C) Speech
   (D) Rehabilitation

3. POLYPS : CORAL :: BEES :

   (A) Flowers
   (B) Colony
   (C) Hive
   (D) Honey

4. PHYSICIAN : PRESCRIPTION :: TEACHER :

   (A) Homework
   (B) Classroom
   (C) Education
   (D) Textbook

5. SPIDER : WEB :: BIRD :

   (A) Deck
   (B) Wood
   (C) Nest
   (D) Wing

6. RIND : ORANGE :: BARK :

   (A) Tree
   (B) Dog
   (C) Forest
   (D) Leaves

7. MITIGATE : ALLEVIATE :: TRAIPSE :

(A) Amble
(B) Run
(C) Accept
(D) Deny

8. DENTIST : DRILL :: ASTRONOMER :

(A) Milky Way
(B) Galaxies
(C) Telescope
(D) Magnification

9. RED : RUDDY :: METAL :

(A) Element
(B) Metallic
(C) Strength
(D) Gray

10. LION : PRIDE :: CAT :

(A) Pod
(B) Murder
(C) Dule
(D) Clowder

11. VIOLIN : PEGBOX :: CLARINET :

(A) Scroll
(B) Piston
(C) Barrel
(D) Cymbal

12. SEISMOLOGY : EARTHQUAKES :: CYTOLOGY :

(A) Cell
(B) Bacteria
(C) Fungi
(D) Tissue

13. TRANSPARENT : CLEAR :: OPAQUE :

(A) White
(B) Heavy
(C) Muddy
(D) Translucent

14. ABSTAIN : INDULGE :: LOOSEN :

(A) Find
(B) Tighten
(C) Yield
(D) Corrupt

15. AIRPLANE : HANGAR :: AUTOMOBILE :

(A) Garage
(B) Travel
(C) Flight
(D) Passenger

16. GRAIN : WOOD :: LUSTER :

(A) Surface
(B) Value
(C) Diamond
(D) Shine

17. TANG : PIQUANCY :: SURREPTITIOUS :

(A) Candid
(B) Garish
(C) Stoic
(D) Clandestine

18. ANACONDA : BOA :: TENNIS :

(A) Racquet
(B) Sport
(C) Court
(D) Serve

19. LENS : MICROSCOPE :: HELMET :

(A) Weapon
(B) Battle
(C) Armor
(D) Head

20. CANARY : ATLANTIC :: COOK :

(A) Arctic
(B) Mediterranean
(C) Pacific
(D) Indian

21. ASSIMILATE : SEGREGATE :: ABATE :

(A) Amplify
(B) Subdue
(C) Allay
(D) Blandish

22. SINGER : MICROPHONE :: PHYSICIAN :

(A) Hippocratic Oath
(B) Stethoscope
(C) Nurse
(D) Surgery

23. BANYAN : TREE :: CHRYSANTHEMUM :

(A) Stem
(B) India
(C) Japan
(D) Flower

24. BOOLEAN : ALGEBRA :: EUCLIDEAN :

(A) Smorgasbord
(B) Geometry
(C) Ghost
(D) Gambling

25. MUZZLE : DOG :: CEREBELLUM :

(A) Brain
(B) Reticular activating system
(C) Amygdala
(D) Electrode

SENTENCE COMPLETIONS (25 QUESTIONS)

Directions: Select the word or set of words that makes the most sense when inserted into the sentence and that best fits the meaning of the sentence as a whole.

26. Around strangers Karen may seem quiet and _____, but once she is around friends and family she is quite _____.

(A) impartial; jaded
(B) lurid; malleable
(C) introverted; loquacious
(D) impious; hostile

27. _____ to an antibiotic means that a microorganism that was formerly _____ to the antibiotic is no longer affected by it.

    (A) Resistance; susceptible
    (B) Synergy; inhibited
    (C) Inhibition; nosocomial
    (D) Suicidal; caustic

28. Before giving an _____ solution, it is necessary to check the medication and dose against the patient's chart.

    (A) ambiguous
    (B) unlikely
    (C) eclectic
    (D) intravenous

29. The humble student received _____ from his teacher and fellow students after winning the state science fair.

    (A) antipathy
    (B) accolades
    (C) ambivalence
    (D) dolefulness

30. The teacher was _____ with the student, as the student was not honest or trustworthy.

    (A) impartial
    (B) understanding
    (C) disenchanted
    (D) elated

31. The next circus performer's act was very _____ because he had to juggle three balls while _____ balancing himself on a tightrope.

    (A) fickle; inadvertently
    (B) complicated; simultaneously
    (C) sufficient; hypothetically
    (D) germane; gradually

32. Her arrogance in the workplace was _____ given how few accomplishments she had achieved.

    (A) justified
    (B) perplexing
    (C) understandable
    (D) apropos

33. We stood in _____ at how we were so easily dwarfed by the _____ sequoia trees.

    (A) bewilderment; versatile
    (B) validation; execrable
    (C) remorse; elusive
    *(D) veneration; gargantuan

34. The amateur _____ hosts a wine tasting party for her friends every few months.

    (A) aficionado
    (B) connoisseur
    (C) sommelier
    (D) apostate

35. While making the icing for the cake, we ran out of blue food coloring, so we had to _____ and use green instead.

    (A) implicate
    (B) substitute
    (C) effervesce
    (D) disseminate

36. Inertia is the _____ to act or change.

    (A) prompt
    (B) drive
    (C) disinclination
    (D) portent

37. Don't be too _____ about the final results of the experiment; something _____ could happen and ruin the project like the test tube falling and shattering on the ground.

    (A) anxious; irreverent
    (B) predisposed; eclectic
    (C) dogmatic; ulterior
    (D) sanguine; unanticipated

38. As a sign of _____, one of the parties scheduled a peaceful conference where each party could negotiate and both reach an agreement.

    (A) hostility
    (B) indifference
    (C) prosperity
    (D) diplomacy

39. The wing of an eagle and the human arm are _____ structures. They differ in function but their anatomy is _____.

    (A) homologous; related
    (B) heterogeneous; stringent
    (C) benign; significant
    (D) simple; blatant

40. After reviewing the protocol from 20 years ago, we determined that it was _____ and that it needed to be revised and updated.

    (A) theoretical
    (B) intangible
    (C) beneficial
    (D) antiquated

41. The _____, which is the second largest portion of the brain, is responsible for controlling _____.

    (A) cerebellum; balance
    (B) cerebrum; language
    (C) cerebellum; respiration
    (D) cerebrum; blood pressure

42. When going from an area of bright sunlight into a dark room, the pupils of your eyes must dilate in order for you to _____ to your changed environment.

    (A) obscure
    (B) differentiate
    (C) adapt
    (D) stimulate

43. One way in which hormones may be _____ from the blood is by excretion into urine or bile.

    (A) celebrated
    (B) eliminated
    (C) replenished
    (D) ratified

44. Because he is so _____, he cannot play harmoniously with the other children in his class and does not have many friends.

    (A) pugnacious
    (B) dubious
    (C) suspicious
    (D) ingenious

45. The accusation of fraud that was printed in the newspaper was _____ and untrue; nonetheless, the organization's reputation was still _____.

    (A) intriguing; pragmatic
    (B) defamatory; besmirched
    (C) astute; commemorative
    (D) prevalent; exalted

46. After the demonstration, Sue realized that the actual product was not the same as what was advertised and she was very _____.

    (A) diversified
    (B) auspicious
    (C) exonerated
    (D) disillusioned

47. We are still _____ about our vacation plans for this year, unlike last year when we were _____ about where we wanted to go.

    (A) vehement; deceptive
    (B) amiss; repressed
    (C) amorphous; resolute
    (D) altruistic; dubious

48. When the doctor left the room, the patient became _____ and aggressive, but when the doctor returned she _____ her composure and became docile once again.

    (A) vicarious; sullied
    (B) supple; promoted
    (C) surly; fostered
    (D) belligerent; regained

49. A person with Type O blood is usually called a _____ donor, since he or she can give blood to a person with any blood type.

    (A) universal
    (B) ambivalent
    (C) confined
    (D) isolated

50. There are many _____ devices that can be used to help us _____ otherwise hard-to-remember concepts.

    (A) automatic; finesse
    (B) mnemonic; recollect
    (C) schematic; respire
    (D) pneumatic; inspire

Answer Key
VERBAL ABILITY

Analogies

1. **D**	6. **A**	11. **C**	16. **C**	21. **A**
2. **B**	7. **A**	12. **A**	17. **D**	22. **B**
3. **D**	8. **C**	13. **C**	18. **B**	23. **D**
4. **A**	9. **B**	14. **B**	19. **C**	24. **B**
5. **C**	10. **D**	15. **A**	20. **C**	25. **A**

Sentence Completion

26. **C**	31. **B**	36. **C**	41. **A**	46. **D**
27. **A**	32. **B**	37. **D**	42. **C**	47. **C**
28. **D**	33. **D**	38. **D**	43. **B**	48. **D**
29. **B**	34. **C**	39. **A**	44. **A**	49. **A**
30. **C**	35. **B**	40. **D**	45. **B**	50. **B**

EXPLANATORY ANSWERS

ANALOGIES

1. **(D)** Humidity is associated with a swamp, and aridity with a desert. This may be considered an analogy of description or characteristic.

2. **(B)** This is an analogy of cause and effect. Just as hypnosis brings about a trance, a stroke may cause paralysis. (If you chose A by mistake, you identified a cause of stroke rather than its effect. Be careful to match the terms appropriately.)

3. **(D)** In this analogy of cause and effect, bees produce honey just as polyps cause or produce coral.

4. **(A)** A physician provides a patient with a prescription to be filled following an appointment, just as a teacher provides a student with homework to be done following a lecture. This is an analogy of association. Answers B, C, and D do not fit the association pattern.

5. **(C)** This is an analogy of association. A spider is housed in its web just as a bird uses a nest for housing.

6. **(A)** In this "part to whole" analogy, the rind is the outer part of an orange, and the bark is the analogous (or corresponding) outer part of a tree. If you mistakenly chose B, you may have made a common error by assuming that bark was a verb rather than a noun.

7. **(A)** This is an analogy of synonyms. Mitigate and alleviate are defined as to make more bearable or less painful, and traipse and amble (answer A) are defined as a relaxed walk. Answer B is an antonym of traipse, while answers C and D are not applicable to the analogy.

8. **(C)** The analogy is worker to tool. An astronomer uses a telescope just as a dentist uses a drill.

9. **(B)** In this grammatical analogy each noun is paired with an adjective derived from it. Ruddy means reddish in color, and metallic means "made from metal" or "metal-like."

10. **(D)** This analogy is one of "part to whole." A lion is part of a pride, or group of lions. Likewise, a cat is part of a clowder, therefore answer D is correct. Answers A through C are terms for other groups of animals (a pod of whales, a murder of crows, and a dule of doves, respectively).

11. **(C)** This is a "whole to part" analogy. A pegbox is part of a violin, just as a barrel is part of a clarinet, therefore answer C is correct. A scroll (answer A) is also part of a violin, while a piston (answer B) is part of a trumpet. A cymbal (answer D) is a percussive instrument and is often part of a drum set.

12. **(A)** This is an analogy of classification. Seismology is the study of earthquakes, just as cytology is the study of the cell (answer A). The study of bacteria (answer B) is bacteriology, the study of fungi (answer C) is mycology, and the study of tissue (answer D) is histology.

13. **(C)** This analogy is based on synonyms. Just as transparent and clear are synonymous, opaque and muddy also have the same or nearly the same meaning.

14. **(B)** This analogy is based on antonyms. Just as abstain and indulge have opposite meanings, loosen and tighten are also antonyms.

15. **(A)** In this analogy of association, an airplane is kept in a hangar and an automobile is kept in a garage.

16. **(C)** This is an analogy of characteristic or description. Grain is a characteristic of wood, and luster is a characteristic of a diamond.

17. **(D)** This analogy is based on synonyms. Tang and piquancy both refer to a sharp, tart, or pungent flavor. Likewise, surreptitious and clandestine (answer D) both refer to secrecy. Candid is an antonym of surreptitious meaning honest. Garish means gaudy and stoic refers to having little emotion. As such, neither of these answers would be a synonym of surreptitious.

18. **(B)** This is a "part to whole" analogy, since an anaconda is one type of boa, and tennis is one type of sport. To help clarify this kind of analogy, think of the group of all boas and the group of all sports as "wholes," of which the anaconda and tennis are merely respective parts.

19. **(C)** This is a "part to whole" analogy. Just as a lens is part of a microscope, a helmet is part of a suit of armor.

20. **(C)** In this geographical analogy, the Canary Islands are located in the Atlantic Ocean and the Cook Islands are located in the Pacific Ocean (answer C).

21. **(A)** This is an analogy of antonyms. Assimilate means to incorporate, while segregate means to separate, just as abate means to reduce while amplify means to increase. Answers B and C are synonyms of abate. Answer D is not applicable to the analogy.

22. **(B)** This is a "worker to tool" analogy. Just as a singer uses a microphone, a physician uses a stethoscope.

23. **(D)** Although the names of two countries are included in the answer selections, this is not a geographical analogy. In this analogy of part to whole, a banyan is one kind of tree; a chrysanthemum is one kind of flower.

24. **(B)** In this "part to whole" analogy, Boolean is a kind of algebra, and Euclidean is a kind of geometry.

25. **(A)** In this "part to whole" analogy, the muzzle is part of a dog, and the cerebellum is part of the brain. It is also necessary to be flexible enough to realize that "muzzle," as used here, means "the forward or projecting part of a dog's head," and not a device used to put over that part of the dog to keep it from barking, biting, or eating.

SENTENCE COMPLETIONS

26. **(C)** We are told that around strangers Karen is quiet, and the placement of the first blank indicates that the correct word will be synonymous with quiet. Because the word "but" comes before the second blank, we know that something contrasting or contradictory happens when she is around family and friends. From this, we can project that the two correct words will be opposites. This eliminates Answers A, B, and D, which leaves Answer C with the words "introverted" (meaning "shy" or "reclusive") and "loquacious" (meaning "talkative") as the correct answer.

27. **(A)** The first blank in this sentence defines a microorganism's NEW reaction to an antibiotic's actions, in which it is "no longer affected." The word "formerly"

preceding the second blank in the sentence provides a clue that there are two contrasting scenarios occurring; thus, the two correct words will most likely have opposite connotations. Accordingly, if the first blank means "impermeable" or "resistant," then the second blank must mean "susceptible" (unprotected or vulnerable). Based on this, Answer A is the best choice for this sentence.

28. **(D)** The words "medication," "dose," and "patient's chart" in this sentence indicate that the correct word will be related to health or medicine. This eliminates Answers A, B, and C, leaving Answer D (intravenous) as the correct response.

29. **(B)** The blank indicates reaction to a science fair win, which is a positive accomplishment. The only answer with a positive connotation is B, accolades, which means praise. Answer A is defined as hostility, answer C as uncertainty or conflicting emotions, and answer D as mournful. Therefore, B is the best answer.

30. **(C)** The blank indicates that the teacher's response to the student is affected by or related to something that the student did that is NOT honest or trustworthy. To be dishonest or untrustworthy has a negative connotation, so we can project that the correct word will have a negative connotation also. This eliminates Answer B (understanding) and Answer D (elated). Answer A (impartial), which means to be fair or without bias, doesn't make sense in this context, so Answer C (disenchanted) is the best answer.

31. **(B)** The word in the first blank most likely is an adjective that describes the circus performer's act of juggling three balls while balancing himself on a tightrope, which is not a simple task. Based on this we can project that the first correct word will mean "hard" or "difficult." Also, the word "very" in this sentence tells us that the performer's act is even more difficult due to some added element or component, indicated by the second blank. Based on these deductions, Answer B is the correct answer, with "complicated" and "simultaneous" as the best match for the sentence context.

32. **(B)** The placement of the blank indicates that the correct response will directly contradict her arrogance because she has had few accomplishments in the workplace. In reading each of the answers back into the sentence, answer B makes sense and is therefore the best choice.

33. **(D)** Given the sentence context, the first blank indicates that an unexpected reaction, possibly amazement or astonishment, is elicited in response to being "so easily dwarfed." This eliminates Answer B. Sequoia trees, noted for their exceptional height as the tallest species of tree, would certainly dwarf a human. Among the remaining choices, Answer D ("veneration" and "gargantuan") provides the best fit for BOTH blanks in the sentence.

34. **(C)** The key to filling in the blank in this sentence is the phrase "wine tasting." Answer C refers to a wine steward or professional (someone who is knowledgeable about wine), and therefore an amateur *sommelier* would be the best fit in the context of the sentence. Answers A and B refer to someone with expertise but do not fit when paired with the "amateur" qualifier. Answer D, defined as someone who renounces a religion, makes no sense in this context.

35. **(B)** The word "instead" in association with the green food coloring in this sentence indicates that an improvised change or solution occurred directly related

to the problem of running out of blue food coloring. This deviation from the blue icing preparation called for a replacement or alternate color to be used. Based on this, the only correct answer is B (substitute).

36. **(C)** Inertia refers to the tendency of a body/object to maintain its state of rest or motion; in other words, to resist change. Therefore, the correct answer is C, disinclination, defined as reluctance or unwillingness. Answers A and B mean to spur on action rather than maintain a current state, while answer D is defined as an omen and would not make sense in this context.

37. **(D)** The word to be placed in the first blank describes an action or reaction regarding the final results that should be avoided. In general, final results from a completed or finished experiment may bring some level of comfort or assuredness. Furthermore, a carefully organized and completed experiment could certainly be ruined by a shattered test tube. An event such as this one would be unexpected and unforeseen, and we can determine that the word in the second blank most likely will have a similar meaning. Based on this, we can eliminate Answers A, B, and C, leaving Answer D (sanguine and unanticipated).

38. **(D)** In this sentence, the correct word will be a symbol or gesture displayed by the scheduling of the peaceful conference—denoting "harmony" and "unity." Furthermore, all we know, based on the sentence, is that during the conference an agreement may be reached following the parties' negotiations. This denotes compromise and consideration. This eliminates Answers A, B, and C, leaving Answer D (diplomacy).

39. **(A)** The first sentence in this item tells us that the wing and the arm have alike or similar structure. However, the word "but" in the second sentence tells us that, although the structures are dissimilar when it comes to function, their anatomy somehow makes them equivalent—just as the first sentence implies. Therefore, the two correct answers should have parallel meanings. The only response that applies is Answer A.

40. **(D)** Based on the sentence context, the revisions and updates that need to be made are in direct response to the protocol being 20 years old, which is an extended time span. Based on this, our response should relate to time or something that results from a long duration of time. The only response that matches is Answer D, "antiquated," which means "outdated," "old-fashioned," or "obsolete."

41. **(A)** The cerebellum is the second largest part of the brain, while the cerebrum is the largest. Therefore, answers B and D can be eliminated. Respiration is controlled by the brain stem, thus eliminating answer C. Answer A is correct.

42. **(C)** The clues in the sentence context suggest that pupil dilation, which occurs when "going from an area of bright sunlight into a dark room," will be associated with an adjustment or transition in the environment. The answer response that best fits the context is Answer C (adapt).

43. **(B)** The phrase "by excretion into urine or bile" tells us that the correct word will be closely related to the disposal or removal of the hormones from the blood. Thus, Answers A, C, and D can be ruled out, leaving Answer B (eliminated), meaning "to remove" or "to purge."

44. **(A)** To play "harmoniously" means to play peacefully or agreeably. The child in this sentence does not have many friends because he "cannot" play harmoniously. This is a clue that the correct word will mean the opposite of harmoniously— "argumentative," "antagonistic," or "combative." Answer A (pugnacious), meaning quarrelsome, is the correct response for this sentence.

45. **(B)** The context of the first blank tells us that the correct word will be closely associated with the word "untrue" or fraudulent. The second blank (describing the organization's reputation resulting from the false fraud accusation) is preceded by the word "still." Since the accusation of fraud has a negative and unflattering connotation, we can assume that the correct word will also have an uncomplimentary tone. In addition, the word "nonetheless" (meaning "in spite of") tells us that this negative reputation will remain regardless of whether the accusation of fraud is untrue or not. Based on these deductions, the best match for the two blanks in this sentence is Answer B.

46. **(D)** Advertisements can often be misleading and exaggerated, which can result in false perceptions, and Sue's previous concept of the product was based on advertisement. However, after the demonstration, her new concept of the product was based on what she was able to see as real. Since the use of the phrase "not the same" tells us that the actual product and its advertisement are opposites, the correct word for the blank most likely describes Sue's disenchantment or disappointment when her previous perceptions or expectations of the product contradicted what was real. Of the words listed in the answer choices given, Answer D (disillusioned) makes the most sense.

47. **(C)** The word "unlike" gives us a clue that the correct words for the two blanks will probably be opposites; the vacation plans for this year are unlike or different compared to last year. Answer C provides the best match for the two blanks. "Amorphous" means vague or indefinite, and "resolute" means fixed, decided, or determined.

48. **(D)** We can tell by the placement of the first blank that the correct word will be synonymous with aggressive (meaning combative or hostile). Also, the patient's behavior described in the first blank is dependent upon the doctor leaving the room. When the doctor returns, however, something happens to the patient's composure, described by the second blank. From the sentence context we can project that a difference or change occurs, resulting in the patient's returning docility. Therefore, the answer choice that provides the best match based on these conclusions is Answer D, belligerent and regained.

49. **(A)** The word in the blank will be an adjective describing the type of donor who is associated with the ability to provide blood regardless of or unrestricted by the recipients' blood type. This type of donor will be able to be used in every instance, which can also be described as general, generic, or undifferentiated. Answer A (universal) best matches the sentence.

50. **(B)** Without the type of devices described in the first blank we might forget or have difficulty bringing back concepts to our mind. Thus, the second blank has to deal with recall, and the context of this sentence is related to memory. By reading each of the answer choices back into the sentence, Answer B (mnemonic and recollect) provides the best match for the sentence.

Biology Review and Practice

TIPS FOR THE BIOLOGY SECTION

The biology section of the PCAT measures your knowledge and understanding of principles and concepts in basic biology (including general biology), microbiology, and human anatomy and physiology. Microbiology, human anatomy, and physiology may not be covered in general pre-pharmacy required biology courses. If you do not feel confident in these areas, you can probably improve your PCAT biology score by reviewing these subjects independently or by taking a course in these subjects.

The biology section of the real PCAT consists of approximately 48 questions (more have been included in this chapter for review purposes). You will have 35 minutes to complete the biology section. Be sure to answer all questions.

BIOLOGY REVIEW OUTLINE

I. **General Biology**
   A. Cellular and Molecular Biology
      i. Structure and function of cells
         1. Four classes of biomolecules
         2. Membranes and membrane transport
      ii. Gene expression and inheritance
         1. Transcription
         2. Translation
         3. Mendelian genetics
            a. Chromosomes
            b. Genes
            c. Traits
            d. Genetic diseases
            e. Phenotype vs. genotype
      iii. Cell division and growth
         1. Mitosis
         2. Meiosis
      iv. Energy transformations

        v.   Metabolism
            1. Glycolysis
            2. Cellular respiration
            3. Chemiosmotic phosphorylation (ATP production)

- B. Diversity of Life Forms
  - i. Phylogenic tree of life
- C. Health
  - i. Nutrition
    1. Proteins
    2. Glucose (energy)
    3. Vitamins
  - ii. Diseases
  - iii. Drugs

II. Microbiology

- A. Microorganisms
  - i. Viruses
  - ii. Bacteria
  - iii. Fungi
- B. Infectious Diseases and Prevention
- C. Microbial Ecology
- D. Medical Microbiology
- E. Immunity

III. Human Anatomy and Physiology

- A. Structure
  - i. Cells
  - ii. Tissue
  - iii. Organs
- B. Systems
  - i. Skeletal/muscular
    1. Axial skeleton
    2. Appendicular skeleton
    3. Bones
    4. Joints
    5. Skeletal muscles
  - ii. Nervous/sensory
    1. Neuron
    2. Central nervous system
    3. Peripheral nervous system
    4. Sensory system
  - iii. Circulatory/respiratory
    1. Blood
    2. Circulation
    3. Blood vessels
    4. Heart anatomy

Answer Sheet

BIOLOGY

1 Ⓐ Ⓑ Ⓒ Ⓓ	26 Ⓐ Ⓑ Ⓒ Ⓓ	51 Ⓐ Ⓑ Ⓒ Ⓓ	76 Ⓐ Ⓑ Ⓒ Ⓓ
2 Ⓐ Ⓑ Ⓒ Ⓓ	27 Ⓐ Ⓑ Ⓒ Ⓓ	52 Ⓐ Ⓑ Ⓒ Ⓓ	77 Ⓐ Ⓑ Ⓒ Ⓓ
3 Ⓐ Ⓑ Ⓒ Ⓓ	28 Ⓐ Ⓑ Ⓒ Ⓓ	53 Ⓐ Ⓑ Ⓒ Ⓓ	78 Ⓐ Ⓑ Ⓒ Ⓓ
4 Ⓐ Ⓑ Ⓒ Ⓓ	29 Ⓐ Ⓑ Ⓒ Ⓓ	54 Ⓐ Ⓑ Ⓒ Ⓓ	79 Ⓐ Ⓑ Ⓒ Ⓓ
5 Ⓐ Ⓑ Ⓒ Ⓓ	30 Ⓐ Ⓑ Ⓒ Ⓓ	55 Ⓐ Ⓑ Ⓒ Ⓓ	80 Ⓐ Ⓑ Ⓒ Ⓓ
6 Ⓐ Ⓑ Ⓒ Ⓓ	31 Ⓐ Ⓑ Ⓒ Ⓓ	56 Ⓐ Ⓑ Ⓒ Ⓓ	81 Ⓐ Ⓑ Ⓒ Ⓓ
7 Ⓐ Ⓑ Ⓒ Ⓓ	32 Ⓐ Ⓑ Ⓒ Ⓓ	57 Ⓐ Ⓑ Ⓒ Ⓓ	82 Ⓐ Ⓑ Ⓒ Ⓓ
8 Ⓐ Ⓑ Ⓒ Ⓓ	33 Ⓐ Ⓑ Ⓒ Ⓓ	58 Ⓐ Ⓑ Ⓒ Ⓓ	83 Ⓐ Ⓑ Ⓒ Ⓓ
9 Ⓐ Ⓑ Ⓒ Ⓓ	34 Ⓐ Ⓑ Ⓒ Ⓓ	59 Ⓐ Ⓑ Ⓒ Ⓓ	84 Ⓐ Ⓑ Ⓒ Ⓓ
10 Ⓐ Ⓑ Ⓒ Ⓓ	35 Ⓐ Ⓑ Ⓒ Ⓓ	60 Ⓐ Ⓑ Ⓒ Ⓓ	85 Ⓐ Ⓑ Ⓒ Ⓓ
11 Ⓐ Ⓑ Ⓒ Ⓓ	36 Ⓐ Ⓑ Ⓒ Ⓓ	61 Ⓐ Ⓑ Ⓒ Ⓓ	86 Ⓐ Ⓑ Ⓒ Ⓓ
12 Ⓐ Ⓑ Ⓒ Ⓓ	37 Ⓐ Ⓑ Ⓒ Ⓓ	62 Ⓐ Ⓑ Ⓒ Ⓓ	87 Ⓐ Ⓑ Ⓒ Ⓓ
13 Ⓐ Ⓑ Ⓒ Ⓓ	38 Ⓐ Ⓑ Ⓒ Ⓓ	63 Ⓐ Ⓑ Ⓒ Ⓓ	88 Ⓐ Ⓑ Ⓒ Ⓓ
14 Ⓐ Ⓑ Ⓒ Ⓓ	39 Ⓐ Ⓑ Ⓒ Ⓓ	64 Ⓐ Ⓑ Ⓒ Ⓓ	89 Ⓐ Ⓑ Ⓒ Ⓓ
15 Ⓐ Ⓑ Ⓒ Ⓓ	40 Ⓐ Ⓑ Ⓒ Ⓓ	65 Ⓐ Ⓑ Ⓒ Ⓓ	90 Ⓐ Ⓑ Ⓒ Ⓓ
16 Ⓐ Ⓑ Ⓒ Ⓓ	41 Ⓐ Ⓑ Ⓒ Ⓓ	66 Ⓐ Ⓑ Ⓒ Ⓓ	91 Ⓐ Ⓑ Ⓒ Ⓓ
17 Ⓐ Ⓑ Ⓒ Ⓓ	42 Ⓐ Ⓑ Ⓒ Ⓓ	67 Ⓐ Ⓑ Ⓒ Ⓓ	92 Ⓐ Ⓑ Ⓒ Ⓓ
18 Ⓐ Ⓑ Ⓒ Ⓓ	43 Ⓐ Ⓑ Ⓒ Ⓓ	68 Ⓐ Ⓑ Ⓒ Ⓓ	93 Ⓐ Ⓑ Ⓒ Ⓓ
19 Ⓐ Ⓑ Ⓒ Ⓓ	44 Ⓐ Ⓑ Ⓒ Ⓓ	69 Ⓐ Ⓑ Ⓒ Ⓓ	94 Ⓐ Ⓑ Ⓒ Ⓓ
20 Ⓐ Ⓑ Ⓒ Ⓓ	45 Ⓐ Ⓑ Ⓒ Ⓓ	70 Ⓐ Ⓑ Ⓒ Ⓓ	95 Ⓐ Ⓑ Ⓒ Ⓓ
21 Ⓐ Ⓑ Ⓒ Ⓓ	46 Ⓐ Ⓑ Ⓒ Ⓓ	71 Ⓐ Ⓑ Ⓒ Ⓓ	96 Ⓐ Ⓑ Ⓒ Ⓓ
22 Ⓐ Ⓑ Ⓒ Ⓓ	47 Ⓐ Ⓑ Ⓒ Ⓓ	72 Ⓐ Ⓑ Ⓒ Ⓓ	97 Ⓐ Ⓑ Ⓒ Ⓓ
23 Ⓐ Ⓑ Ⓒ Ⓓ	48 Ⓐ Ⓑ Ⓒ Ⓓ	73 Ⓐ Ⓑ Ⓒ Ⓓ	98 Ⓐ Ⓑ Ⓒ Ⓓ
24 Ⓐ Ⓑ Ⓒ Ⓓ	49 Ⓐ Ⓑ Ⓒ Ⓓ	74 Ⓐ Ⓑ Ⓒ Ⓓ	99 Ⓐ Ⓑ Ⓒ Ⓓ
25 Ⓐ Ⓑ Ⓒ Ⓓ	50 Ⓐ Ⓑ Ⓒ Ⓓ	75 Ⓐ Ⓑ Ⓒ Ⓓ	100 Ⓐ Ⓑ Ⓒ Ⓓ

Practice Questions

100 Questions

Directions: Select the best answer to each of the following questions.

1. Which of the following is the fluid medium of the nucleus?

   (A) Chloroplasm
   (B) Golgi complex
   (C) Nucleoplasm
   (D) Nucleolus

2. A newly discovered bacterium is found to infect animals and cause a reduction in muscle contractions. Symptoms include labored breathing, difficulty swallowing, and slowed physical movement. All animals presenting these symptoms tested positive for the presence of this bacterium.

   Further studies reveal that the bacterium secretes a toxin while in the host. The toxin is called "Toxin β." The toxin enters muscle cells and binds to ATP synthase, blocking the active sites where new ATP is formed. Based on the mode of action of how the toxin works, which of the following options best describes where the toxin localizes in the muscle cells?

   (A) Mitochondrial matrix
   (B) Outer membrane of the mitochondria
   (C) Cytoplasm
   (D) Nucleus

3. Which of the following describes Stage 1 of sleep?

   (A) Characterized by drowsiness. The eyes may be closed, but the person is able to hear nearby activity.
   (B) Characterized by alternating periods of muscle tension and relaxation. Heart rate slows and body temperature drops.
   (C) Little body movement, vivid dreaming.
   (D) Known as delta sleep. Breathing and heart rate slows.

4. Different types of proteins are directed to different locations in a cell according to how they function. Their subcellular localization is determined by

   (A) entry into transport vesicles.
   (B) binding to receptor proteins.
   (C) binding to motor proteins.
   (D) localization signals in the proteins.

5. Human conception is a complex process that results in the combination of sperm and egg to form a zygote. Fertility issues can occur in females and can include a lack of egg viability, a lack of egg release, or a thyroid disorder that affects the menstrual cycle. Males can also possess fertility issues.

   If a male is infertile, the first step is to test his ejaculate. The seminal fluid of the semen is tested for qualities such as pH and sugar content. Then, the sperm is quantified and observed for qualitative characteristics (e.g., swimming ability, morphology). If an infertile male has morphologically abnormal sperm, what is likely the reasoning for this abnormality?

   (A) Seminal fluid with a pH that is too low or too high
   (B) Seminal fluid with low sugar content
   (C) Abnormal function of the spermatogonia cells
   (D) Abnormal function of the prostate gland

6. The number and size of organelles in a cell correlate with that cell's function. For example, muscle cells typically have a high number of mitochondria to keep up with the demand for ATP used in muscle contractions.

   Three cell types, A-C, were evaluated for the size of the smooth and rough endoplasmic reticulum. The data was collected and ranked from highest (1) to lowest (3). The data is shown in the table below. Based on the data in the table below, which of the following conclusions is true?

	Smooth Endoplasmic Reticulum	Rough Endoplasmic Reticulum
Cell type A	1	2
Cell type B	3	1
Cell type C	2	3

   (A) Cell type B produces a large quantity of fatty acids and other lipids.
   (B) Cell type C produces a large quantity of fatty acids and other lipids.
   (C) Cell type B produces a large quantity of proteins that are secreted from the cell.
   (D) Cell type A produces a large quantity of proteins that are secreted from the cell.

7. You are an endocrinologist who is testing a new drug to replace testosterone in males with low testosterone. The results of your trial suggest the drug is effective. Which of the following describes your drug?

   (A) Your drug is binding to signal receptors at the surface of a cell.
   (B) Your drug is binding to the little testosterone present in a cell.
   (C) Your drug forms a hormone receptor complex and moves to the nucleus.
   (D) Your drug locates to the surface of the mitochondria.

8. In this organelle, sugar side chains on proteins and lipids are modified.

   (A) Rough endoplasmic reticulum
   (B) Golgi complex
   (C) Nuclear lamella
   (D) Smooth endoplasmic reticulum

9. The relationship of microorganisms with one another and with their environment is called

   (A) micronology.
   (B) micrologies.
   (C) microbial ecologies.
   (D) biologies.

10. How much time is required for an adult human to produce detectable antibodies in the blood during a primary immune response?

    (A) 8 weeks
    (B) 6 weeks
    (C) 4 weeks
    (D) 1 week

11. The peptide bond formed between amino acids in a protein involves the

    (A) amino and the carboxyl groups.
    (B) central carbon and the carboxyl group.
    (C) amino and the variable R-groups.
    (D) hydrogen and the variable R-groups.

12. The pigment that is responsible for giving skin its color is called

    (A) epidermis.
    (B) melanin.
    (C) dermis.
    (D) subcutaneous layer.

13. In general, enzymes are used by a cell to

    (A) increase the energy required to start a chemical reaction.
    (B) decrease the energy required to start a chemical reaction.
    (C) disrupt a chemical reaction.
    (D) bypass a chemical reaction.

14. The sugar found in DNA has _____ carbons.

    (A) three
    (B) four
    (C) five
    (D) six

15. Which part of a cell produces ribonucleoproteins such as ribosomes?

    (A) Nuclear envelope
    (B) Chromosomes
    (C) Nucleoplasm
    (D) Nucleolus

16. A clouding of the lens of the eye that causes blurred vision is known as

    (A) exetis.
    (B) dermatitis.
    (C) cataracts.
    (D) pink eye.

17. The Centers for Disease Control and Prevention reports that 1/3 of American adults are obese or overweight. Obesity is often linked to a myriad of health issues such as diabetes, stroke, and heart attack. Overeating, or consuming more calories than the body needs, is the most common cause of obesity. However, a small portion of overweight adults has this condition due to an imbalance of hormones. Which of the following glands can explain obesity in this population?

    (A) Thyroid gland
    (B) Pineal gland
    (C) Parathyroid gland
    (D) Thymus gland

18. The theory of spontaneous generation states that

    (A) microorganisms arise from lifeless matter.
    (B) evolution has taken place in large animals.
    (C) humans have generated from apes.
    (D) viruses are degenerative forms of bacteria.

19. What metal ion is responsible for the binding of oxygen gas to hemoglobin?

    (A) Magnesium
    (B) Manganese
    (C) Copper
    (D) Iron

20. Rhodopsin is an important protein in the cell membrane of photoreceptor cells. What vitamin is important for the function of rhodopsin?

    (A) Vitamin D
    (B) Vitamin E
    (C) Vitamin A
    (D) Vitamin C

21. The spleen is primarily involved with which of the following systems?

    (A) Immune
    (B) Digestive
    (C) Endocrine
    (D) Reproductive

22. Fluoride deficiency problems include:

    (A) anemia.
    (B) muscle weakness.
    (C) osteoporosis.
    (D) hair loss.

23. The long chain of carbons and hydrogens that form the "tails" of phospholipids are

    (A) hydrophobic.
    (B) hydrophilic.
    (C) both hydrophobic and hydrophilic.
    (D) neither hydrophobic nor hydrophilic.

24. Diffusion is the

    (A) movement of molecules of one substance through the molecules of another substance from regions of lower concentration to regions of higher concentration by means of an outside energy source.
    (B) movement of molecules of one substance through the molecules of another substance from regions of higher concentration to regions of lower concentration by means of an outside energy source.
    (C) movement of molecules of one substance through the molecules of another substance from regions of lower concentration to regions of higher concentration by means of the molecules' own kinetic energy.
    (D) movement of molecules of one substance through the molecules of another substance from regions of higher concentration to regions of lower concentration by means of the molecules' own kinetic energy.

25. In eukaryotes, DNA is

    (A) naked.
    (B) bound by histone proteins to form chromatin.
    (C) transcribed into messenger RNA while in a condensed state.
    (D) may be a single-stranded molecule.

26. Which of the following is a polysaccharide stored in the liver?

    (A) Glycogen
    (B) Starch
    (C) Cellulose
    (D) Chitin

27. The influenza virus is an example of a negative-stranded RNA virus. What does this term mean?

    (A) Negative-stranded RNA viruses can only enter a host cell that is undergoing mitosis.
    (B) Negative-stranded RNA viruses contain DNA that must be transcribed into mRNA before a protein can be made.
    (C) Negative-stranded RNA viruses contain RNA in the form of mRNA that can be used to make a protein.
    (D) Negative-stranded RNA viruses contain RNA that must be copied into mRNA in order to make a protein.

28. What is a health risk associated with exposure to UV radiation?

    (A) Infection
    (B) Cancer
    (C) Reduced immune function
    (D) Blood-borne disease

29. Organic molecules, at the very least, must be composed of

    (A) hydrogen.
    (B) carbon.
    (C) carbon and hydrogen.
    (D) carbon, hydrogen, and oxygen.

30. Crossing over of homologous chromosomes occurs during what phase of meiosis?

    (A) Prophase I
    (B) Metaphase II
    (C) Anaphase I
    (D) Telophase II

31. Progression through the cell cycle is regulated by the oscillations in the concentrations of which types of molecules?

    (A) Suppressor proteins
    (B) Cyclin-dependent kinases
    (C) Cyclins
    (D) Tubulin

32. The chemical component of a nucleotide that forms hydrogen bonds with another nucleotide on the complementary strand of DNA is the

    (A) amino group.
    (B) phosphate group.
    (C) deoxyribose sugar.
    (D) nitrogenous base.

33. At the end of meiosis, the ploidy level of the resulting cells

    (A) remains the same.
    (B) is cut in half.
    (C) doubles.
    (D) triples.

34. The process of splitting glucose into two molecules of pyruvate while creating ATP is called

    (A) the Krebs cycle (the citric acid cycle).
    (B) the electron transport chain.
    (C) glycolysis.
    (D) fermentation.

35. The stage in cell division marked by chromosome separation is

    (A) anaphase.
    (B) metaphase.
    (C) prophase.
    (D) telophase.

36. The lac operon is usually in the _____ position and is activated by a(n) _____ molecule.

    (A) on; repressor
    (B) off; repressor
    (C) on; inducer
    (D) off; inducer

37. How many total chromosomes are found in human somatic cells?

    (A) 12
    (B) 23
    (C) 46
    (D) 92

38. According to the Centers for Disease Control and Prevention, approximately 25% of the population experiences sleep disorders on a regular basis. In general, a sleep disorder is the inability of a person to progress through the stages of sleep. To help diagnose and treat a sleep disorder, a patient participates in a sleep trial where their sleep is monitored all night.

    After completion of a sleep trial, a patient is told that his/her sleep disorder is associated with Stage 3 of sleep. Which of the following best describes this stage?

    (A) Characterized by drowsiness. The eyes may be closed, but the person is able to hear nearby activity.
    (B) Characterized by alternating periods of muscle tension and relaxation. Heart rate slows and body temperature drops.
    (C) Little body movement, vivid dreaming.
    (D) Known as delta sleep. Breathing and heart rate slows.

39. The main role of apoptosis is to

    (A) remove damaged or diseased cells from tissue.
    (B) remove old or damaged organelles within a cell.
    (C) repair unfolded or misfolded proteins within a cell.
    (D) repair damaged DNA within a cell.

40. The amount of energy needed to carry out basic body functions when you are at rest is known as

    (A) intermediate metabolism.
    (B) complex metabolism.
    (C) catabolic metabolism.
    (D) basal metabolism.

41. Which of the following cells excavate bone cavities?

    (A) Osteoclasts
    (B) Osteoblasts
    (C) Osteomasts
    (D) Osteocytes

42. How do large molecules like glucose enter a cell?

    (A) Large molecules pass through the cell plasma membrane via a channel protein.
    (B) Large molecules pass through the cell plasma membrane via a transporter protein.
    (C) Large molecules pass directly through the cell plasma membrane.
    (D) Large molecules are never allowed to enter a cell.

43. Osteoporosis is a condition in which mature bone weakens, becomes brittle, and is slowly or rarely replaced. People with osteoporosis are often slow to recover from bone breaks or fractures and can even display height decline due to loss of bone in the spine.

    A mutation in which of the following cell types would lead to osteoporosis-like symptoms in a person?

    (A) Osteoclasts
    (B) Osteocytes
    (C) Osteoblasts
    (D) Osteomasts

44. The bones of the skeleton articulate with each other at

    (A) the appendicular skeleton.
    (B) the joints.
    (C) the axial skeleton.
    (D) cartilage.

45. Ball and socket, plane, gliding, hinge, and condylar are all types of

(A) bones.
(B) muscles.
(C) cartilage.
(D) joints.

46. During which stage of the cell cycle is DNA replicated?

(A) G_1 phase
(B) S phase
(C) G_2 phase
(D) M phase

47. In 2014, an outbreak of the Ebola virus caused fever, organ failure and even death in Senegal, West Africa. Recent studies on primates may provide evidence for a new, effective treatment. Researchers injected Ebola-infected monkeys with siRNA, or small interfering RNA. This single stranded nucleotide enters infected cells and binds to the viral mRNA preventing it from binding to ribosomes. The virus is then unable to replicate and the disease progression stops.

Based on the research described above, what specific step in the life cycle of the Ebola virus is blocked by the siRNA?

(A) Viral DNA replication
(B) Viral RNA replication
(C) Viral transcription
(D) Viral translation

48. What is the function of the middle ear?
(A) It contains hair cells that detect specific frequencies of sound.
(B) It transmits sound vibrations to the tympanic membrane.
(C) It amplifies sound transmitted to the cochlea.
(D) It externally collects sound waves from the environment.

49. Blood is delivered to the heart from the lungs by the

(A) renal veins.
(B) pulmonary veins.
(C) mitral arteries.
(D) pulmonary arteries.

50. A mutation in DNA that changes an adenine to a cytosine is an example of

(A) a frame shift mutation.
(B) a point mutation.
(C) a deletion mutation.
(D) an insertion mutation.

51. What is another name for red blood cells?

    (A) Erythrocytes
    (B) Leukocytes
    (C) Lymphocytes
    (D) Basophils

52. Which of the following is found in gram-positive bacteria?

    (A) Pseudomurein
    (B) Sterol-rich membranes
    (C) Peptidoglycan
    (D) Amniotransports

53. What is the role of oxygen in cellular respiration?

    (A) Oxygen provides electrons for the electron transport chain.
    (B) Oxygen provides hydrogen ions for the production of ATP.
    (C) Oxygen is an electron acceptor for the electron transport chain.
    (D) Oxygen is an electron acceptor for the citric acid cycle.

54. The primary function of platelets involves

    (A) blood formation.
    (B) blood clotting.
    (C) metabolism.
    (D) defense against infections.

55. What is not a primary function of white blood cells?

    (A) Phagocytosis
    (B) Proteolysis
    (C) Antibody formation
    (D) Oxygenation

56. Albumin is a storage protein found in

    (A) the blood.
    (B) cardiac muscle cells.
    (C) skin cells.
    (D) lymphatic fluid.

57. The movement of an action potential along the axon of a neuron is caused by the opening and closing of what type of voltage-gated, membrane channels?

    (A) Sodium and potassium
    (B) Potassium and calcium
    (C) Calcium and sodium
    (D) Sodium, potassium, and calcium

58. Diaphragm contraction aids in what step of respiration?

    (A) Inhalation
    (B) Exhalation
    (C) Oxygen exchange in red blood cells
    (D) Carbon dioxide exchange in red blood cells

59. Bacterial meningitis affects what part of the body?

    (A) The nervous system
    (B) The respiratory system
    (C) The urinary tract
    (D) The integumentary system

60. What components do all viruses possess?

    (A) Nucleic acids only
    (B) Protein coat only
    (C) Protein coat and nucleic acids
    (D) Protein coat, nucleic acids, and plasma membrane

61. The process in which two bacteria exchange DNA via a pilus is called

    (A) translation.
    (B) transduction.
    (C) conjugation.
    (D) transformation.

62. How are carbohydrates digested?

    (A) By amylases in the mouth and small intestines
    (B) By pepsin and HCL acid in the stomach
    (C) By lipases in the small intestine
    (D) By nucleases in the stomach

63. What role do bile salts play in the digestion of complex fats?

    (A) They emulsify lipids by converting large masses of fat molecules into smaller masses.
    (B) They activate enzymes that digest fat.
    (C) They cleave the bonds releasing fatty acids and other small lipids.
    (D) The mechanism is unknown.

64. What is the name of the thin, mucus-secreting epithelial membrane that lines the interior surface of the eyelid?

    (A) Tarsal plate
    (B) Lacrimal gland
    (C) Conjunctiva
    (D) Sclera

65. Prions are disease-causing agents that are composed of

    (A) DNA only.
    (B) protein only.
    (C) proteins and DNA.
    (D) proteins, DNA, and a plasma membrane.

66. The term "oral cavity" refers to the

    (A) stomach.
    (B) intestine.
    (C) mouth.
    (D) liver.

67. Bacteria that are transmitted via insect fall into which of the following categories?

    (A) Contact transmission
    (B) Fluid transmission
    (C) Vector transmission
    (D) Airborne transmission

68. Most nutrients are absorbed in which organ of the digestive system?

    (A) Esophagus
    (B) Stomach
    (C) Small intestine
    (D) Large intestine

69. Animal viruses are classified into taxonomic groups based on

    (A) their type of genetic material.
    (B) the kind of cells they infected.
    (C) their replication strategy.
    (D) whether they are naked or enveloped.

70. Prokaryotes that thrive in extremely high temperatures are considered to be

    (A) bacteria.
    (B) archaea.
    (C) fungi.
    (D) protists.

71. What is the primary function of the gallbladder?

    (A) To store gastrin
    (B) To store bile
    (C) To synthesize insulin
    (D) To store amylase

72. Rumen bacteria that live in the digestive tracts of animals such as cows are

    (A) antagonists.
    (B) pathogens.
    (C) anaerobes.
    (D) aerobes.

73. Which of the following enhance(s) the intestinal absorption of fatty acids?

    (A) Bile salts
    (B) Amylase
    (C) Hydrochloric acid
    (D) Pepsin

74. A sample of blood of three males, Mark, Richard, and Steve, was taken at rest and a second sample was taken after each watched a scary movie clip. Based on the data in the table below, who hyperventilated when they saw the scary movie clip?

	Blood pH at rest	Blood pH after
Mark	7.4	7.2
Richard	7.4	7.4
Steve	7.4	7.6

    (A) Mark
    (B) Richard
    (C) Steve
    (D) No one hyperventilated

75. Immunity that includes the production of new antibodies is called

    (A) acquired immunity.
    (B) natural immunity.
    (C) rapid-response immunity.
    (D) innate immunity.

76. Which endocrine gland(s) controls circadian rhythms?

    (A) The parathyroid glands
    (B) The pineal gland
    (C) The adrenal glands
    (D) The ovaries or testes

77. Antibiotic resistance has become a major issue in the field of medicine. Pathogenic bacteria such as *Staphylococcus aureus* have evolved and are no longer affected by the commonly used antibiotic penicillin.

    To help combat this resistance issue, you decide to create a variety of new, experimental antibiotics. The use of which of the following new antibiotics would be an ineffective treatment against a resistant strain of *S. aureus*?

    (A) An experimental antibiotic that targeted peptidoglycan production
    (B) An experimental antibiotic that targeted binary fission
    (C) An experimental antibiotic that targeted ribosome function
    (D) An experimental antibiotic that targeted DNA polymerase function

78. Which of the following drugs is considered to be a depressant?

    (A) Alcohol
    (B) Nicotine
    (C) Amphetamines
    (D) Cocaine

79. Koch's postulate defines the criterion used to demonstrate that

    (A) an organism is a heterotrophy.
    (B) an organism causes a specific disease.
    (C) a disease-causing organism also has harmless variants.
    (D) organisms that lack cell walls undergo lyses in hypotonic solutions.

Figure 1 is needed to answer question 80.

Figure 1.

80. Figure 1 illustrates a typical neuron. Which number on the figure indicates where impulses from other neurons are received?

   (A) 1
   (B) 2
   (C) 3
   (D) 4

81. What neurotransmitter causes an increase in skeletal muscle contractions?

   (A) Nitric oxide
   (B) Acetylcholine
   (C) Norepinephrine
   (D) Serotonin

82. Which of the following is(are) responsible for the removal and destruction of erythrocytes?

   (A) Liver
   (B) Gallbladder
   (C) Kidneys
   (D) Pancreas

83. Which of the following human body parts is vestigial?

   (A) Stomach
   (B) Spinal chord
   (C) Appendix
   (D) Pancreas

84. Which of the following nutrients has the highest caloric value per gram?

    (A) Protein
    (B) Glucose
    (C) Fat
    (D) Carbohydrates

85. _____ is a condition where a person eats a great deal of food and then vomits or uses other purging methods.

    (A) Binge-eating disorder
    (B) Bulimia nervosa
    (C) Anorexia nervosa
    (D) Disordered-eating pattern

86. Many animal viruses contain a membrane-like envelope structure that includes viral proteins protruding from a lipid bilayer. When do viruses acquire an envelope?

    (A) During the entry of the virus into the host cell
    (B) During the removal of the viral proteins inside the host cell
    (C) During replication of the virus inside the host cell
    (D) During the exiting of the virus from the host cell

87. Which of the following ecological terms best describes a virus in relation to the cell that it infects?

    (A) Mutualist
    (B) Parasite
    (C) Obligate parasite
    (D) Symbiotic partner

88. Which of the following diseases/disorders is caused by a fungal pathogen?

    (A) Phenomena
    (B) Common cold
    (C) Ringworm
    (D) Malaria

89. The Rh factor in blood is a

    (A) protein.
    (B) carbohydrate.
    (C) blood cell.
    (D) nuclear acid.

90. In _____ drug dependence, the user's body needs the drug to avoid the discomfort of withdrawal.

    (A) physical
    (B) psychological
    (C) sociological
    (D) medical

91. If Y represents yellow (dominant color) and y represents green (recessive color), which of the following crosses would be expected to result in 75 percent yellow offspring?

    (A) Yy × yy
    (B) YY × yy
    (C) Yy × Yy
    (D) Yy × YY

92. _____ is the process in which energy is released as electrons pass through a series of electron acceptors to either oxygen or another inorganic compound.

    (A) Oxidative phosphorylation
    (B) Phosphorylation
    (C) Photosynthetic phosphorlyation
    (D) Substrate-level phosphorylation

93. Blue (B) is the dominant color for the Figbird, whereas white (b) is the alternative recessive color. When a homozygous blue bird is crossed with a homozygous white bird, what percentage of the offspring is expected to be white?

    (A) 0
    (B) 25
    (C) 50
    (D) 100

94. Blue (B) is the dominant color for the Figbird, whereas white (b) is the alternative recessive color. When a homozygous blue bird is crossed with a homozygous white bird, what percentage of the offspring is expected to be blue heterozygous?

    (A) 0
    (B) 25
    (C) 50
    (D) 100

95. Which of the following provide(s) daylight color vision and is (are) responsible for visual acuity?

    (A) Rods
    (B) Cones
    (C) Optic disc
    (D) Retina

96. During an inflammation response, white blood cells are recruited to the site of inflammation by what signal?

    (A) Antibodies
    (B) Excess carbon dioxide in the blood
    (C) Cytokines
    (D) Growth factor

97. A person who is heterozygous at the gene locus related to a disorder, but shows no signs of the disorder, is called a(n) _____ of the disorder.

    (A) infector
    (B) carrier
    (C) infection
    (D) holder

98. Which of the following molecules is read and interpreted by a ribosome to create a new protein?

    (A) DNA
    (B) Messenger RNA
    (C) Ribosomal RNA
    (D) Gene

99. Sickle-cell anemia develops in individuals who inherit two copies of a recessive gene(s). If a man with sickle-cell anemia marries a woman who does not have the disease but is a carrier of it, what percentage of their offspring is expected to have the disease or to be a carrier of it?

    (A) 25
    (B) 50
    (C) 75
    (D) 100

100. The fluidity of cell membranes is due to the nature of which of the following molecules?

    (A) Proteins
    (B) Phospholipids
    (C) 5-carbon sugars
    (D) Nucleic acids

Answer Key
BIOLOGY

1. **C**	26. **A**	51. **A**	76. **B**
2. **A**	27. **D**	52. **C**	77. **A**
3. **A**	28. **B**	53. **C**	78. **A**
4. **D**	29. **C**	54. **B**	79. **B**
5. **C**	30. **A**	55. **D**	80. **A**
6. **C**	31. **C**	56. **A**	81. **B**
7. **C**	32. **D**	57. **A**	82. **A**
8. **B**	33. **B**	58. **A**	83. **C**
9. **C**	34. **C**	59. **A**	84. **C**
10. **D**	35. **A**	60. **C**	85. **B**
11. **A**	36. **D**	61. **C**	86. **B**
12. **B**	37. **C**	62. **A**	87. **C**
13. **B**	38. **D**	63. **A**	88. **C**
14. **C**	39. **A**	64. **C**	89. **A**
15. **D**	40. **D**	65. **B**	90. **A**
16. **C**	41. **A**	66. **C**	91. **C**
17. **A**	42. **B**	67. **C**	92. **A**
18. **A**	43. **C**	68. **C**	93. **A**
19. **D**	44. **B**	69. **C**	94. **D**
20. **C**	45. **D**	70. **B**	95. **B**
21. **A**	46. **B**	71. **B**	96. **C**
22. **C**	47. **D**	72. **C**	97. **B**
23. **A**	48. **C**	73. **A**	98. **B**
24. **D**	49. **B**	74. **C**	99. **D**
25. **B**	50. **B**	75. **D**	100. **B**

EXPLANATORY ANSWERS

1. **(C)** Nucleoplasm, meaning protoplasm of the nucleus, is the fluid medium of the nucleus.

2. **(A)** The active sites of ATP synthase function in the matrix of the mitochondria.

3. **(A)** Stage 1 of sleep is characterized by drowsiness and the eyes may be closed, but the person is able to hear nearby activity. Stage 2 of sleep is characterized by light sleep and alternating periods of muscle tension and relaxation; the heart rate slows and body temperature drops. Stage 3 of sleep is known as delta sleep; breathing and heart rate slows. Stage 4 of sleep is the deepest stage of delta sleep and is the stage during which it is the most difficult to rouse the sleeper; the stage when the body produces growth hormone and repairs itself from injuries. During the final stage, REM sleep, there is little body movement and vivid dreaming.

4. **(D)** The destination of proteins in a cell is dependent upon the order of amino acids that makes up the signal, or localization, sequence. The signal sequence is a part of the amino acid sequence of the protein.

5. **(C)** Spermatogonia cells produce sperm via meiosis. Issues with these cells may lead to abnormally shaped sperm. If you were considering answer D, this is incorrect because the prostate produces seminal fluid, not the sperm.

6. **(C)** A cell with an extensive rough endoplasmic reticulum would be producing proteins that are secreted from the cell. Ribosomes that translate messenger RNAs that encode secretory proteins bind to the rough endoplasmic reticulum and the protein being synthesized enters the lumen of the rough endoplasmic reticulum. The proteins destined for secretion move to the Golgi vesicles that, ultimately, fuse with the cell membrane releasing the protein from the cell.

7. **(C)** If your drug is mimicking testosterone, then it would bind to testosterone's receptor and move into the nucleus.

8. **(B)** The Golgi complex modifies carbohydrate chains of glycosylated proteins and lipids. The original sugar chain is added in the endoplasmic reticulum first, and then it is modified in the Golgi.

9. **(C)** No explanation needed.

10. **(D)** In general, it takes approximately one week (or within one week), for an adult human to produce detectable antibodies in the blood during a primary immune response.

11. **(A)** No explanation needed.

12. **(B)** There are specialized cells in the deepest level of the epidermis, or outer layer of the skin, that produce a pigment called melanin. Melanin is responsible for giving color to skin.

13. **(B)** All chemical reactions must overcome a certain amount of energy in order to begin, called the "activation energy." Enzymes reduce the activation energy needed, therefore encouraging the chemical reaction to occur.

14. **(C)** The sugar found in DNA is deoxyribose, and it is a 5-carbon sugar.

15. **(D)** The nucleolus, a small area within the nucleus, is where ribonucleoproteins such as ribosomes are produced.

16. **(C)** No explanation needed.

17. **(A)** The thyroid gland (answer A) produces thyroid hormone that controls metabolism. The pineal gland (answer B) affects sleep, the parathyroid gland (answer C) controls calcium in the blood, and the thymus gland (answer D) is involved in the immune system.

18. **(A)** The theory of spontaneous generation states that certain living things arose from vital forces present in living or nonliving decomposers.

19. **(D)** Iron is the atom at the center of the heme groups found within hemoglobin proteins on red blood cells. Oxygen binds to the iron.

20. **(C)** No explanation needed.

21. **(A)** The spleen collects and kills certain types of pathogenic bacteria making it part of the immune system.

22. **(C)** No explanation needed.

23. **(A)** No explanation needed.

24. **(D)** No explanation needed.

25. **(B)** Eukaryotic DNA is bound by histones and condensed to form chromatin. The regions of the DNA that are transcribed into RNA are not condensed.

26. **(A)** Glycogen is stored in the liver. Starch (B) and cellulose (C) are polysaccharides stored in plant cells. Chitin (D) is a polysaccharide found in insect exoskeletons and in the cell walls of fungi.

27. **(D)** No explanation needed.

28. **(B)** UV radiation can damage DNA, leading to cancer.

29. **(C)** No explanation needed.

30. **(A)** Crossing over occurs during prophase I of meiosis, the stage where the homologous chromosomes first interact with one another.

31. **(C)** The cyclin concentrations of a cell cycle in dividing cells. Cyclin concentrations are greatest in the M phase. Protein kinases and cyclins blend to form a mitosis-promoting complex that activates other proteins leading to initiation of the M phase.

32. **(D)** When paired, the nitrogenous bases of adenine and thymine form two hydrogen bonds, while the bases of cytosine and guanine form three hydrogen bonds.

33. **(B)** Meiosis is a process of cell division comprising two nuclear divisions in succession. It results in four gametocytes, each containing half the number of chromosomes (B) as the parent cell.

34. **(C)** No explanation needed.

35. **(A)** The stages of cellular division include prophase, metaphase, anaphase, and telophase. During prophase (C) the chromosomes condense, the nuclear membrane deteriorates, and the spindle microtubules attach to the chromosomes. During metaphase the chromosomes move to the center of the cell. During anaphase (A) each kinetochore divides, and the chromosomes separate. During telophase (D) the nuclear membrane reforms around each new daughter cell's nucleus.

36. **(D)** The lac operon is usually in the off position and is activated by an inducer molecule.

37. **(C)** Human somatic, or nonreproductive, cells are diploid and contain 46 total chromosomes, or 23 pairs.

38. **(D)** Stage 3 of sleep is known as delta sleep; breathing and heart rate slows. Stage 1 of sleep is characterized by drowsiness and the eyes may be closed, but the person is able to hear nearby activity. Stage 2 of sleep is characterized by light sleep and alternating periods of muscle tension and relaxation; the heart rate slows and body temperature drops. Stage 4 of sleep is the deepest stage of delta sleep and is the stage during which is it most difficult to rouse the sleeper; the stage when the body produces growth hormone and repairs itself from injuries. During the final stage, REM sleep, there is little body movement and vivid dreaming.

39. **(A)** Apoptosis, or programmed cell death, occurs when a cell (1) has DNA damage beyond repair, (2) is infected, or (3) is old or unnecessary.

40. **(D)** No explanation needed.

41. **(A)** In the bone remolding cycle, osteoclasts (A) are cells that remove bone, and osteoblasts (B) are cells that form bone. Choices C and D are irrelevant.

42. **(B)** Large molecules like glucose cannot pass directly through the phospholipid bilayer. Instead, they require membrane transport proteins to allow passage. Channel proteins (A) typically move small ions.

43. **(C)** In the bone remodeling cycle, osteoclasts (A) are cells that remove bone, and osteoblasts (C) are cells that form bone. Choices B and D are irrelevant.

44. **(B)** Joints (B) are the place of union between two or more bones whereas cartilage (D) is a type of connective tissue with a solid elastic matrix. Choices A and C are irrelevant.

45. **(D)** No explanation needed.

46. **(B)** The G phases (A) and (C) are periods of growth. The M phase (D) is the stage where DNA condenses, the nuclear envelop dissolves, chromosomes are divided, and two new cells form.

47. **(D)** mRNA binds to ribosomes during translation, or protein production. If siRNA binds to mRNA, it would prevent translation from occurring.

48. **(C)** The middle ear amplifies the sound energy transmitted to the cochlea.

49. **(B)** To answer this question correctly, it is important to remember two principles: (1) arteries carry blood away from the heart, while veins carry blood to the heart; and (2) the pulmonary circulation consists of blood vessels that transport blood to the lungs and then to the heart. Therefore, the correct choice is pulmonary veins (B), not pulmonary arteries (D). Choices A and C are irrelevant.

50. **(B)** A point mutation is the change of one nucleotide to another nucleotide in DNA.

51. **(A)** No explanation needed.

52. **(C)** In gram-positive bacteria, peptidoglycan is found within the cell wall.

53. **(C)** No explanation needed.

54. **(B)** No explanation needed.

55. **(D)** Answers A through C are primary functions of white blood cells, while D is not.

56. **(A)** Protein in the blood is composed of albumin and globulin, with albumin being the most abundant serum protein. The total quantity of albumin is two to three times the level of globulin. Choices B, C, and D are irrelevant.

57. **(A)** Sodium and potassium channels are opened and closed as voltage changes during an action potential in neurons.

58. **(A)** The diaphragm pulls air into the lungs upon contraction. When it relaxes, air is forced out of the lungs.

59. **(A)** No explanation needed.

60. **(C)** No explanation needed.

61. **(C)** Transduction (B) occurs when bacteriophages inject new DNA into a bacterium. Transformation (D) is when a bacterium takes up free DNA from the environment. Option (A) is not a means of DNA exchange between bacteria.

62. **(A)** Carbohydrates are digested by amylases in the mouth and small intestines. Pepsin digests proteins, lipase lipids, and nucleases nucleic acids.

63. **(A)** Before lipases can act on the fat that enters the small intestine, they must first be broken down into smaller fat globules. This emulsification process is carried out by bile salts.

64. **(C)** The tarsal plates (A) are made of dense fibrous connective tissue and are important in maintaining the shape of the eyelids. The lacrimal gland (B) secretes lacrimal fluid through the ducts into the conjunctival sac of the upper eye. The answer is (C), the conjunctiva is the thin, mucus-secreting epithelial membrane that lines the interior surface of the eyelid.

65. **(B)** Prions are misfolded proteins that cause diseases like Mad Cow Disease.

66. **(C)** No explanation needed.

67. **(C)** Insects carry, or vector, the pathogen and therefore spread disease. This process is called vector transmission. Contact transmission (A) requires direct contact with the pathogen (e.g., touching). Fluid transmission (B) requires that the pathogen contact the host via fluid (e.g., saliva), and airborne transmission (D) includes pathogen movement to the host on air current (e.g., cough).

68. **(C)** The esophagus (A) is a passage for food from the mouth to the stomach and does not absorb any nutrients. The stomach (B) mostly absorbs sugars. The small intestine (C) absorbs most nutrients. The large intestine (D) absorbs mostly water.

69. **(C)** Animal viruses are classified on the basis of their replication strategy.

70. **(B)** Archaea. Bacteria (A) are prokaryotes but do not live in extreme environments. Options (C) and (D) are eukaryotes, not prokaryotes.

71. **(B)** The gallbladder serves as a reservoir for bile (B). Bile aids in the emulsification of fats. The beta cells of the pancreas produce insulin (C), not the gallbladder. Choices A and D are irrelevant.

72. **(C)** Because rumen bacteria live inside the digestive tracts where there is little oxygen, these bacteria are anaerobic (C), not aerobic (D). They are also symbiotic with the cow, not antagonistic (A) or pathogenic (B).

73. **(A)** Bile salts enhance the intestinal absorption of fatty acids. The other three choices are involved in the digestion of food.

74. **(C)** The answer is Steve (C) because his pH increased. The pH of the blood will increase after hyperventilating due to a low level of carbon dioxide.

75. **(D)** Options A through C all describe the same thing, immunity that a person is born with. Only innate immunity (D) involves the production of new antibodies.

76. **(B)** No explanation needed.

77. **(A)** Penicillin targets peptidoglycan in the cell wall of gram-positive bacteria. A bacterium with resistance to penicillin would not respond to an experimental antibiotic with the same mode of action.

78. **(A)** All other options (B through D) are stimulants.

79. **(B)** Koch's postulate defines the criterion used to demonstrate that an organism is responsible for causing a specific disease.

80. **(A)** Impulses from other neurons are picked up by dendrites (A).

81. **(B)** No explanation needed.

82. **(A)** No explanation needed.

83. **(C)** Vestigial means that the organ or tissue is of no known use in modern man. All other options are needed for humans to survive, but the appendix is not.

84. **(C)** No explanation needed.

85. **(B)** Bulimia nervosa is an eating disorder in which a person eats a great deal of food and then vomits or uses other purging methods. Anorexia nervosa is an eating disorder in which individuals do not eat enough to maintain body function at a normal level. Individuals with binge-eating disorder eat large amounts of food frequently and repeatedly. Disordered-eating patterns occur when concerns about dieting, food restriction, fear of becoming overweight, and dissatisfaction with body image interfere with normal daily life.

86. **(B)** Viruses obtain their envelope by budding through host cell membranes at sites where viral proteins have been inserted.

87. **(C)** Viruses require the help of a host cell in order to replicate. This definition makes it an obligate parasite.

88. **(C)** Phenomena (A) is caused by a bacterium, the common cold (B) is caused by a virus, and malaria (D) is caused by a protist carried by a mosquito.

89. **(A)** No explanation needed.

90. **(A)** Physical drug dependence results when an individual's body needs a drug to avoid withdrawal. Psychological drug dependence occurs when the drug is constantly on the user's mind and he or she feels an overwhelming need to use the drug often. Answer C is a nonsense answer.

91. **(C)** The best way to solve this problem is to find the cross that will most likely result in 75 percent yellow offspring given that yellow is dominant over green. After making your selection from the four possible choices, you should perform the cross by using a Punnett square. For example, let's cross choice C (Yy and Yy):

	Y	y
Y	YY	Yy
y	Yy	yy

YY = homozygous yellow;
Yy = heterozygous yellow;
yy = green

This cross will result in 75 percent yellow offspring.
To check the other choices, set up each of them in a Punnett square. Choice A will result in 50 percent yellow and 50 percent green. Choice B will result in 100 percent yellow offspring. Choice D will result in 100 percent yellow.

92. **(A)** Oxidative phosphorylation is the process in which energy is released as electrons pass through a series of electron acceptors to either oxygen or another inorganic compound.

93. **(A)** A homozygous (having the same pair) blue bird is represented by BB, and a homozygous white bird is represented by bb. Cross the two in the following Punnett square:

	b	b
B	Bb	Bb
B	Bb	Bb

Bb = blue

A cross between a homozygous blue bird (BB) and a homozygous white bird (bb) will result in 0 percent white birds.

94. **(D)** Follow the same procedure as in question 93:

	b	b
B	Bb	Bb
B	Bb	Bb

Bb = blue

A cross between a homozygous blue bird and a homozygous white bird will result in 100 percent blue heterozygous (Bb) birds, 0 percent white birds.

95. **(B)** Cones (B) provide daylight color vision and are responsible for visual acuity. Rods (A) respond to dim light for black-and-white vision. The optic disc (C) is a small region of the retina where the fibers of the ganglion neurons exit from the eyeball. The retina (D) is the inner layer of eyeball, and it contains the rods and cones.

96. **(C)** Cytokines are released by damaged or inflamed cells. The cytokines act as a signal molecule on the surface of endothelial cells that line blood vessels. Those cells then attract white blood cells to the site of inflammation. Antibodies (A) can be involved during inflammation but they do not recruit white blood cells. Excess carbon dioxide in the blood (B) is not associated with an inflammatory response. Growth factors (D) are signal molecules that promote cell growth and can be released by macrophages during an inflammatory response. However, they do not recruit white blood cells.

97. **(B)** No explanation needed.

98. **(B)** No explanation needed.

99. **(D)** Set up the cross between the individual carrying the disease (Ss) and the individual with the disease (ss):

	S	s
s	Ss	ss
s	Ss	ss

Ss = carrier of disease;
ss = have the disease

Therefore, 100 percent are expected to either be a carrier or have the disease.

100. **(B)** No explanation needed.

Chemistry Review and Practice

TIPS FOR THE CHEMISTRY SECTION

The chemistry section of the PCAT consists of approximately 48 questions. You will have 35 minutes to complete the chemistry section. To prepare for the chemistry section of the PCAT, review textbooks and notes used in chemistry courses. General chemistry, organic chemistry, and biochemistry questions are asked.

GENERAL CHEMISTRY REVIEW OUTLINE

  I. **Matter and the Periodic Table**
    A. Three states of matter
       1. Solid
       2. Liquid
       3. Gas
    B. Chemical and physical properties
    C. Elements, compounds, and mixtures
    D. Metals and nonmetals
    E. Electrolytes and nonelectrolytes
    F. Sizes of atoms
    G. Electronegativity
    H. Phase changes

 II. **Simple mathematics**
    A. Density
    B. Percent composition
    C. Average atomic weight
    D. Conversions (e.g., English and metric systems; see Appendix)

III. **Atomic structure**
    A. Atomic particles
       1. Protons
       2. Neutrons
       3. Electrons
    B. Atomic number

C. Atomic mass (atomic weight)

D. Molecular weight

E. Formula weight

F. Isotopes

G. Allotropes

H. Moles and Avogadro's number

IV. **Oxidation and reduction**

A. Oxidation number

B. Formal charge

C. Oxidizing agents

D. Reducing agents

V. **Balancing equations**

A. Simple equations

B. Redox equations

VI. **Solutions**

A. Concentration

1. Molarity

2. Molality

3. Percent composition

4. Mole fraction

B. Dilution of solutions

C. Colligative properties

1. Depression of vapor pressure

2. Elevation of boiling point

3. Depression of freezing point

4. Osmosis

D. Solubility rules

VII. **Gas laws**

A. Boyle's law

B. Charles's law

C. Ideal gas law

D. Dalton's law of partial pressure

E. Real gases

F. Effusion and diffusion

VIII. **Bonding**

A. Ionic

B. Covalent

C. Polar covalent

D. Intermolecular forces

1. Hydrogen bonding

2. Van der Waals forces

IX. Stoichiometry and equations
  A. Molar relationships
  B. Volume relationships
  C. Limiting reagent
  D. Percent yield

X. Nomenclature and writing formulas

XI. Molecular geometry
  A. Hybridization
  B. Bond angles
  C. Dipole moment

XII. Resonance

XIII. Electromagnetic spectrum
  A. Quantum theory and quantum numbers
  B. Electron configuration
  C. Lewis dot structures

XIV. Calorimetry
  A. Specific heat
  B. Heat capacity

XV. Acids and bases
  A. Definitions–Arrhenius, Brönsted-Lowry (conjugate pairs), Lewis
  B. Strengths of acids and bases
  C. pH
  D. Neutralization
  E. Buffers
  F. Acidic, basic, and amphoteric oxides

XVI. Kinetics
  A. First-order reactions
  B. Second-order reactions
  C. Half-life
  D. Determination of reaction orders
  E. Graphs

XVII. Equilibrium
  A. Equilibrium constants
    1. Acid
    2. Base
    3. Solubility product
    4. Complex ion formation
  B. Le Châtelier's Principle

XVIII. Electrochemistry
  A. Electrolytic and galvanic cells
  B. Oxidation and reduction
  C. Anode and cathode

XIX. Radioactivity
  A. Nuclear particles
  B. Balancing equations
  C. Fission
  D. Fusion

ORGANIC CHEMISTRY REVIEW OUTLINE

I. Formulas for families
  A. RCOOH, carboxylic acid, etc.
  B. General formulas for families (e.g., alkanes are C_nH_{2n+2})
  C. Empirical, molecular, and structural formulas
  D. Hybridization states of carbon

II. Physical properties of various organic families

III. Nomenclature

IV. Isomerism
  A. Geometric
  B. Optical
    1. Enantiomer
    2. Diastereomer
    3. Stereocenter
    4. Racemic mixture

V. Examples of simple reactions
  A. Addition
    1. Electrophilic addition to alkenes/alkynes
    2. Nucleophilic addition to carbonyl compounds
  B. Substitution
    1. Electrophilic substitution of benzene compounds
    2. Nucleophilic substitution of alkyl halides, acid derivatives
    3. Alpha substitution of carbonyl compounds
  C. Oxidation
    1. Cleavage of alkenes/alkynes
    2. Alcohols
  D. Reduction
    1. Alkenes/alkynes
    2. Carbonyl compounds

    E. Elimination

    F. Free-radical substitution

    G. Condensations of carbonyl compounds

       1. Aldol condensation

       2. Claisen condensation

VI. Resonance

    A. Benzene

    B. Cations, anions

    C. Radicals

VII. Spectroscopy

    A. Infrared (IR)

    B. Nuclear magnetic resonance (NMR)

BIOCHEMISTRY REVIEW OUTLINE

I. DNA, RNA

    A. Structures

    B. Processes

       1. Transcription

       2. Translation

       3. Replication

II. Lipids

    A. Structures

    B. Processes

       1. Storage, triglycerides

       2. Energy production, beta oxidation

       3. Membrane formation

       4. Steroid hormones

III. Proteins

    A. Levels of structure

       1. Primary

       2. Secondary

       3. Tertiary

       4. Quaternary

    B. Processes

       1. Synthesis, translation

       2. Degradation, digestion

IV. Carbohydrates

    A. Structures

    B. Processes

       1. Glycolysis, citric acid cycle, oxidative phosphorylation

       2. Gluconeogenesis

Answer Sheet
CHEMISTRY

1 Ⓐ Ⓑ Ⓒ Ⓓ	26 Ⓐ Ⓑ Ⓒ Ⓓ	51 Ⓐ Ⓑ Ⓒ Ⓓ	76 Ⓐ Ⓑ Ⓒ Ⓓ
2 Ⓐ Ⓑ Ⓒ Ⓓ	27 Ⓐ Ⓑ Ⓒ Ⓓ	52 Ⓐ Ⓑ Ⓒ Ⓓ	77 Ⓐ Ⓑ Ⓒ Ⓓ
3 Ⓐ Ⓑ Ⓒ Ⓓ	28 Ⓐ Ⓑ Ⓒ Ⓓ	53 Ⓐ Ⓑ Ⓒ Ⓓ	78 Ⓐ Ⓑ Ⓒ Ⓓ
4 Ⓐ Ⓑ Ⓒ Ⓓ	29 Ⓐ Ⓑ Ⓒ Ⓓ	54 Ⓐ Ⓑ Ⓒ Ⓓ	79 Ⓐ Ⓑ Ⓒ Ⓓ
5 Ⓐ Ⓑ Ⓒ Ⓓ	30 Ⓐ Ⓑ Ⓒ Ⓓ	55 Ⓐ Ⓑ Ⓒ Ⓓ	80 Ⓐ Ⓑ Ⓒ Ⓓ
6 Ⓐ Ⓑ Ⓒ Ⓓ	31 Ⓐ Ⓑ Ⓒ Ⓓ	56 Ⓐ Ⓑ Ⓒ Ⓓ	81 Ⓐ Ⓑ Ⓒ Ⓓ
7 Ⓐ Ⓑ Ⓒ Ⓓ	32 Ⓐ Ⓑ Ⓒ Ⓓ	57 Ⓐ Ⓑ Ⓒ Ⓓ	82 Ⓐ Ⓑ Ⓒ Ⓓ
8 Ⓐ Ⓑ Ⓒ Ⓓ	33 Ⓐ Ⓑ Ⓒ Ⓓ	58 Ⓐ Ⓑ Ⓒ Ⓓ	83 Ⓐ Ⓑ Ⓒ Ⓓ
9 Ⓐ Ⓑ Ⓒ Ⓓ	34 Ⓐ Ⓑ Ⓒ Ⓓ	59 Ⓐ Ⓑ Ⓒ Ⓓ	84 Ⓐ Ⓑ Ⓒ Ⓓ
10 Ⓐ Ⓑ Ⓒ Ⓓ	35 Ⓐ Ⓑ Ⓒ Ⓓ	60 Ⓐ Ⓑ Ⓒ Ⓓ	85 Ⓐ Ⓑ Ⓒ Ⓓ
11 Ⓐ Ⓑ Ⓒ Ⓓ	36 Ⓐ Ⓑ Ⓒ Ⓓ	61 Ⓐ Ⓑ Ⓒ Ⓓ	86 Ⓐ Ⓑ Ⓒ Ⓓ
12 Ⓐ Ⓑ Ⓒ Ⓓ	37 Ⓐ Ⓑ Ⓒ Ⓓ	62 Ⓐ Ⓑ Ⓒ Ⓓ	87 Ⓐ Ⓑ Ⓒ Ⓓ
13 Ⓐ Ⓑ Ⓒ Ⓓ	38 Ⓐ Ⓑ Ⓒ Ⓓ	63 Ⓐ Ⓑ Ⓒ Ⓓ	88 Ⓐ Ⓑ Ⓒ Ⓓ
14 Ⓐ Ⓑ Ⓒ Ⓓ	39 Ⓐ Ⓑ Ⓒ Ⓓ	64 Ⓐ Ⓑ Ⓒ Ⓓ	89 Ⓐ Ⓑ Ⓒ Ⓓ
15 Ⓐ Ⓑ Ⓒ Ⓓ	40 Ⓐ Ⓑ Ⓒ Ⓓ	65 Ⓐ Ⓑ Ⓒ Ⓓ	90 Ⓐ Ⓑ Ⓒ Ⓓ
16 Ⓐ Ⓑ Ⓒ Ⓓ	41 Ⓐ Ⓑ Ⓒ Ⓓ	66 Ⓐ Ⓑ Ⓒ Ⓓ	91 Ⓐ Ⓑ Ⓒ Ⓓ
17 Ⓐ Ⓑ Ⓒ Ⓓ	42 Ⓐ Ⓑ Ⓒ Ⓓ	67 Ⓐ Ⓑ Ⓒ Ⓓ	92 Ⓐ Ⓑ Ⓒ Ⓓ
18 Ⓐ Ⓑ Ⓒ Ⓓ	43 Ⓐ Ⓑ Ⓒ Ⓓ	68 Ⓐ Ⓑ Ⓒ Ⓓ	93 Ⓐ Ⓑ Ⓒ Ⓓ
19 Ⓐ Ⓑ Ⓒ Ⓓ	44 Ⓐ Ⓑ Ⓒ Ⓓ	69 Ⓐ Ⓑ Ⓒ Ⓓ	94 Ⓐ Ⓑ Ⓒ Ⓓ
20 Ⓐ Ⓑ Ⓒ Ⓓ	45 Ⓐ Ⓑ Ⓒ Ⓓ	70 Ⓐ Ⓑ Ⓒ Ⓓ	95 Ⓐ Ⓑ Ⓒ Ⓓ
21 Ⓐ Ⓑ Ⓒ Ⓓ	46 Ⓐ Ⓑ Ⓒ Ⓓ	71 Ⓐ Ⓑ Ⓒ Ⓓ	96 Ⓐ Ⓑ Ⓒ Ⓓ
22 Ⓐ Ⓑ Ⓒ Ⓓ	47 Ⓐ Ⓑ Ⓒ Ⓓ	72 Ⓐ Ⓑ Ⓒ Ⓓ	97 Ⓐ Ⓑ Ⓒ Ⓓ
23 Ⓐ Ⓑ Ⓒ Ⓓ	48 Ⓐ Ⓑ Ⓒ Ⓓ	73 Ⓐ Ⓑ Ⓒ Ⓓ	98 Ⓐ Ⓑ Ⓒ Ⓓ
24 Ⓐ Ⓑ Ⓒ Ⓓ	49 Ⓐ Ⓑ Ⓒ Ⓓ	74 Ⓐ Ⓑ Ⓒ Ⓓ	99 Ⓐ Ⓑ Ⓒ Ⓓ
25 Ⓐ Ⓑ Ⓒ Ⓓ	50 Ⓐ Ⓑ Ⓒ Ⓓ	75 Ⓐ Ⓑ Ⓒ Ⓓ	100 Ⓐ Ⓑ Ⓒ Ⓓ

Practice Questions

100 Questions

Directions: Select the best answer to each of the following questions.

1. What is the percentage of hydrogen, H, present in dimethyl ether, C_2H_6O?
   (C = 12 amu, H = 1 amu, O = 16 amu)

   (A) 2
   (B) 13
   (C) 52
   (D) 35

2. Calculate the formula weight, in atomic mass units (amu), of the salt ammonium sulfate, $(NH_4)_2SO_4$. (S = 32 amu, O = 16 amu, N = 14 amu, H = 1 amu)

   (A) 72
   (B) 132
   (C) 128
   (D) 114

3. The mass of 1 mole of copper (Cu) atoms equals 63.55 grams. What is the weight, in grams, of one atom of Cu?
   (Avogadro's number = 6×10^{23})

   (A) 1.06×10^{-24}
   (B) 9.47×10^{-23}
   (C) 9.47×10^{-21}
   (D) 1.06×10^{-22}

4. The classification of macromolecules as lipids is primarily based on the

   (A) cellular function of the molecule.
   (B) nonpolarity of the molecule.
   (C) absence of phosphate groups.
   (D) presence of peptide bonds.

5. How many neutrons are contained in the following atom of the element scandium: $^{45}_{21}Sc$?

   (A) 21
   (B) 66
   (C) 45
   (D) 24

6. Which of the following statements is NOT true concerning DNA?

   (A) It contains deoxyribonucleotides.
   (B) It contains adenine, guanine, cytosine, and thymine.
   (C) It exists as a double helix in the cell.
   (D) It is commonly found in the cytoplasm of animal cells.

7. Which of the following is NOT a nuclear reaction?

   (A) A sodium atom becomes a sodium ion.
   (B) A uranium atom becomes a barium atom and a krypton atom.
   (C) A thorium atom releases a gamma particle.
   (D) An iodine atom becomes a different isotope of iodine.

8. If the volume of a sample of gas at 1 atm and 25°C is reduced and the temperature remains constant, then

   (A) pressure will decrease.
   (B) gas particles will slow down.
   (C) Boyle's law will be demonstrated.
   (D) Charles's law will be demonstrated.

9. Which of the following theories would describe the covalent bond in water as the overlap of a half-filled 1s orbital with a half-filled sp^3 orbital?

   (A) Molecular Orbital Theory
   (B) Valence Shell Electron Pair Repulsion Theory (VSEPR)
   (C) Valence Bond Theory
   (D) Kinetic Molecular Theory

10. Which of the following statements describes a chemical property?

   (A) Liquid water is converted to water vapor by application of heat.
   (B) Salt, NaCl, dissolves in water.
   (C) A stone displaces its volume in a liquid.
   (D) Milk sours more readily at room temperature than in the refrigerator.

11. Proteins are important biological molecules involved in catalyzing reactions (enzymes) and in providing rigidity/support, among other things. Genetic mutations that result in changes in the primary structure of proteins can be harmful (or fatal) to the cell. For example, in the disorder phenylketonuria (PKU), a mutation in the gene coding for the enzyme phenylalanine hydroxylase results in irreversible mental retardation in newborns if undiagnosed. For this reason, a laboratory test (blood or urine analysis) is performed shortly after birth and dietary adjustments are made if PKU is diagnosed. Such adjustments are effective at preventing the damage associated with this disease.

The primary structure of proteins is

(A) the order of the amino acids in the polymer.
(B) the result of hydrogen bonding between amino acids.
(C) irrelevant to the protein's function.
(D) destroyed by denaturation.

12. When the following equation is balanced with the smallest set of whole numbers, what is the coefficient of H_2SO_4?

___Na_2CO_3 + ___H_2SO_4 → ___$NaHSO_4$ + ___H_2O + ___CO_2

(A) 1
(B) 2
(C) 3
(D) 5

13. What is the oxidation number of sulfur, S, in H_2SO_3?

(A) 2
(B) 4
(C) 5
(D) 6

14. What is the reducing agent in the following equation?

$$Zn + CuSO_4 \rightarrow ZnSO_4 + Cu$$

(A) Zn
(B) $CuSO_4$
(C) $ZnSO_4$
(D) Cu

15. RNA differs from DNA in that it

(A) cannot base-pair.
(B) doesn't contain phosphate groups.
(C) is not used to synthesize new molecules of itself.
(D) contains uracil rather than thymine found in DNA.

16. In the following reaction, how many moles of O_2 are necessary to react with 5 moles of NH_3? (O = 16 amu, N = 14 amu, H = 1 amu)

$$4NH_3 + 5O_2 \rightarrow 4NO + 6H_2O$$

(A) 4.0
(B) 5.0
(C) 5.5
(D) 6.3

17. How many liters of oxygen gas, O_2, will react completely with 3.5 liters of carbon disulfide gas, CS_2, in the following reaction?

$$CS_2 + 2O_2 \rightarrow CO_2 + 2SO_2$$

(A) 14.0
(B) 3.5
(C) 7.0
(D) 1.8

18. In the following reaction, how many grams of H_2O are produced from 17.0 g of NH_3? (O = 16 amu, N = 14 amu, H = 1 amu)

$$4\ NH_3 + 5\ O_2 \rightarrow 4\ NO + 6\ H_2O$$

(A) 1.5
(B) 18
(C) 27
(D) 2.4

19. In the following reaction, how many liters of NO are produced from 1.70 g of NH_3 at standard temperature and pressure conditions? (O = 16 amu, N = 14 amu, H = 1 amu)

$$4\ NH_3 + 5\ O_2 \rightarrow 4\ NO + 6\ H_2O$$

(A) 2.24
(B) 1.70
(C) 8.96
(D) 0.026

20. In the following reaction, how many molecules of NO are produced from 0.17 g of NH_3? (O = 16 amu, N = 14 amu, H = 1 amu)

$$4\ NH_3 + 5\ O_2 \rightarrow 4\ NO + 6\ H_2O$$

(A) 6.0×10^{21}
(B) 1.4×10^{22}
(C) 4.0×10^{23}
(D) 2.9×10^{23}

21. A 100-milliliter sample of oxygen, O_2, is collected over water at 25°C and 750 mm Hg pressure. The pressure of water vapor at 25°C is 23.76 mm Hg. Which of the following equations is correct to calculate the number of grams of oxygen collected? (R = 0.082 L-atm/K-mole)

(A) $750\,\text{mm}\left(100\,\text{ml}\right) = \dfrac{x}{16\,\text{g/mole}}\left(\dfrac{0.082\ \text{L-atm}}{\text{K-mole}}\right)\left(25°\text{C}\right)$

(B) $\dfrac{726.24\,\text{mm}\left(0.100\,\text{liter}\right)}{760\,\text{mm/atm}} = \dfrac{16\,\text{g/mole}}{x}\left(\dfrac{0.082\ \text{L-atm}}{\text{K-mole}}\right)\left(25°\text{C}\right)$

(C) $\dfrac{750\,\text{mm}\left(100\,\text{ml}\right)}{760\,\text{mm/atm}} = \dfrac{x}{32\,\text{g/mole}}\left(\dfrac{0.082\ \text{L-atm}}{\text{K-mole}}\right)\left(298\text{K}\right)$

(D) $\dfrac{726.24\,\text{mm}\left(0.100\,\text{liter}\right)}{760\,\text{mm/atm}} = \dfrac{x}{32\,\text{g/mole}}\left(\dfrac{0.082\ \text{L-atm}}{\text{K-mole}}\right)\left(298\text{K}\right)$

22. What is the molarity (M) of a solution prepared by dissolving 1.8 grams of sugar, $C_6H_{12}O_6$, in 1000 milliliters of solution? (O = 16 amu, C = 12 amu, H = 1 amu)

(A) 0.01
(B) 1.80
(C) 0.0018
(D) 0.10

23. How many grams of nitrogen gas, N_2, are present in a bulb of volume 1.0 liter, at 27°C and 1 atmosphere? (R = 0.082 liter-atm/K-mole, N = 14 amu)

(A) 7.9×10^{-2}
(B) 1.0×10^{5}
(C) 1.1
(D) 8.4×10^{-3}

24. How many milliliters of 5.0 M, sodium hydroxide, NaOH, solution must be used to prepare 200 milliliters of 2.5 M solution?

(A) 440
(B) 36
(C) 500
(D) 100

25. A variety of laboratory methods are used to separate components of a mixture. Common among those is distillation. Industrially, distillation is used in petroleum refineries to separate the organic components found in crude petroleum. More than 100 operating refineries in the United States purify millions of barrels of crude petroleum each year. Gasoline, a mixture of organic compounds, is a commodity of increasing concern as a result of its cost and the environmental impact of its combustion products. Distillation separates the components of mixtures based on boiling point—the lowest boiling component evaporates at the lowest temperature, its vapor is removed and condensed, thus isolating that component from the mixture. This process continues to isolate the next lowest boiling component, and so on.

Which of the following compounds would be expected to have the highest boiling point?

(A)

(B)

(C)

(D)

26. How many milliliters of 2.0 M lithium hydroxide, LiOH, solution are necessary to neutralize 10 milliliters of 3.0 M sulfuric acid, H_2SO_4, according to the following equation?

$$2 \text{ LiOH} + H_2SO_4 \rightarrow Li_2SO_4 + 2H_2O$$

(A) 60
(B) 30
(C) 15
(D) 12

27. A bubble of gas (1.4 mL) is at the bottom of a lake where the temperature and pressure are 7° C and 2.0 atmospheres, respectively. The temperature and pressure at the surface of the lake are 27° C and 1.0 atmosphere. What is the volume, in milliliters, of a gas bubble at the surface of the lake?

(A) 2.6
(B) 3.0
(C) 0.75
(D) 0.65

28. Ammonia, NH_3, and oxygen, O_2, are gases at standard temperature and pressure. They are combined to produce nitrous oxide gas, NO, and water vapor. How many liters of NO can be produced at 27°C and 2.0 atmospheres from 1.7 g of NH_3? (O = 16 amu, N = 14 amu, H = 1 amu, R = 0.082 liter-atm/K-mole).

$$4NH_3 + 5O_2 \rightarrow 4NO + 6H_2O$$

(A) 2.2
(B) 1.2
(C) 4.0
(D) 0.8

29. About 50% of the dry biomass on earth is glucose. Glucose is a carbohydrate produced in plants from water and carbon dioxide. When animals eat plants, polymers of glucose are hydrolyzed to release free glucose molecules. After absorption in the digestive tract, glucose travels via the blood to the tissues and is transported into the cells. Within cells, glucose is oxidized with the concomitant production of energy, stored in adenosine triphosphate (ATP) molecules. A variety of cellular processes are involved in this transformation including glycolysis, the citric acid cycle (Krebs Cycle), and oxidative phosphorylation.

The process by which glucose is converted to two molecules of pyruvic acid is called

(A) oxidative phosphorylation.
(B) the citric acid cycle.
(C) gluconeogenesis.
(D) glycolysis.

30. Specify the absolute configuration of each chiral center in:

(A) 2R
(B) 2S
(C) 2R, 3R
(D) 2S, 3S

31. The specific heat of copper, Cu, is 0.385 joule per gram ° C. What is the heat capacity, in joules per ° C, of 10.0 grams of copper?

(A) 0.03
(B) 15.4
(C) 3.85
(D) 38.9

32. All of the following are uses of lipids EXCEPT

(A) hormones.
(B) energy production.
(C) cell membrane construction.
(D) gene composition.

33. Name the following molecule.

(A) 3-ethylenehexane
(B) (E)-3-propyl-2-pentene
(C) (Z)-3-ethyl-2-hexene
(D) (E)-3-ethyl-2-hexene

Use the periodic table to answer questions 34, 35, 37–43.

H																	He
Li	Be											B	C	N	O	F	Ne
Na	Mg											Al	Si	P	S	Cl	Ar
K	Ca	Sc	Ti	V	Cr	Mn	Fe	Co	Ni	Cu	Zn	Ga	Ge	As	Se	Br	Kr
Rb	Sr	Y	Zr	Nb	Mo	Tc	Ru	Rh	Pd	Ag	Cd	In	Sn	Sb	Te	I	Xe
Cs	Ba	La	Hf	Ta	W	Re	Os	Ir	Pt	Au	Hg	Tl	Pb	Bi	Po	At	Rn
Fr	Ra	Ac	Rf	Ha	Sg	Ns	Hs	Mt									

Ce	Pr	Nd	Pm	Sm	Eu	Gd	Tb	Dy	Ho	Er	Tm	Yb	Lu
Th	Pa	U	Np	Pu	Am	Cm	Bk	Cf	Es	Fm	Md	No	Lr

34. Radium undergoes beta decay producing what element?

$$^{228}_{88}Ra \rightarrow ^{\ \ 0}_{-1}e + ?$$

(A) Fr
(B) Rn
(C) Ac
(D) Ra

35. The electron configuration for the sulfide ion, S^{2-}, is

    (A) $1s^2 2s^2 2p^6 3s^2 3p^6$.
    (B) $1s^2 2s^2 2p^6 3s^2 3p^4$.
    (C) $1s^2 2s^2 2p^6 3s^2 3p^2$.
    (D) $1s^2 2s^2 2p^6 3s^2 3p^6 4s^2$.

36. Protein function is intimately linked to the three-dimensional conformation assumed by the protein in aqueous solution. A loss of that conformation ordinarily results in a loss of function. Extreme changes in temperature or pH can cause these changes because the intermolecular forces responsible for the protein's conformation are adversely affected. An important intermolecular force involved is hydrogen bonding. When hydrogen bonding is disrupted, the protein's secondary and tertiary structure is affected. A protein's secondary structure involves hydrogen bonding between the partial negative oxygen of a peptide bond and the hydrogen covalently bound to the nitrogen of another peptide bond. The tertiary structure involves hydrogen bonding between polar side chains of amino acids and the water molecules within the cell.

    An example of secondary structure in proteins includes a

    (A) tetramer.
    (B) peptide bond.
    (C) beta sheet.
    (D) double helix.

37. Which specie below has the valence shell electron configuration of $3s^2 3p^2$?

    (A) Mg^{2+}
    (B) Si
    (C) C
    (D) Si^{2-}

38. How many unshared electrons are on the phosphorus atom in the Lewis dot structure for PCl_5?

    (A) 5
    (B) 2
    (C) 0
    (D) 8

39. What is the formal charge on the carbon atom in the carbonate ion, CO_3^{2-}?

    (A) 0
    (B) +1
    (C) −1
    (D) +4

40. The compound with the greatest amount of ionic bonding character is

   (A) CO_2
   (B) Li_2O
   (C) CH_4
   (D) NH_3

41. What is the molecular geometry of the silicon hydride, SiH_4, molecule?

   (A) Linear
   (B) Bent
   (C) Tetrahedral
   (D) Trigonal pyramid

42. What is the approximate value of the bond angle for the H-S-H bond in hydrogen sulfide, H_2S?

   (A) 105°
   (B) 120°
   (C) 180°
   (D) 90°

43. What is the hybridization state of the aluminum (Al) atom in $AlCl_3$?

   (A) sp
   (B) sp^2
   (C) sp^3
   (D) sp^3d^2

44. The synthesis of protein directly involves all of the following EXCEPT

   (A) amino acids.
   (B) DNA.
   (C) ribosomes.
   (D) RNA.

45. Adenosine triphosphate (ATP) is an important source of chemical energy in the cell and is produced

   (A) directly during translation.
   (B) from NADH and $FADH_2$ through oxidative phosphorylation (aka the electron transport chain).
   (C) in the cell nucleus.
   (D) from DNA.

46. What is the product of the following reaction?

1. BH_3
2. H_2O_2, OH^-

(A)

(B)

(C)

(D)

47. Which of the following molecules has a dipole moment of zero?

(A) CO_2
(B) H_2O
(C) HF
(D) NH_3

48. In the process of replication

(A) the DNA duplex does not melt (unwind).
(B) the two resulting DNA molecules are identical.
(C) both new DNA molecules are synthesized discontinuously.
(D) the raw material nucleotides are carried by tRNA.

49. Which of the following sets of quantum numbers is possible?

(A) $n = 2$, $\ell = 0$, $m_\ell = 1$, $m_s = +\frac{1}{2}$
(B) $n = 1$, $\ell = 1$, $m_\ell = 0$, $m_s = -\frac{1}{2}$
(C) $n = 3$, $\ell = 2$, $m_\ell = -1$, $m_s = +\frac{1}{2}$
(D) $n = 2$, $\ell = 1$, $m_\ell = 1$, $m_s = -1$

50. What reagent would accomplish the following conversion?

$$CH_3CH_2CHO \rightarrow CH_3CH_2CH_2OH$$

(A) PCC (pyridinium chlorochromate)
(B) $NaBH_4$
(C) H_2
(D) $KMnO_4$

51. What is a product of the following reaction?

NH$_2$

Br$_2$, FeBr$_3$

(A) NHBr

(B) NH$_2$

Br

(C) NH$_2$

Br

(D) NO$_2$

52. Proteins are used to catalyze biological reactions. Their three-dimensional shape and function are determined by their amino acid sequence. That sequence is coded in the nucleotide sequence of the cell's genes, the DNA. However, proteins are not synthesized directly from the DNA genetic sequence. The information in DNA is first used to synthesize RNA. The nucleotide sequence of the RNA is then used to dictate the amino acid sequence in the resultant proteins. Changes in the DNA sequence may result in changes in the amino acid sequence of the protein ultimately produced. These changes can adversely affect the protein's function—particularly if the amino acid changes are in the protein's active site.

The process by which an RNA molecule is synthesized based on the nucleotide sequence in DNA is called

(A) transcription.
(B) translation.
(C) replication.
(D) respiration.

53. The major kind of lipid found in cell membranes is

(A) triglycerides.
(B) phospholipids.
(C) waxes.
(D) starch.

54. Which of the following types of RNA carries amino acids to the ribosome for protein synthesis?

    (A) mRNA
    (B) rRNA
    (C) tRNA
    (D) aRNA

55. What is the half life, in seconds, for a first-order reaction having a rate constant of 6.93×10^2 per second?

    (A) $1.0 \times 10^{+1}$
    (B) 1.0×10^{-3}
    (C) 1.0×10^{-1}
    (D) $1.0 \times 10^{+5}$

56. What functional group is formed by the following reaction?

    $$CH_3OH + (CH_3)_2CHCOBr \rightarrow$$

    (A) Ester
    (B) Acid
    (C) Acid anhydride
    (D) Ketone

57. What is the structure of the starting material if, after the addition of potassium permanganate, the products are carbon dioxide and acetone?

    (A)   (B)

    (C)   (D)

58. What is the equilibrium constant for the following reaction when $[H_2] = 0.25$ M, $[I_2] = 0.25$ M and $[HI] = 0.50$ M?

    $$H_2 + I_2 \leftrightarrow 2HI$$

    (A) 4.0
    (B) 0.25
    (C) 8.0
    (D) 0.13

59. Which of the following changes will NOT cause the reaction equilibrium shown below to shift toward the products on the right?

$$Heat + N_2O_4(g) \leftrightarrow 2NO_2 (g)$$

(A) A decrease in temperature
(B) Addition of more N_2O_4
(C) Removal of some NO_2
(D) An increase in temperature

60. What reagent is needed for the following conversion?

$$CH_3CH_2CH(CH_3)CO_2H \rightarrow CH_3CH_2CH(CH_3)CH_2OH$$

(A) $NaBH_4$
(B) H_2
(C) $LiAlH_4$
(D) $KMnO_4$

61. What is the major product of the following elimination?

(A) (B)

(C) (D)

OC(CH₃)₃

62. What kind of condensation reaction is demonstrated by the following reaction under basic conditions?

(A) Claisen
(B) Williamson
(C) Michael
(D) Aldol

63. What are the monomeric units of peptides and proteins?

    (A) Amino acids
    (B) Aminoalcohols
    (C) Aminals
    (D) β–hydroxyacids

64. Which of the following is a resonance structure of

    (A)   (B)

    (C)   (D)

65. What is the pH of a solution having a hydroxide ion concentration, $[OH^-]$, equal to 0.01 M?

    (A) 2
    (B) 10
    (C) 12
    (D) 14

66. The intermolecular force that holds the two strands of DNA in a helical form is called

    (A) van der Waal's forces.
    (B) covalent bonding.
    (C) hydrogen bonding.
    (D) dipole-dipole interactions.

67. The infrared spectrum of a substance has a strong absorption at 3300 cm^{-1} and at 1700 cm^{-1}. What functional group is present in the substance?

    (A) Ester
    (B) Alcohol
    (C) Acid
    (D) Aldehyde

68. Which statement describes triglycerides?

    (A) They are stored in smooth muscle.
    (B) Basic hydrolysis yields soap.
    (C) They are triesters of glucose.
    (D) Their long carbon chains are used to generate ATP via gluconeogenesis.

69. Which of the following statements is true concerning the acid-base reaction below?

$$NH_3 + H_2O \rightarrow NH_4^+ + OH^-$$

    (A) The equilibrium lies far to the left.
    (B) Water is acting as a base.
    (C) Ammonium is the conjugate base of ammonia.
    (D) Hydroxide is the conjugate acid of water.

70. What is the hydroxide ion concentration, $[OH^{-1}]$, in 2.50 M $Mg(OH)_2$?

    (A) 2.50 M
    (B) 1.25 M
    (C) 5.00 M
    (D) 7.25 M

71. Which structure for a compound with the formula $C_9H_{10}O$ is consistent with the following ^1H NMR data?

    δ 1.4 ppm, triplet, 3H
    δ 4.1 ppm, quartet, 2H
    δ 7.0 ppm, doublet, 2H
    δ 7.8 ppm, doublet, 2H
    δ 9.8 ppm, singlet, 1H

(A) CHO

(B) CH₂OH

(C) CHO

(D) CHO

72. Organic compounds found in food may be used as energy sources for cells. They may alternatively be used to synthesize cofactors like NAD^+ and FAD. Different biochemical processes are used to oxidize organic compounds depending on the class of compound. Many of the enzymes in these processes require cofactors to facilitate catalysis. The biochemical processes include glycolysis and beta oxidation. Both of these processes result in the production of acetylCoA molecules which are further oxidized in the citric acid cycle (Krebs Cycle) producing substrate-level ATP and reduced cofactors, NADH and $FADH_2$. The reduced cofactors then result in the production of more ATP through oxidative phosphorylation (the electron transport chain).

    Beta oxidation is a metabolic pathway involving the oxidation of

    (A) polysaccharides.
    (B) nucleic acids.
    (C) fatty acids.
    (D) polypeptides.

73. If the value of K_A for an acid, HY, is 5×10^{-5}, what is the value of K_B for the conjugate ion, Y^{-1}?

    (A) 2.0×10^{-10}
    (B) 2.0×10^{-8}
    (C) 2.0×10^{-18}
    (D) 2.0×10^{-20}

74. Which of the following weak acids is the strongest acid? (The ionization constants are given.)

		K_A
(A)	Benzoic acid	6.5×10^{-5}
(B)	Nitrous acid	4.5×10^{-4}
(C)	Formic acid	1.7×10^{-4}
(D)	Acetic acid	1.8×10^{-5}

75. Which is a product of the following reaction?

(A)

(B)

(C)

(D)

76. Which of the following compounds is insoluble in water?

(A) NaOH
(B) NH$_4$Cl
(C) LiNO$_3$
(D) CaCO$_3$

77. Amino acids used in translation come from

(A) biosynthesis reactions.
(B) digestion of dietary fats.
(C) degradation of cellular nucleic acids.
(D) the citric acid cycle.

78. Which of the following slightly soluble salts is the most soluble? (The solubility product constants are given.)

	K_{sp}
(A) Copper (II) sulfide	6.0×10^{-37}
(B) Nickel (II) sulfide	1.4×10^{-24}
(C) Silver chloride	1.6×10^{-10}
(D) Lead (II) chromate	2.0×10^{-14}

79. Which of the following complex ions is the most stable? (The formation constants, K_f, are given.)

	K_f
(A) $Ag(NH_3)_2^{+1}$	1.5×10^7
(B) $Zn(NH_3)_4^{2+}$	2.0×10^9
(C) HgI_4^{2-}	2.0×10^{30}
(D) $Cd(CN)_4^{2-}$	7.1×10^{16}

80. Proteins are polymers of alpha amino acids. The "alpha" designation indicates that the carboxylic acid and amine functional groups are covalently bonded to the same carbon, the alpha carbon. Proteins in the food eaten by the organism are hydrolyzed to smaller peptides and free amino acids through digestive processes. Amino acids are then absorbed in the gastrointestinal tract and transported to the tissues via the blood. The amino acids needed for protein synthesis may be biosynthesized or salvaged from the degradation of proteins within the cells. Protein synthesis is a complex process involving nucleic acids and individual amino acids. During this process, the alpha amino group of one amino acid is condensed with the alpha carboxylic acid of a second amino acid. This condensation continues until the final protein has been synthesized. A shortage of the requisite amino acids can adversely impact protein synthesis and/or the amino acid sequence of resultant proteins.

Proteins are composed of twenty amino acids that

(A) are joined by glycosidic bonds.
(B) differ in the identity of a group at the alpha carbon.
(C) are all essential.
(D) are not water soluble.

81. In which of the following solutions will aluminum hydroxide, $Al(OH)_3$, be the LEAST soluble?

(A) H_2O
(B) 0.5 M $Al(NO_3)_3$
(C) 1.6 M NaOH
(D) 0.3 M HCl

82. Molecular polarity affects solubility. The adage "like dissolves like" describes solubility patterns. Polar molecules are soluble in polar solvents and nonpolar molecules are soluble in nonpolar solvents. For example, when using oil-based paint, turpentine (a nonpolar solvent) is required for cleanup. Water is a polar solvent ubiquitous in biological tissues. Polar biological molecules are soluble in water, while nonpolar biological molecules are not. In order to solubilize nonpolar molecules in an aqueous environment, surfactants are required. Surfactants are molecules with both nonpolar and polar areas allowing them to solubilize nonpolar molecules as well as interact favorably with water. Biological surfactants include the bile acids and the lipoproteins. The water solubility of the major classes of biomolecules (proteins, lipids, carbohydrates, and nucleic acids) varies and is governed by the polarity of each.

Which of the following molecules is a lipid?

(A)

(B)

(C)

(D)

Use the following table of standard reduction potentials to answer questions 83–84.

			$emf°$
Li^+ (aq) + e^-	$\rightarrow$	Li (s)	-3.05
Ca^{2+} (aq) + $2e^-$	$\rightarrow$	Ca (s)	-2.87
Zn^{2+} (aq) + $2e^-$	$\rightarrow$	Zn (s)	-0.76
Sn^{+2} (aq) + $2e^-$	$\rightarrow$	Sn (s)	-0.14
$2 H^+$ (aq) + $2e^-$	$\rightarrow$	H_2 (g)	0.00
Cu^{2+} (aq) + $2e^-$	$\rightarrow$	Cu (s)	$+0.34$
Fe^{3+} (aq) + e^-	$\rightarrow$	Fe^{2+}	$+0.77$
Br_2 (ℓ) + $2e^-$	$\rightarrow$	$2 Br^{-1}$	$+1.07$

83. In the following overall reaction:
$$Zn (s) + Cu^{+2} \rightarrow Zn^{2+} + Cu (s)$$
which partial reaction shows the reagent that is oxidized?

(A) Zn^{2+} (aq) + $2e^- \rightarrow$ Zn (s)
(B) Cu^{2+} (aq) + $2e^- \rightarrow$ Cu (s)
(C) Zn (s) $\rightarrow Zn^{2+}$ (aq) + $2e^-$
(D) Cu (s) $\rightarrow Cu^{2+}$ (aq) + $2e^-$

84. Which of the following species is the strongest reducing agent?

(A) Li^+
(B) Br_2
(C) Br^{-1}
(D) Li

85. Which of the following statements describes the reaction which occurs at the cathode in an electrochemical cell?

(A) The cathode is the electrode at which electrons are lost and oxidation occurs.
(B) The cathode is the electrode at which electrons are lost and reduction occurs.
(C) The cathode is the electrode at which electrons are gained and oxidation occurs.
(D) The cathode is the electrode at which electrons are gained and reduction occurs.

86. Which of the following reactions is an oxidation?

(A) $CH_3CH_2OH \rightarrow CH_2 = CH_2$
(B) $CH_2 = CH_2 \rightarrow CH_3CH_3$
(C) $CH_2Br–CH_2Br \rightarrow HCCH$
(D) $CH_2 = CH_2 \rightarrow CH_2Br–CH_2Br$

87. Which of the following groups is expected to have the greatest 1,3-diaxial energy in a monosubstituted cyclohexane?

    (A) Methyl
    (B) Ethyl
    (C) Isopropyl
    (D) t-Butyl

88. Food products are frequently labeled as containing no saturated fats and/or no trans fats. Studies have shown a correlation between the risk for cardio-vascular disease and dietary content of these types of fats. Saturated fats and trans fats have higher melting points than unsaturated naturally-occurring fats and cis fats. This is true because the carbon chains of saturated and trans fats are able to participate in a larger number of hydrophobic interactions (van der Waal's or London forces) compared to cis unsaturated fats. An increased number of van der Waal's interactions between molecules means more energy is needed to disrupt them in the melting process.

    Which of the following formulas represents an unsaturated compound?

    (A) C_2H_6
    (B) C_3H_6
    (C) C_2H_6O
    (D) CH_3Cl

89. How many different structural isomers can be formed by the compound having the molecular formula C_4H_9Cl?

    (A) 1
    (B) 2
    (C) 3
    (D) 4

90. How many different compounds (ignoring stereoisomers) can be formed by the monochlorination of pentane?

    (A) 1
    (B) 2
    (C) 3
    (D) 4

91. What is the name of the following compound?

(A) 5-Bromo-3,4-dimethyloctane
(B) 4-Bromo-2-ethyl-3-methylheptane
(C) 4-Bromo-6-ethyl-5-methylheptane
(D) 4-Bromo-5,6-dimethyloctane

92. A stereocenter is one to which are attached

(A) four groups that are the same.
(B) three groups that are the same, one group that is different.
(C) four groups that are different.
(D) two groups that are the same, and another two groups which are the same yet different from the first two groups.

93. The two formulas shown below represent

$$CH_3 \quad CH_3 \qquad\qquad CH_3 \quad Cl$$
$$\diagdown \quad \diagup \qquad\qquad\qquad \diagdown \quad \diagup$$
$$C = C \qquad\qquad\qquad C = C$$
$$\diagup \quad \diagdown \qquad\qquad\qquad \diagup \quad \diagdown$$
$$Cl \quad\quad Cl \qquad\qquad\qquad Cl \quad\quad CH_3$$

(A) constitutional isomers.
(B) a racemic mixture.
(C) enantiomers.
(D) diastereomers.

94. The carbon atom in methane, CH_4, has the hybridization

(A) sp.
(B) sp^2.
(C) sp^3.
(D) sp^3d^2.

95. The carbon atom in ethylene, $H_2C = CH_2$, has the hybridization

(A) sp.
(B) sp^2.
(C) sp^3.
(D) sp^3d^2.

96. Oxidation of the secondary alcohol 2-propanol

$$CH_3-CH-CH_3$$
$$|$$
$$OH$$

yields:

(A) ethanol.
(B) propanone.
(C) propanal.
(D) dimethyl ether.

97. Which of the following compounds is the most water soluble?

(A) Ethyl ether, $CH_3CH_2OCH_2CH_3$
(B) Ethyl chloride, CH_3CH_2Cl
(C) Ethane, CH_3CH_3
(D) Benzene, C_6H_6

98. After reaction workup, the reaction of the Grignard reagent, methyl magnesium bromide, CH_3MgBr, with the aldehyde, acetaldehyde, CH_3CHO, produces as a product

(A) methyl ethyl ether.
(B) 2-propanol.
(C) 1-propanol.
(D) dimethyl ketone.

99. Which of the following is true concerning the dehydration of an alcohol?

(A) It may occur through an SN2 mechanism.
(B) It may occur through an E1 mechanism with a primary alcohol.
(C) It may occur through an SN1 mechanism with a tertiary alcohol.
(D) It may occur through an E1 mechanism with a tertiary alcohol.

100. A mixture of equal amounts of a pair of enantiomers is called a

(A) pair of diastereomers.
(B) conformational mixture.
(C) meso compound.
(D) racemic mixture.

Answer Key
CHEMISTRY

1. **B**	26. **B**	51. **C**	76. **D**
2. **B**	27. **B**	52. **A**	77. **A**
3. **D**	28. **B**	53. **B**	78. **C**
4. **B**	29. **D**	54. **C**	79. **C**
5. **D**	30. **B**	55. **B**	80. **B**
6. **D**	31. **C**	56. **A**	81. **C**
7. **A**	32. **D**	57. **B**	82. **A**
8. **C**	33. **C**	58. **A**	83. **C**
9. **C**	34. **C**	59. **A**	84. **D**
10. **D**	35. **A**	60. **C**	85. **D**
11. **A**	36. **C**	61. **B**	86. **D**
12. **B**	37. **B**	62. **D**	87. **D**
13. **B**	38. **C**	63. **A**	88. **B**
14. **A**	39. **A**	64. **B**	89. **D**
15. **C**	40. **B**	65. **C**	90. **C**
16. **D**	41. **C**	66. **C**	91. **A**
17. **C**	42. **A**	67. **C**	92. **C**
18. **C**	43. **B**	68. **B**	93. **D**
19. **A**	44. **B**	69. **A**	94. **C**
20. **A**	45. **B**	70. **C**	95. **B**
21. **D**	46. **C**	71. **C**	96. **B**
22. **A**	47. **A**	72. **C**	97. **A**
23. **C**	48. **B**	73. **A**	98. **B**
24. **D**	49. **C**	74. **B**	99. **D**
25. **D**	50. **B**	75. **A**	100. **D**

EXPLANATORY ANSWERS

1. **(B)** Percentage equals part divided by whole times 100.

$$\frac{Part}{Whole} \times 100 = \%$$

$$\frac{6\,H}{C_2H_6O} \times 100 = \frac{6}{46} \times 100 = 13\%$$

2. **(B)** A formula weight (or molecular weight) is calculated by adding the number of atoms of each element multiplied by its atomic mass, or weight; a total weight in atomic mass units for $(NH_4)_2SO_4$.

$$
\begin{array}{lll}
2N = 2(14) & = & 28 \\
8H = 8(1) & = & 8 \\
1S = 1(32) & = & 32 \\
4O = 4(16) & = & \underline{64} \\
& & 132 \text{ amu}
\end{array}
$$

3. **(D)** Use the factor-label method to calculate the weight of one atom of Cu.

Avogadro's number $\cong 6 \times 10^{23}$ atoms = 1 mole

63.55 g Cu = 1 mole

$$\frac{63.55\,g}{1\,mole} \times \frac{1\,mole}{6 \times 10^{23}\,atoms} = 10.59 \times 10^{-23} = 1.06 \times 10^{-22}\,g$$

4. **(B)** The feature that all lipids share is that they are poorly water soluble (hydrophobic or nonpolar) due to extensive numbers of carbon-hydrogen bonds. The functions of lipids are varied and include incorporation into cell membranes, energy storage in adipose tissue, and the steroid hormones.

5. **(D)** In the symbol, 45 is the mass number, or atomic weight (number of protons plus number of neutrons), and 21 is the atomic number (number of protons) of scandium, Sc. Subtracting 21 from 45 gives the number of neutrons, 24.

6. **(D)** DNA is contained in the nucleus of animal cells (eucaryotes).

7. **(A)** Nuclear reactions are reactions involving the nucleus. When a sodium atom becomes a sodium ion, an electron is lost from the valence shell of sodium (not from the nucleus). All of the other reactions are nuclear reactions. Option (B) is an example of fission (two nuclei are produced from one). Emission of gamma particles and conversion of one isotope of an element into another are both nuclear processes.

8. **(C)** If the volume of a gas is reduced (and the temperature remains constant), then the pressure must increase. This is stated formally in Boyle's law ($P_1V_1 = P_2V_2$). The movement of the gas particles is dependent on the temperature so (B) is not correct. Charles's law has to do with changes in volume and temperature ($V_1/T_1 = V_2/T_2$).

9. **(C)** The Valence Bond Theory is a theory concerning how atoms share electrons in covalent bonds. It views covalent bonds as being the overlap of an atomic orbital from each of the involved atoms. The Molecular Orbital Theory is also a theory of covalent bonding but it views the covalent bonding in molecules as being the addition of the individual atoms' atomic orbitals creating new orbitals that encompass the molecule (called molecular orbitals) that replace the atomic orbitals. The Valence Shell Electron Pair Repulsion Theory is used to predict the geometry of molecules and says that the electron pairs around a central atom in a molecule will spread out as far as possible. The Kinetic Molecular Theory is the theory that brings together the observed properties of gases.

10. **(D)** Physical changes are illustrated by answers A, B, and C. Most physical changes are reversible. For example, water vapor can be converted back to liquid water by cooling, salt can be separated from water by evaporating the water, and the volume of the liquid returns to its original volume when the stone is removed. Answer D, however, represents a chemical change. Once milk sours, the original chemicals present in the milk are converted to new compounds and the change is not reversible. Some chemical changes are reversible, but most are not.

11. **(A)** With respect to proteins, primary structure is the sequence of amino acids in the protein, secondary structure is localized patterns that arise due to hydrogen bonding between peptide bonds in the protein, tertiary structure is the overall folding pattern of the protein, and quaternary structure is the association of multiple proteins (not all proteins exhibit quaternary structure). All of the levels of structure are important in the protein's function. Denaturation disrupts the noncovalent interactions in the protein (secondary through quaternary structure), but the primary structure (which involves covalent bonds) is not affected.

12. **(B)** The coefficient of H_2SO_4 is 2 as shown in the balanced equation below:
$$Na_2CO_3 + 2H_2SO_4 \rightarrow 2\,NaHSO_4 + H_2O + CO_2$$

13. **(B)** The oxidation number of hydrogen, H, in a compound is +1, except when that element is present as a hydride [eg., LiH (–1)], and the oxidation number of oxygen, O, in a compound is –2, except when that element is present as a peroxide [eg., Na_2O_2 (–1)].

$$\begin{array}{cc} +2 & -6 \\ 2(+1) & 3(-2) \\ \multicolumn{2}{c}{H_2SO_3} \end{array}$$

Since sulfurous acid, H_2SO_3, is a neutral compound, the sum of the oxidation numbers for hydrogen, sulfur, and oxygen must equal zero; +2 (for H) plus +4 (for S) combine with –6 (for O) to equal zero.

14. **(A)** Oxidation is the loss of electrons; the substance oxidized is the reducing agent. Reduction is the gain of electrons; the substance reduced is the oxidizing agent. In the given equation, Zn loses electrons while Cu^{2+} gains electrons. Thus, Zn^0 (which is oxidized to Zn^{2+}) is the reducing agent; Cu^{2+} (which is reduced to Cu^0) is the oxidizing agent.

$$Zn + CuSO_4 \rightarrow ZnSO_4 + Cu$$
$$Zn^0 \rightarrow Zn^{2+} + 2\ e^-$$
$$Cu^{2+} + 2\ e^- \rightarrow Cu$$

15. **(C)** RNA (ribonucleic acid) and DNA (deoxyribonucleic acid) are both polymers of nucleotides (nucleotides are composed of a purine or pyrimidine base, a ribose or deoxyribose sugar, and a phosphate). The purines in both RNA and DNA are named guanine and adenine. Both RNA and DNA contain the pyrimidine cytosine but only RNA contains the pyrimidine uracil and only DNA contains the pyrimidine thymine. Base-pairing refers to hydrogen bonding between nucleotides so both RNA and DNA are capable of base-pairing. The synthesis of RNA molecules is called transcription and uses the nucleotide sequence in DNA as a template for synthesis. The synthesis of DNA is called replication and uses the nucleotide sequence in DNA as a template for synthesis.

16. **(D)** The coefficients of the reactants and products in a balanced equation represent *volume* for gases, as well as *molecules* and *moles*. These are the only direct relationships involving coefficients that exist in a balanced equation. Use the factor-label method to calculate the number of moles of oxygen formed when the reaction begins with 4 moles of ammonia.

$$4NH_3(g) + 5O_2(g) \rightarrow 4NO(g) + 6H_2O(g)$$

Two fractions are possible from the relationship that 4 moles NH_3 require 5 moles O_2:

$$\frac{4 \text{ moles } NH_3}{5 \text{ moles } O_2} \qquad \frac{5 \text{ moles } O_2}{4 \text{ moles } NH_3}$$

Having 5 moles of NH_3, multiply by the appropriate fraction so that only moles of O_2 remain.

$$5 \text{ moles } NH_3 \ \times \frac{5 \text{ moles } O_2}{4 \text{ moles } NH_3} = 6.3 \text{ moles } O_2$$

17. **(C)** Refer to the explanation for question 16.

18. **(C)** Convert 17.0 g of NH_3 to moles NH_3:

$$17.0 \text{ g} \times \frac{1 \text{ mol } NH_3}{17.0 \text{ g } NH_3} = 1 \text{ mol } NH_3$$

Use the coefficients in the equation to find moles of H_2O:

$$1 \text{ mol NH}_3 \times \frac{6 \text{ mol H}_2\text{O}}{4 \text{ mol NH}_3} = 1.5 \text{ mol H}_2\text{O}$$

Convert mol H_2O to grams H_2O:

$$1.5 \text{ mol H}_2\text{O} \times \frac{18 \text{ g H}_2\text{O}}{1 \text{ mol H}_2\text{O}} = 27 \text{ g H}_2\text{O}$$

19. **(A)** Follow the same method as shown in the explanation to problem 18, except convert from moles NO to liters NO. Remember, 1 mole of any gas at standard temperature and pressure, STP, 0°C and 1 atm, occupies 22.4 liters.

$$\underline{\text{g NH}_3} \rightarrow \underline{\text{moles NH}_3} \rightarrow \underline{\text{moles NO}} \rightarrow \underline{\text{liters NO}}$$

$\underline{\text{g NH}_3}$

17.0 g NH_3

$\underline{\text{moles NH}_3}$

$$\frac{1.70 \text{ g}}{17 \text{ g/mole}} = 0.10 \text{ mole NH}_3$$

$\underline{\text{moles NO}}$

$$0.10 \text{ mole NH}_3 \times \frac{4 \text{ moles NO}}{4 \text{ moles NH}_3} = 0.10 \text{ mole NO}$$

$\underline{\text{liters NO}}$

$$0.10 \text{ mole NO} \times \frac{22.4 \text{ liters NO}}{1 \text{ mole NO}} = 2.24 \text{ liters NO}$$

20. **(A)** Follow the same method as shown in the explanations to problems 18 and 19, except convert from moles NO to molecules NO. Remember, 1 mole of any substance contains 6×10^{23} particles.

$$\underline{\text{g NH}_3} \rightarrow \underline{\text{moles NH}_3} \rightarrow \underline{\text{moles NO}} \rightarrow \underline{\text{molecules NO}}$$

$\underline{\text{g NH}_3}$

0.17 g NH_3

$\underline{\text{moles NH}_3}$

$$\frac{0.17 \text{ g NH}_3}{17 \text{ g/mole}} = 0.01 \text{ mole NH}_3$$

$\underline{\text{moles NO}}$

$$0.01 \text{ mole NH}_3 \times \frac{4 \text{ moles NO}}{4 \text{ moles NH}_3} = 0.01 \text{ mole NO}$$

$\underline{\text{molecules NO}}$

$$0.01 \text{ mole NO} \times \frac{6 \times 10^{23} \text{ molecules NO}}{1 \text{ mole NO}} = 6 \times 10^{21} \text{ molecules NO}$$

21. **(D)** The equation used to solve the problem is

$$PV = nRT$$

The symbol P is pressure in atmospheres, V is volume in liters, n is number of moles, which equals grams/molar mass, R is the gas constant, and T is temperature in Kelvin. Because the oxygen is collected over water, both water and oxygen contribute to the pressure of the gas. The contribution of water, 23.76 mm, must be subtracted from the total pressure, 750 mm, in order to determine the pressure contributed by the oxygen, 726.24 mm. Pressure must be converted to atmospheres, volume converted to liters, and temperature converted to Kelvin. In addition, oxygen is a diatomic gas and, consequently, its molar mass is 32 amu.

22. **(A)** Molarity is defined as moles of solute divided by liters of solution.

$$M = \frac{\text{moles of solute}}{\text{liters of solution}} = \frac{\text{g/mol. wt.}}{\text{liters of solution}}$$

Sugar, $C_6H_{12}O_6$, has a molecular weight of 180 g/mole. Substitute 1.8 g, 180 g/mole, and 1.0 L into the above equation to obtain the molarity of the solution.

$$M = \frac{1.8 \text{ g}/180 \text{ g}/\text{mole}}{1.0 \text{ L}} = 0.01 \frac{\text{mole}}{\text{liter}} = 0.01M$$

23. **(C)** The ideal gas law, PV = nRT, or

$$PV = \frac{\# \text{g}}{\text{mol. wt.}}(RT)$$

is used to solve this problem. Pressure is used in atmospheres, volume in liters, and temperature in Kelvin. Moles of gas is represented by n, which equals grams divided by molecular weight. The molar mass of nitrogen is 28 grams/mole since nitrogen is a diatomic molecule, N_2. Substituting the given data into the above formula gives:

$$1 \text{ atm}\left(1.0 \text{ liter}\right) = \frac{x}{28 \text{ grams/mole}}\left(0.082\frac{\text{L-atm}}{\text{K-mole}}\right)(273+27) \text{ K}$$

$$x = 1.1 \text{ g}$$

24. **(D)** In a dilution problem, # moles of solute before dilution = # moles of solute after dilution. Therefore

$$\begin{array}{ll}
\text{Molarity} \times \text{volume} & = \text{Molarity} \times \text{volume} \\
\text{(before dilution)} & \text{(after dilution)} \\
2.5 \frac{\text{moles}}{\text{L}} \times 0.2 \text{ L} & = 5.0 \frac{\text{moles}}{\text{L}} \times \text{volume}
\end{array}$$

$$0.100 \text{ L} = \text{volume}$$

To prepare the 2.5 M solution of NaOH, dilute 100 mL of the 5.0 M solution to 200 mL.

25. **(D)** Boiling point is based on molecular weight (how heavy the molecule is) and the strength of the intermolecular forces of attraction that occur between molecules. The heavier the molecule, the more energy will be required to get

it into the gaseous state and the boiling point will increase. The stronger the intermolecular forces of attraction between molecules, the more energy it will take to break these forces and liberate the molecules in the gas form so the higher the boiling point. All of the selections have about the same molecular weight so the determining factor will be the strength of the intermolecular forces possible in a sample of each. Since the molecule in choice (D) has an alcohol functional group that can hydrogen bond (the strongest of all the available intermolecular forces) with other alcohol functional groups on nearby molecules, it will have the highest boiling point. Remember that in order for a molecule to be capable of hydrogen bonding, it must have a hydrogen atom covalently attached to a small electronegative element (N, O, halogen)—so the molecule in choice (D) is the only one capable of hydrogen bonding.

26. **(B)** Neutralization is the reaction of acid plus base to produce salt plus water.

$$2LiOH + H_2SO_4 \rightarrow Li_2SO_4 + 2H_2O$$

The balanced equation shows that twice as many moles of LiOH are needed to completely react with H_2SO_4. Given the volume and molarity of the sulfuric acid, 10 mL of 3 M H_2SO_4, calculate the number of moles of sulfuric acid.

$$M = \frac{\text{\# moles}}{\text{\# liters}} \qquad 3M = \frac{\text{\#moles}}{0.01\ L} \qquad \text{\# moles } H_2SO_4 = 0.03$$

Multiply the moles of acid by 2 (factor-label method from balanced equation) to determine the number of moles of lithium hydroxide.

$$0.03 \text{ mole } H_2SO_4 \times \frac{2 \text{ moles LiOH}}{1 \text{ mole } H_2SO_4} = 0.06 \text{ mole LiOH}$$

Finally, determine the volume of lithium hydroxide necessary to contain that number of moles of 2 M lithium hydroxide.

$$M = \frac{\text{\#moles}}{\text{\#liters}} \qquad 2M = \frac{0.06 \text{ mole}}{\text{\#liters}} \qquad \text{\#liters LiOH} = 0.03 \ (30 \text{ mL})$$

27. **(B)** The bubble at the bottom of the lake has a volume of 1.4 mL at $(7 + 273)K$ and 2.0 atm pressure. To determine the volume of the bubble at the surface of the lake at $(27 + 273)K$ and 1.0 atm pressure, use the equation shown below.

$$\frac{P_1V_1}{T_1} = \frac{P_2V_2}{T_2} = \frac{2.0 \text{ atm } (1.4 \text{ mL})}{280 \text{ K}} = \frac{1 \text{ atm } V_2}{300 \text{ K}} \qquad V_2 = 3.0 \text{ mL}$$

Since pressure and volume are present on both sides of the equation, any pressure or volume term (atm, psi, mL, liters, etc.) can be used as long as the term is the same on both sides of the equation. The pressure units cancel, and the volume term is part of the answer.

Also, one can predict that the volume of the gas bubble will increase since, as temperature rises, volume increases, and as pressure decreases, volume increases.

28. **(B)** This problem involves calculating the number of liters of NO produced at STP, 0°C, and 1.0 atm, and converting that volume to the new volume at 27°C and 2.0 atm.

$$4 \, NH_3 \, (g) + 5 \, O_2 \, (g) \rightarrow 4 \, NO \, (g) + 6 \, H_2O \, (g)$$

$$\underline{g \, NH_3} \rightarrow \underline{moles \, NH_3} \rightarrow \underline{moles \, NO} \rightarrow \underline{liters \, NO \, at \, STP}$$

$$1.7 \qquad \frac{1.7}{17} = 0.10 \qquad \frac{0.10(4)}{4} = 0.10 \qquad 0.10(22.4) = 2.2 \, L$$

After finding the volume at STP, convert this volume to the volume at 2.0 atm and (27 + 273)K.

$$\frac{P_1 V_1}{T_1} = \frac{P_2 V_2}{T_2} = \frac{1.0 \, atm \, (2.2 \, L)}{(0+273) \, K} = \frac{2.0 \, atm \, V_2}{(27+273) \, K}$$

$$V_2 = 1.2 \, L \, at \, 27°C \, and \, 2.0 \, atm$$

An alternative solution involves use of the ideal gas law equation, $PV = nRT$.

$$(2.0 \, atm)V = \frac{1.7 \, g}{17 \, g/mole}\left(0.082 \frac{L\text{-}atm}{K\text{-}mole}\right)(27 + 273) \, K$$

$$V = 1.2 \, liters \, at \, 27°C \, and \, 2.0 \, atm$$

29. **(D)** In glycolysis, one glucose molecule (6 carbons) is converted to two pyruvic acid molecules (3 carbons each). The pyruvic acid molecules are then converted to acetyl coenzyme A molecules that enter the citric acid cycle for oxidation. Gluconeogenesis is the synthesis of glucose from noncarbohydrate precursors. Oxidative phosphorylation is the oxidation of reduced cofactors (NADH, $FADH_2$) from glycolysis and the citric acid cycle coupled to the phosphorylation of ADP to ATP.

30. **(B)** To determine absolute configuration of a chiral center (a carbon with four different groups attached to it), prioritize the four groups according to atomic number. Place the fourth priority group pointed away from you and look at the priorities of the other three groups. If their priority of 1, 2, 3 is arranged clockwise, the chiral center is designated as R and if counterclockwise, S. In this molecule, there is only one chiral center and the chlorine will be priority 1, the isopropyl group will be priority 2, the methyl will be priority 3, and the hydrogen will be priority 4. Directing the hydrogen away from you places the other three groups in a counterclockwise priority order. Note: Since the iso-propyl and the methyl groups begin with a carbon, determining their priorities requires a look at the atoms the first carbon of each group is attached to. In the case of the isopropyl group, the first carbon of that group is attached to a hydrogen and two carbons, whereas the first carbon in the methyl group is attached to three hydrogens. Because the isopropyl carbon is attached to carbons that have a higher atomic number than the hydrogens of the methyl group, the isopropyl group has a higher priority than the methyl group.

31. **(C)** The heat capacity, C, of a substance equals the specific heat, s, times the mass of the material, m.

$$C = ms$$

$$C = 10.0 \text{ g} \left(0.385 \frac{J}{g°C} \right) = 3.85 \text{ J/°C}$$

32. **(D)** See the answer to question 4. Genes are composed of DNA.

33. **(C)** When naming alkenes, find the longest carbon chain that includes the double bond. In this case, it's 6 carbons with the double bond at carbon 2, so immediately you know that either (C) or (D) is correct. To assign E or Z to the double bond, prioritize the two groups at each end of the double bond according to atomic number (as described in question 30). If the alkene has both its priority 1 groups on the same side of the double bond, it is designated as a Z alkene as is the case with this molecule. If the two priority 1 groups are on opposite sides of the double bond, it is designated E.

34. **(C)** To balance nuclear equations, the mass numbers on each side of the equation must be equal and the atomic numbers on each side of the equation must be equal. For the given equation, the atomic number of the element produced would have to be 89, meaning the element's symbol would be the one right of Ra in the periodic table.

35. **(A)** The correct electron configuration for the sulfide ion, S^{2-}, is $1s^2 2s^2 2p^6 3s^2 3p^6$. The letters s, p, d, and f indicate the type of orbital. The number in front of the symbols, as in 1s, indicates the number of the orbital, in this case 1. The superscript, as in $1s^2$, indicates the number of electrons present in the orbital, in this case 2. The electron configuration for the sulfur atom, S, which is $1s^2 2s^2 2p^6 3s^2 3p^4$, shows the 16 electrons present in the atom. The sulfur ion, S^{2-}, has two more electrons in the p orbital: $1s^2 2s^2 2p^6 3s^2 3p^6$.

36. **(C)** See question 11. The two most common examples of secondary structure are alpha helices and beta (pleated) sheets. A tetramer would be an example of quaternary structure, and peptide bonds are what connect amino acids so they are involved in the primary structure. A double helix refers to the arrangement of DNA molecules (which aren't proteins).

37. **(B)** The correct specie is in the third row and the second box in the p block. Si^{2-} would have the same valence shell electron configuration as sulfur and Mg^{2+} would have the same valence shell electron configuration as neon.

38. **(C)** Draw the Lewis structure of the molecule by adding up the valence electrons for the atoms in the formula. Phosphorus has 5 and each chlorine has 7. That's a total of 40 valence electrons to distribute. Place the phosphorus in the center and arrange the chlorines symmetrically around it using a pair of electrons to attach each chlorine atom to the central phosphorus. Now, complete the octet for each chlorine by adding 6 unshared electrons on each. That uses up all of the valence electrons so there are no unshared electrons on the phosphorus atom.

39. **(A)** The formal charge on a bonded atom equals the number of valence electrons in the nonbonded atom minus the number of nonbonded electrons in the bonded atom minus one-half the number of bonding electrons in the bonded atom.

The number of valence electrons in the nonbonded atom (Lewis dot formula) $\quad\quad\quad .\overset{.}{C}. = 4$

The number of nonbonded electrons in the bonded atom (Lewis dot structure) $\quad\quad =\overset{|}{C}- \quad\quad = 0$

One-half the number of bonding electrons in the bonded atom $\quad\quad =\overset{|}{C}- \quad\quad \frac{1}{2}(8) = 4$

The formal charge on a bonded atom $\quad\quad\quad\quad 4 - 0 - 4 = 0$

40. **(B)** The farther two elements are from each other in the periodic table, one being a metal and the other a nonmetal, the more ionic the bond between them. Consequently, of the compounds listed, Li_2O has the most ionic bond.

For the other compounds, CO_2, CH_4, and NH_3, the bonding is covalent because the atoms are close to each other and the compounds are nonmetals. Although hydrogen, H, may be located a distance from carbon, C, and from nitrogen, N, this element is an anomaly and has unique properties.

41. **(C)** The molecular geometry of SiH_4, like that of CH_4, is tetrahedral. Carbon is above silicon in the periodic table; consequently, if the same number of bonds is formed by the 4 hydrogen atoms to the central atom, Si or C, the geometry of the molecule is the same. If there are 2 bonding electron pairs around the central atom, as in BeF_2, the molecule is linear. If there are 3 bonding electron pairs around the central atom, as in BF_3, the molecule is trigonal planar. With 4 bonding electron pairs, as in SiH_4 or CH_4, the molecule is tetrahedral. In the molecule NH_3, there are 4 electron pairs but 1 is a nonbonding pair (only 3 hydrogen atoms), and the molecule is described as being a trigonal pyramid. In H_2O, there are 4 electron pairs but only 2 pairs participate in bonding to the 2 hydrogen atoms, and the molecule is bent.

42. **(A)** The molecule H_2S has the same geometry as does H_2O, which is bent. Sulfur, S, is under oxygen, O, in the periodic table and has the same number of atoms bonded to it, two hydrogens in each case. A bent molecule has a bond angle of about 105°, a trigonal pyramid an angle of 107°, a tetrahedron an angle of 109°, a trigonal planar molecule an angle of 120°, and a linear molecule an angle of 180°.

43. **(B)** The molecule $AlCl_3$, a trigonal planar molecule, has sp^2 hybridization. The linear molecule BeF_2 is sp hybridized. The tetrahedral CH_4, as well as the trigonal pyramid, NH_3, and the bent molecule, H_2O, are all sp^3 hybridized.

44. **(B)** Protein synthesis (translation) involves the covalent connection of amino acids associated with the cellular structure called the ribosome. Several types of RNA are involved in the process: mRNA (messenger RNA) provides the "instructions" for the amino acid sequence, rRNA (ribosomal RNA) is part of

the ribosome structure, and tRNA (transfer RNA) brings the appropriate amino acids to the ribosome for incorporation into the growing protein.

45. **(B)** See explanation for question 29.

46. **(C)** These reagents represent hydroboration-oxidation, which is a method of hydrating an alkene (adding the components of water across the double bond). It occurs with anti-Markovnikov regiochemistry (meaning the H goes on the more highly substituted carbon of the alkene and the OH goes on the less highly substituted carbon of the alkene) and with syn stereochemistry (meaning the new H and OH add to the ring from the same side and will therefore be cis to each other). The other method of hydration of alkenes, oxymercuration-demercuration, occurs with Markovnikov regiochemistry and anti-stereochemistry.

47. **(A)** The dipole moment is a measure of the polarity of a molecule, that is, one part of the molecule is partially positive and one part partially negative. The greater the dipole moment, the more polar a molecule is. Carbon dioxide, CO_2, has a dipole moment of zero because the molecule is linear with carbon in the middle and one oxygen atom on either side of the carbon. Although each individual C – O bond is polar, the two bonds balance each other to produce a nonpolar molecule.

   H_2O, HF, and NH_3 are all polar molecules. The water molecule is bent with the electrons being drawn toward the oxygen. The hydrogen fluoride molecule is linear, but the H – F bond is polar with the electrons drawn toward the fluorine. The ammonia molecule is trigonal pyramidal with the electrons drawn toward the nitrogen.

48. **(B)** Replication is the process whereby DNA is duplicated. The DNA duplex unwinds to expose its nucleotide sequence and new DNA molecules are synthesized complementary to each of the exposed DNA molecules resulting in two molecules of DNA having identical nucleotide sequences. Since the involved synthetic enzymes (DNA polymerases) can synthesize new DNA in only one direction and since the two DNA molecules composing the original duplex are antiparallel to each other, only one of the new DNA molecules can be synthesized continuously (without interruption). The other new DNA molecule is synthesized in pieces (called Okazaki fragments) or discontinuously.

49. **(C)** The allowed values for the quantum numbers of electrons are: n may be any whole number; 1 may be from zero up to n–1; m_ℓ may be from negative ℓ through zero to positive ℓ; and m_s may be either –½ or +½. Answer C is the only set containing four allowed values.

50. **(B)** The conversion of an aldehyde to an alcohol is a reduction. Hydride donors like $NaBH_4$ and $LiAlH_4$ are used to perform this reduction. H_2 is used to reduce alkenes and alkynes. PCC and $KMnO_4$ are both oxidizing agents.

51. **(C)** Bromine with $FeBr_3$ is used to accomplish electrophilic aromatic substitution on arene rings. A bromine atom will substitute for a hydrogen on the

ring. The ring already has an amino group on it and an amino group is an ortho,para director (and also an activator by electron donation through resonance) so choice (C) is correct.

52. **(A)** Transcription is the synthesis of RNA, translation is the synthesis of protein, replication is the synthesis of DNA, and respiration is the oxidation of molecules for energy production.

53. **(B)** The first three options are lipids. Triglycerides are the lipids found in adipose tissue and waxes are used to coat fruits or animal hair. Starch is not a lipid; it is a carbohydrate.

54. **(C)** See question 44.

55. **(B)** In a first-order reaction, the half-life, that is, the length of time for one-half of the concentration to be reacted, is dependent only on the rate constant, not on the original concentration. If the rate constant, k, is 6.93×10^2 / sec, the length of time needed for one-half of the starting material to be reacted is

$$4t_{1/2} = \frac{0.693}{k}$$

$$t_{1/2} = \frac{0.693}{6.93 \times 10^2 \text{ / sec}} = 1.0 \times 10^{-3} \text{ sec}$$

56. **(A)** When an alcohol reacts with an acid halide, an ester results through nucleophilic acyl substitution. All acid derivatives (acid halides, anhydrides, esters, and amides) undergo this type of reaction. In questions like this using condensed formulas, it is always a good idea to draw the line-bond structure before selecting an answer so that you can see clearly what types of functional groups are present (they are sometimes hard to see in a condensed structure).

57. **(B)** When potassium permanganate is added to an alkene or an alkyne, oxidative cleavage occurs. In the case of alkenes, the double bond is cut and each carbon of the double bond becomes doubly bonded to an oxygen atom. If any products are aldehydes, then they are further oxidized to carboxylic acids and if any resulting carboxylic acids are one-carbon acids, they are further oxidized to carbon dioxide. For alkynes, oxidative cleavage cuts the triple bond and both carbons of the triple bond become carboxylic acid groups. Again, if any one-carbon acids are formed, they are further oxidized to carbon dioxide.

58. **(A)** An equilibrium constant may be written for the following reaction. An equilibrium constant is equal to the product of the products divided by the product of the reactants, each raised to the power as indicated in the balanced equation.

$$H_2 + I_2 \leftrightarrow 2\,HI \qquad K = \frac{[HI]^2}{[I_2][H_2]} \qquad K = \frac{(0.5)^2}{(0.25)(0.25)} = 4$$

59. **(A)** According to Le Châtelier's Principle, any stress applied to a system in equilibrium will cause the equilibrium to shift so as to relieve the stress. For example, in the given system:

$$\text{Heat} + N_2O_4 \text{ (g)} \leftrightarrow 2NO_2 \text{ (g)}$$

think of heat as one of the reactants. An increase in any reactant concentration on the left will cause the equilibrium to shift to the right, to the products. An increase in the product concentration on the right will cause the equilibrium to shift left, to the reactants. A decrease in any reactant concentration will cause the equilibrium to shift to the left. A decrease in any product concentration will cause the equilibrium to shift to the right. Therefore, a decrease in temperature or heat will cause the reaction to shift to the left, NOT to the right.

An increase in the concentration of N_2O_4, a decrease in the concentration of NO_2, and an increase in temperature will all cause the equilibrium to shift to the right.

60. **(C)** The conversion of a carboxylic acid to an alcohol is a reduction. Hydride-reducing agents are used to reduce carboxylic acids but $NaBH_4$ (a hydride reducing agent) is a mild hydride donor and is not powerful enough to reduce an acid. See question 50.

61. **(B)** Potassium t-butoxide is a strong base and is used to perform an E2 elimination by causing the removal of HI on this alkyl halide, creating an alkene. The most stable alkene will predominate. Remember, trans alkenes are more stable than cis alkenes, and more highly substituted alkenes are more stable than less highly substituted ones.

62. **(D)** When aldehydes and ketones condense in the presence of a base and either a beta-hydroxy carbonyl compound or an alpha beta-unsaturated carbonyl compound (as in this case) results, an aldol condensation has occurred. A Claisen condensation involves an ester, a Williamson is used to make an ether, and a Michael is the reaction between an enolate and an alpha beta-unsaturated carbonyl compound.

63. **(A)** Proteins and peptides are polymers of amino acids joined by amide bonds (called peptide bonds).

64. **(B)** Resonance structures have the same atom connections but different placements of pi and unshared electrons. Only choice (B) has all of the atoms in the same place.

65. **(C)** The acidity of a solution can be measured by determining the pH or the pOH.

$$\text{pH} = -\log [H^+] \qquad \text{pOH} = -\log [OH^-]$$

The pH and pOH values are related by the following equations:

$$\text{pH} + \text{pOH} = 14 \text{ and } [H^+][OH^-] = 10^{-14}$$

Calculating the pH when the $[OH^-] = 0.01$ M gives

$$\text{pOH} = -\log [OH^-] = -\log (10^{-2}) = -(-2) = 2$$

$$\text{pH} + 2 = 14$$

$$\text{pH} = 12$$

66. **(C)** The DNA helix is composed of two molecules of DNA (strands) that are intertwined and held together by hydrogen bonding between the purine and pyrimidine bases of each strand. This type of hydrogen bonding is called base-pairing.

67. **(C)** The most important infrared (IR) absorptions are around 3000 cm^{-1} for O-H or N-H, around 2100 cm^{-1} for triple bonds, and around 1600–1700 cm^{-1} for double bonds. The only functional group that would have bands at both 3300 and 1700 is the acid.

68. **(B)** Triglycerides are lipids stored in adipose tissue. They are triesters of glycerol with three fatty acids (long-chain carboxylic acids). Basic hydrolysis of triglycerides (i.e., reaction with water and base, also called saponification) yields glycerol and three molecules of deprotonated fatty acid (also called soap). These fatty acids can be liberated from adipose tissue for beta-oxidation that results in the production of ATP.

69. **(A)** Since ammonia is a weak base, the equilibrium would lie to the left for the deprotonation of water. In this reaction, water is acting as an acid. Ammonium is the conjugate acid of ammonia and hydroxide is the conjugate base of water.

70. **(C)** Magnesium hydroxide, $Mg(OH)_2$, is a strong base. Strong bases ionize completely.

$$Mg(OH)_2 \rightarrow Mg^{2+} + 2OH^-$$

From the balanced equation above, we see that, for every 1 mole of magnesium hydroxide, 2 moles of hydroxide ion are formed. If the concentration of magnesium hydroxide is 2.5 M, or 2.5 moles/L, then the concentration of the hydroxide ion, $[OH^-]$, is 2×2.5 M = 5.0 M, that is, 5.0 moles/L.

Strong acids also ionize completely and their concentrations are calculated in the same manner as shown above for $Mg(OH)_2$. A balanced equation for hydrochloric acid, HCl, is shown below.

$$HCl \rightarrow H^+ + Cl^-$$

71. **(C)** ^{1}H NMR gives information about the hydrogens in a molecule. Since there are five signals, there are five kinds of hydrogen in the molecule. Choice (A) can be excluded since the molecule has only four kinds of hydrogen and choice (D) can be excluded since the molecule has seven kinds of hydrogen. After comparing the number of signals in the spectrum to the number of different kinds of hydrogen in the molecule, look at the splitting pattern and integration information. Simple splitting patterns follow the n + 1 rule meaning that the splitting pattern for a group of hydrogens will be equal to the number of neighboring hydrogens (those on an adjacent carbon) plus one. For example, a triplet indicates that the hydrogens represented by that signal have two neighboring hydrogens, and a quartet indicates that the hydrogens represented by that signal have three neighboring hydrogens. Since the data include a triplet that integrates for 3H and a quartet that integrates for 2H, there must be an ethyl group, meaning choice (C) is the answer.

72. **(C)** Beta oxidation refers to the series of reactions that results in the oxidation of the carbons of fatty acids resulting in ATP synthesis (through oxidative phosphorylation). Polysaccharides (after conversion to monosaccharides) are oxidized through glycolysis followed by the citric acid cycle resulting in ATP synthesis.

73. **(A)** The constant K_B may be defined for the Y^{-1} ion, a base. The base, Y^{-1}, reacts with water, which is the acid, and an equilibrium expression for a base can be written.

$$Y^{-1} + H_2O \leftrightarrow HY + OH^{-1} \qquad K_B = \frac{[HY][OH^{-1}]}{[Y^{-1}]}$$

Since water is present in large excess in a dilute solution, its concentration does not change significantly, and therefore its concentration is included in the constant K_B.

The relationship that exists between K_A and K_B is as follows:

$$(K_A)(K_B) = K_w = 1 \times 10^{-14}$$

where K_w is the ionization constant for water.

Substituting the given K_A value for HY, 5×10^{-5}, into the above equation gives a value of 2×10^{-10} for K_B.

74. **(B)** The larger the value of the equilibrium constant, K_A, the greater the amount of products, the greater the amount of ionization of the acid (or base), or the stronger the acid (or base). See the equation below for acetic acid, a weak acid.

$$HAc \leftrightarrow H^+ + Ac^- \qquad K_A = \frac{[H^+][Ac^-]}{[HAc]}$$

Of the acids listed, nitrous acid (HNO_2) has the largest ionization constant and is the strongest acid. Conversely, the smaller the equilibrium constant, the weaker the acid (or base).

75. **(A)** When a Grignard reagent reacts with an ester, a tertiary alcohol results. The Grignard reagent first attacks the ester converting it into a ketone by nucleophilic acyl substitution (see question 56) but a second Grignard reagent attacks the ketone carbonyl resulting in an alcohol after protonation.

76. **(D)** Calcium carbonate, $CaCO_3$ (marble), is insoluble in water. The other compounds—NaOH, NH_4Cl, and $LiNO_3$—are all water soluble. The solubility rules include the following:

All salts formed with the alkali metals, for example, any member of the lithium family, are soluble.

All ammonium salts (NH_4^+) and all nitrate salts (NO_3^-) are soluble.

Many chlorides (Cl^-), bromides (Br^-), and iodides (I^-) are soluble.

Many sulfates (SO_4^{2-}) are soluble.

77. **(A)** One source of amino acids for protein synthesis is cellular biosynthesis (the other source is dietary protein).

78. **(C)** The larger the value of K_{sp}, the more silver and chloride ions are present in solution and hence the more soluble the salt. Of the salts listed, silver chloride is the most soluble.

79. **(C)** The formation constant for the formation of a complex ion, K_f, may be defined for the silver ammonia complex, $Ag(NH_3)_2^{+1}$, as shown below.

$$Ag^{+1} + 2NH_3 \leftrightarrow Ag(NH_3)_2^{+1} \qquad K_f = \frac{\left[Ag(NH_3)_2^{+1}\right]}{\left[Ag^{+1}\right]\left[NH_3\right]^2}$$

The concentration of each of the species in the equation is raised to the power shown in the balanced equation. As can be seen from the equation above, K_f will have a large value when the concentration of the complex ion, $[Ag(NH_3)_2^{+1}]$, is high. When much complex ion is formed the ion must be stable. Hence the largest value for the formation complex, 2.0×10^{30} for HgI_4^{-2}, gives the most stable ion.

80. **(B)** Proteins are polymers of amino acids joined by peptide bonds, a kind of amide bond. The different amino acids differ in a group attached to the alpha carbon (the carbon to which the amine and acid groups are attached)—this group is often called the side chain. The term "essential," when used in reference to amino acids, specifically means amino acids that cannot be biosynthesized and are therefore essential in the diet.

81. **(C)** Aluminum hydroxide, $Al(OH)_3$, dissolves in water to produce aluminum ions, Al^{+3}, and hydroxide ions, OH^{-1}.

$$Al(OH)_3 \text{ (s)} \leftrightarrow Al^{+3} \text{ (aq)} + 3OH^{-1} \text{ (aq)}$$

An equilibrium exists in solution between undissolved aluminum hydroxide, $Al(OH)_3$ (s), and dissolved aluminum hydroxide, Al^{+3} (aq) + $3OH^{-1}$ (aq).

Dissolving aluminum hydroxide in either **B**, 0.5 M $Al(NO_3)$, or **C**, 1.6 M NaOH, will decrease its solubility relative to its solubility in water. Since aluminum nitrate, $Al(NO_3)$, is a soluble salt, the concentration of the aluminum ion, Al^{+3}, will be 0.5 M (0.5 mole/ liter) in a solution of 0.5 M $Al(NO_3)_3$.

$$Al(NO_3)_3 \text{ (s)} \quad \rightarrow \quad Al^{+3} \text{ (aq)} \quad + \quad 3NO_3^{-1} \text{ (aq)}$$

$$\frac{0.5 \text{ mole}}{\text{liter}} \qquad \frac{0.5 \text{ mole}}{\text{liter}} \qquad \frac{3(0.5 \text{ mole})}{\text{liter}}$$

In the same way, the concentration of the hydroxide ion, OH^{-1}, in a solution of 1.6 M sodium hydroxide, NaOH (s), a soluble base, will be 1.6 M.

$$NaOH \text{ (s)} \quad \rightarrow \quad Na^{+1} \text{ (aq)} \quad + \quad OH^{-1} \text{ (aq)}$$

$$\frac{1.6 \text{ moles}}{\text{liter}} \qquad \frac{1.6 \text{ moles}}{\text{liter}} \qquad \frac{1.6 \text{ moles}}{\text{liter}}$$

Both the aluminum and hydroxide ions result in solution from dissolving solid aluminum hydroxide in water. According to LeChâtelier's Principle, increasing the concentration of either ion on the right side of the equation will shift the equilibrium to the left and decrease the solubility of $Al(OH)_3$ (s). Therefore, the presence of aluminum ions in the aluminum nitrate solution and the presence of hydroxide ions in the sodium hydroxide solution decrease the solubility of aluminum hydroxide in either of these solutions. The concentration of hydroxide in the sodium hydroxide solution is 1.6 M which is larger than the concentration of the aluminum ion, 0.5 M, in the aluminum nitrate solution. The 1.6 M sodium hydroxide solution will decrease the solubility of aluminum hydroxide more than the 0.5 M aluminum nitrate solution will.

Adding solid aluminum hydroxide to the 0.3 M hydrochloric acid, HCl, will increase the solubility of the aluminum hydroxide relative to its solubility in water, since the hydroxide ion concentration would be reduced by reacting with the hydrogen ion, H^{+1}, of the hydrochloric acid, HCl, and the equilibrium would shift to the right. More aluminum hydroxide would dissolve.

82. **(A)** Lipids are nonpolar molecules meaning they have lots of carbon-hydrogen bonds (which are nonpolar) and very few, if any, polar bonds (like carbon-oxygen, nitrogen-hydrogen, or oxygen-hydrogen bonds).

83. **(C)** Oxidation is the loss of electrons; reduction is the gain of electrons. The oxidizing agent is the material reduced, and the reducing agent is the material oxidized.

    In the given reaction between zinc and the ion Cu^{2+}:

    $$Zn + Cu^{2+} \rightarrow Zn^{2+} + Cu$$

    Zn is oxidized because it has lost electrons to form Zn^{2+} as in answer C, and consequently is the reducing agent. The ion Cu^{2+} has gained electrons to form copper, Cu, and is the oxidizing agent.

84. **(D)** Refer to the answer given to question 83. The reducing agent is the species that loses electrons, Li or Br^{-1}. The equation with the more negative value for emf^0 indicates the species with the greater tendency to lose electrons, Li. The equation with the more positive value indicates the species with the greater tendency to gain the electrons, Br_2.

85. **(D)** An electrochemical cell is made up of two electrodes connected in solution and by wires. One of the chemical species in solution loses electrons, the process of oxidation, to an electrode, the anode. Oxidation occurs at the anode. The electrons travel from the anode, through the wire, to the cathode where another species in solution gains the electrons, the process of reduction, supplied by the cathode. Reduction occurs at the cathode.

86. **(D)** An oxidation results in a net loss of electron density. Oxidation numbers can be used to "follow" electrons. For organic compounds, assign each carbon an oxidation number by giving a +1 for each bond to hydrogen and a –1 for each bond to an element more electronegative than carbon (i.e., O, N, halogens). So, in answer A, the reactant has 2 carbons. One carbon has an oxidation number of –3; the other has an oxidation number of –1 for a total of –4. The product also has 2 carbons and each has an oxidation number of –2 for

a total of −4. Neither an oxidation nor a reduction has occurred. (If the oxidation number goes up, an oxidation has occurred; if the oxidation number goes down, a reduction has occurred.) In answer D, the reactant has an oxidation number of −4 and the product has an oxidation number of −2, which represents an increase (−4 is smaller than −2), so an oxidation has occurred.

87. **(D)** 1,3-diaxial energy is a function of steric bulk: The bigger the group, the greater the steric energy.

88. **(B)** The formula, C_3H_6, is one for either an alkene or a cycloalkane, both of which are unsaturated. The formula C_2H_6 represents an alkane; the formula C_2H_6O represents a fully saturated compound and could be dimethyl ether or ethyl alcohol; the formula CH_3Cl represents an alkyl halide, methyl chloride.

89. **(D)** Four different structural isomers can be formed by C_4H_9Cl.

$CH_3 - CH_2 - CH_2 - CH_2 - Cl$	1-chlorobutane
$CH_3 - CH_2 - CHCl - CH_3$	2-chlorobutane
$(CH_3)_2 - CH - CH_2Cl$	1-chloro-2-methylpropane
$(CH_3)_3 - C - Cl$	2-chloro-2-methylpropane

90. **(C)** Draw pentane and then draw it again substituting a chlorine atom for one of the hydrogens. Now draw it again substituting a different hydrogen with a chlorine atom. See how many different compounds can be drawn by this method. If in doubt about whether a structure you've drawn is different from a previous one, name your structures. If they have the same name, they are the same compound. The three compounds that can be formed from this monochlorination are 1-chloropentane, 2-chloropentane, and 3-chloropentane (4-chloropentane is actually 2-chloropentane, and 5-chloropentane is actually 1-chloropentane).

91. **(A)** Pick the longest straight chain for the base name of the alkane, in this case octane. Next, name each of the substituents, two methyl groups and one bromo group. Give each substituent the lowest possible number and arrange the substituents in alphabetical order. The name is 5-bromo-3,4-dimethyloctane.

    The base names are listed below for the straight-chain alkanes with the general formula C_nH_{2n+2}. The names of compounds in other families can be derived from these names by using the proper suffix.

1 Carbon	methane
2 Carbons	ethane
3 Carbons	propane
4 Carbons	butane
5 Carbons	pentane
6 Carbons	hexane
7 Carbons	heptane
8 Carbons	octane
9 Carbons	nonane
10 Carbons	decane

92. **(C)** A stereocenter is an atom to which four different groups are attached. The different groups may be atoms such as the chlorine atom, Cl, or the bromine atom, Br, or they may be groups of atoms such as the methyl group, CH_3, or the ethyl group, CH_3CH_2. The underlined C in the following molecule, 2-bromo-2-chlorobutane, is a stereocenter.

$$
\begin{array}{c}
CH_3 \\
| \\
Cl - \underline{C} - CH_2 - CH_3 \\
| \\
Br
\end{array}
$$

93. **(D)** The two molecules pictured in question 93 have carbon-carbon double bonds. It is not possible to freely rotate around a carbon-carbon double bond as it is around a carbon-carbon single bond. Therefore, when a carbon-carbon double bond is present in a compound, two different compounds, geometric isomers, exist. In the example shown in question 93, the two chlorine atoms are on the same side of the double bond in one compound and on opposite sides of the double bond in the other compound. One could just as easily compare the positions of the two methyl groups relative to the carbon-carbon double bond and arrive at the same conclusion.

Racemic mixture – Refer to the explanation for question 100.

Enantiomers are a form of stereoisomers, i.e., compounds which have the same atom connections but different spatial (3D) arrangements. Enantiomers are two compounds having the same four different groups bonded to the stereocenter in each compound, but because of the different positions in which these groups are placed relative to each other, i.e., because of different configurations, they are nonsuperimposable mirror images. Enantiomers are identical in almost all their physical and chemical properties. The Fischer projections of enantiomers of 1-chloro-1-iodoethane are shown below.

$$
\begin{array}{c}
CH_3 \\
| \\
H - C - Cl \\
| \\
I
\end{array}
\qquad\qquad
\begin{array}{c}
CH_3 \\
| \\
Cl - C - H \\
| \\
I
\end{array}
$$

Diastereomers are also a form of stereoisomers. They are stereoisomers which are not enantiomers. Diastereomers are two compounds, each having at least two different stereocenters or E/Z isomers of alkenes (refer to explanation for question 33). The diastereomers have the arrangement of the four different groups at one of the stereocenters identical in both molecules but the arrangement of another four different groups at the other stereocenter different in both compounds. In other words, diastereomers with two stereocenters have the same configuration at one of the stereocenters but opposite configurations at the other stereocenter. Diastereomers are nonsuperimposable and have different physical and chemical properties. The Fischer projections of one pair of diastereoisomers of 2-bromo-3-chlorobutane are shown below.

94. **(C)** Refer to the explanation for question 43.

95. **(B)** The carbon atom in ethylene has four pairs of electrons around it.

Based upon the explanation given to questions 41, 42, and 43, one might expect the hybridization to be sp^3. However, when a multiple bond such as the carbon-carbon double bond in ethylene is present, the multiple bond is considered as one set of electrons for the purpose of determining hybridization. The carbon atom is considered to have three sets of electrons around it and consequently has sp^2 hybridization.

96. **(B)** Oxidation may be defined as the loss of hydrogen. Oxidation of the secondary alcohol results in the loss of the two underlined hydrogen atoms, one bonded to the carbon atom and one bonded to the oxygen atom. A double bond forms between the two atoms which lost the hydrogen atoms. The product is a ketone.

97. **(A)** Water-soluble compounds are substances whose structures are most like the structure of water. An ether, alkyl chloride, alkane, and benzene are given as possible answers. Ethyl ether or diethyl ether contains an oxygen atom, as does water. The hydrogen atoms in water are capable of hydrogen bonding to the oxygen atom in the ether, just as they can hydrogen bond to other water molecules.

Of the compounds listed, ether is not only the most soluble in water; it is the only one that is slightly soluble. The other functional groups are totally water insoluble.

98. **(B)** A Grignard reagent reacts with an aldehyde to produce, upon subsequent workup with water, a secondary alcohol. The reaction consists of addition across the carbon-oxygen double bond, with the alkyl group from the Grig-

nard reagent adding to the carbon atom and hydrogen adding to the oxygen atom. The methyl of the Grignard reagent adds to the carbon atom of the double bond and the hydrogen adds to the oxygen to produce 2-propanol.

$$
\underset{\substack{\text{acetaldehyde}\\\text{or ethanal}}}{CH_3 - \overset{\overset{\textstyle O}{\|}}{C} - H} \quad \xrightarrow[\text{2. H}_2\text{O}]{\text{1. CH}_3\text{MgBr}} \quad \underset{\text{2-propanol}}{CH_3 - \overset{\overset{\textstyle OH}{|}}{\underset{\underset{\textstyle CH_3}{|}}{C}} - H}
$$

99. **(D)** Dehydration of an alcohol yields an alkene. Alkenes are made by elimination reactions. Therefore, answers A and C can be eliminated since those mechanisms are for substitution reactions. E1 involves a carbocation intermediate so would only occur through the more stable tertiary carbocation from a tertiary alcohol.

100. **(D)** Each member of a pair of enantiomers rotates plane polarized light to an equal extent but in opposite directions. If one enantiomer rotates plane polarized light +42°, the other enantiomer of the pair rotates the light −42°. When the two enantiomers are mixed together in equal amounts, the mixture does not rotate plane polarized light and is called a racemic mixture (Answer D). A conformational mixture is a mixture of conformers, i.e., structures that differ from each other only in orientation of groups but that can be converted into each other by rotation around a carbon-carbon single bond. A meso compound is one in which the molecule can be visualized as two parts which are nonsuperimposable mirror images of each other, i.e., a pair of enantiomers in one molecule. Refer to the answer to question 93 for an explanation of diastereomers.

CHAPTER 7

Quantitative Ability Review and Practice

TIPS FOR THE QUANTITATIVE ABILITY SECTION

The quantitative ability section of the PCAT consists of approximately 48 math problems. You will have 45 minutes to complete the quantitative ability section. This section is the one that most students say they are unable to finish. Therefore, it is important that you pace yourself and answer all questions. There are 100 questions in this section to give you sufficient practice.

Currently, the use of calculators during the PCAT is prohibited. Therefore, it is important to brush up on your math skills!

QUANTITATIVE ABILITY REVIEW OUTLINE

I. **Basic mathematic calculations**

II. **Whole numbers and their operations**
   A. Addition of negative and positive integers
   B. Subtraction of negative and positive integers
   C. Multiplication of negative and positive integers
   D. Division of negative and positive integers
   E. Absolute value
   F. Factorial
   G. Order of operations

III. **Fractions**
   A. Adding fractions
   B. Subtracting fractions
   C. Multiplying fractions
   D. Dividing fractions
   E. Comparing fractions: Which is larger or smaller?

IV. Decimals
   A. Adding decimals
   B. Subtracting decimals
   C. Multiplying decimals
   D. Dividing decimals

V. Percentages
   A. Calculating percents
   B. Adding percentages
   C. Subtracting percentages
   D. Multiplying percentages
   E. Dividing percentages
   F. Percent increase and decrease (percent change)
   G. Simple and compound interest

VI. Converting percents, fractions, and decimals
   A. Converting fractions to percents
   B. Converting percents to fractions
   C. Converting fractions to decimals
   D. Converting decimals to fractions
   E. Converting percents to decimals
   F. Converting decimals to percents

VII. Ratios and proportions

VIII. Powers and exponents

IX. Logarithms
   A. Base 10 and natural logarithm
   B. Solving equations with logarithms or exponents
   C. Laws of logarithms
      1. Addition
      2. Subtraction
      3. Multiplication
      4. Division

X. Roots and radicals
   A. Square root
   B. Cube root
   C. Addition of radicals
   D. Subtraction of radicals
   E. Multiplying radicals

XI. Statistics
  A. Mean
  B. Median
  C. Mode
  D. Probability

XII. Basic Algebra
  A. Simplifying variable expressions
  B. Factoring
  C. Slope of a line
  D. Linear equations
  E. Quadratic equations and the discriminant
  F. Rational equations
  G. Logarithmic equations

XIII. Precalculus
  A. Functions and graphs
  B. Domain, range, symmetry
  C. Inverse functions
  D. Linear functions
  E. Quadratic functions
  F. Rational functions and asymptotes
  G. Function composition
  H. Distance formula, Midpoint formula
  I. Circle equations, completing the square
  J. Average rate of change
  K. Graphing via transformations (shifting, stretching, compressing, reflecting)
  I. Piecewise functions

XIV. Calculus
  A. Derivatives of functions
  B. Product Rule, Quotient Rule
  C. Limits
  D. Slope of a tangent line to a curve
  E. Instantaneous rate of change
  F. Integrals of functions
  G. Area under a curve
  H. Inflection points and concavity

XV. Operations concerning the conversion of basic units of measure
  (see Appendix)

XVI. Word-problem solving—analytical reasoning

XVII. Interpretation of graphs and figures

XVIII. Probabilities
A. Venn diagrams and set operations
B. Counting combinations
C. Counting permutations
D. Calculating probabilities of indepedent events

Answer Sheet
QUANTITATIVE ABILITY

1 Ⓐ Ⓑ Ⓒ Ⓓ	26 Ⓐ Ⓑ Ⓒ Ⓓ	51 Ⓐ Ⓑ Ⓒ Ⓓ	76 Ⓐ Ⓑ Ⓒ Ⓓ
2 Ⓐ Ⓑ Ⓒ Ⓓ	27 Ⓐ Ⓑ Ⓒ Ⓓ	52 Ⓐ Ⓑ Ⓒ Ⓓ	77 Ⓐ Ⓑ Ⓒ Ⓓ
3 Ⓐ Ⓑ Ⓒ Ⓓ	28 Ⓐ Ⓑ Ⓒ Ⓓ	53 Ⓐ Ⓑ Ⓒ Ⓓ	78 Ⓐ Ⓑ Ⓒ Ⓓ
4 Ⓐ Ⓑ Ⓒ Ⓓ	29 Ⓐ Ⓑ Ⓒ Ⓓ	54 Ⓐ Ⓑ Ⓒ Ⓓ	79 Ⓐ Ⓑ Ⓒ Ⓓ
5 Ⓐ Ⓑ Ⓒ Ⓓ	30 Ⓐ Ⓑ Ⓒ Ⓓ	55 Ⓐ Ⓑ Ⓒ Ⓓ	80 Ⓐ Ⓑ Ⓒ Ⓓ
6 Ⓐ Ⓑ Ⓒ Ⓓ	31 Ⓐ Ⓑ Ⓒ Ⓓ	56 Ⓐ Ⓑ Ⓒ Ⓓ	81 Ⓐ Ⓑ Ⓒ Ⓓ
7 Ⓐ Ⓑ Ⓒ Ⓓ	32 Ⓐ Ⓑ Ⓒ Ⓓ	57 Ⓐ Ⓑ Ⓒ Ⓓ	82 Ⓐ Ⓑ Ⓒ Ⓓ
8 Ⓐ Ⓑ Ⓒ Ⓓ	33 Ⓐ Ⓑ Ⓒ Ⓓ	58 Ⓐ Ⓑ Ⓒ Ⓓ	83 Ⓐ Ⓑ Ⓒ Ⓓ
9 Ⓐ Ⓑ Ⓒ Ⓓ	34 Ⓐ Ⓑ Ⓒ Ⓓ	59 Ⓐ Ⓑ Ⓒ Ⓓ	84 Ⓐ Ⓑ Ⓒ Ⓓ
10 Ⓐ Ⓑ Ⓒ Ⓓ	35 Ⓐ Ⓑ Ⓒ Ⓓ	60 Ⓐ Ⓑ Ⓒ Ⓓ	85 Ⓐ Ⓑ Ⓒ Ⓓ
11 Ⓐ Ⓑ Ⓒ Ⓓ	36 Ⓐ Ⓑ Ⓒ Ⓓ	61 Ⓐ Ⓑ Ⓒ Ⓓ	86 Ⓐ Ⓑ Ⓒ Ⓓ
12 Ⓐ Ⓑ Ⓒ Ⓓ	37 Ⓐ Ⓑ Ⓒ Ⓓ	62 Ⓐ Ⓑ Ⓒ Ⓓ	87 Ⓐ Ⓑ Ⓒ Ⓓ
13 Ⓐ Ⓑ Ⓒ Ⓓ	38 Ⓐ Ⓑ Ⓒ Ⓓ	63 Ⓐ Ⓑ Ⓒ Ⓓ	88 Ⓐ Ⓑ Ⓒ Ⓓ
14 Ⓐ Ⓑ Ⓒ Ⓓ	39 Ⓐ Ⓑ Ⓒ Ⓓ	64 Ⓐ Ⓑ Ⓒ Ⓓ	89 Ⓐ Ⓑ Ⓒ Ⓓ
15 Ⓐ Ⓑ Ⓒ Ⓓ	40 Ⓐ Ⓑ Ⓒ Ⓓ	65 Ⓐ Ⓑ Ⓒ Ⓓ	90 Ⓐ Ⓑ Ⓒ Ⓓ
16 Ⓐ Ⓑ Ⓒ Ⓓ	41 Ⓐ Ⓑ Ⓒ Ⓓ	66 Ⓐ Ⓑ Ⓒ Ⓓ	91 Ⓐ Ⓑ Ⓒ Ⓓ
17 Ⓐ Ⓑ Ⓒ Ⓓ	42 Ⓐ Ⓑ Ⓒ Ⓓ	67 Ⓐ Ⓑ Ⓒ Ⓓ	92 Ⓐ Ⓑ Ⓒ Ⓓ
18 Ⓐ Ⓑ Ⓒ Ⓓ	43 Ⓐ Ⓑ Ⓒ Ⓓ	68 Ⓐ Ⓑ Ⓒ Ⓓ	93 Ⓐ Ⓑ Ⓒ Ⓓ
19 Ⓐ Ⓑ Ⓒ Ⓓ	44 Ⓐ Ⓑ Ⓒ Ⓓ	69 Ⓐ Ⓑ Ⓒ Ⓓ	94 Ⓐ Ⓑ Ⓒ Ⓓ
20 Ⓐ Ⓑ Ⓒ Ⓓ	45 Ⓐ Ⓑ Ⓒ Ⓓ	70 Ⓐ Ⓑ Ⓒ Ⓓ	95 Ⓐ Ⓑ Ⓒ Ⓓ
21 Ⓐ Ⓑ Ⓒ Ⓓ	46 Ⓐ Ⓑ Ⓒ Ⓓ	71 Ⓐ Ⓑ Ⓒ Ⓓ	96 Ⓐ Ⓑ Ⓒ Ⓓ
22 Ⓐ Ⓑ Ⓒ Ⓓ	47 Ⓐ Ⓑ Ⓒ Ⓓ	72 Ⓐ Ⓑ Ⓒ Ⓓ	97 Ⓐ Ⓑ Ⓒ Ⓓ
23 Ⓐ Ⓑ Ⓒ Ⓓ	48 Ⓐ Ⓑ Ⓒ Ⓓ	73 Ⓐ Ⓑ Ⓒ Ⓓ	98 Ⓐ Ⓑ Ⓒ Ⓓ
24 Ⓐ Ⓑ Ⓒ Ⓓ	49 Ⓐ Ⓑ Ⓒ Ⓓ	74 Ⓐ Ⓑ Ⓒ Ⓓ	99 Ⓐ Ⓑ Ⓒ Ⓓ
25 Ⓐ Ⓑ Ⓒ Ⓓ	50 Ⓐ Ⓑ Ⓒ Ⓓ	75 Ⓐ Ⓑ Ⓒ Ⓓ	100 Ⓐ Ⓑ Ⓒ Ⓓ

Practice Questions

100 Questions

Directions: Select the best answer to each of the following questions.

1. Given the function $f(x) = \dfrac{x^2 + 5x + 2}{x^3 + 9}$, compute $\dfrac{dy}{dx}$.

(A) $\dfrac{(x^3 + 9)(2x + 5) + (x^2 + 5x + 2)(3x^2)}{(x^3 + 9)^2}$

(B) $\dfrac{(x^3 + 9)(2x + 5) - (x^2 + 5x + 2)(3x^2)}{(x^3 + 9)^2}$

(C) $\dfrac{(x^2 + 5x + 2)(3x^2) - (x^3 + 9)(2x + 5)}{(x^3 + 9)^2}$

(D) $\dfrac{2x + 5}{5x^2}$

For questions 2–3, consider the data shown in the table below.

Cause of Death	# of deaths
Accidents and adverse effects	590
Homicide and legal intervention	230
Suicide	142
Malignant neoplasms	55
Diseases of heart	335
Human immunodeficiency virus infection	29
Congenital anomalies	115
Chronic obstructive pulmonary diseases	114
Pneumonia and influenza	111
Cerebrovascular diseases	35
All other causes	244

2. What percentage of deaths were due to suicide or congenital anomalies?

   (A) 14.85%
   (B) 10.85%
   (C) 12.85%
   (D) 16.85%

3. What percentage of deaths were NOT due to malignant neoplasms?

   (A) 97.25%
   (B) 2.75%
   (C) 55%
   (D) 45%

4. John has $9.00 in quarters and dimes. He has twice as many dimes as quarters. How many quarters does he have?

   (A) 25
   (B) 30
   (C) 35
   (D) 20

5. Simplify the expression $\dfrac{x^2 - 12x + 35}{x - 5}$.

   (A) $x + 7$
   (B) $x - 19$
   (C) $x - 7$
   (D) $x + 19$

For questions 6–8, consider the given graph of the function $y = f(x)$.

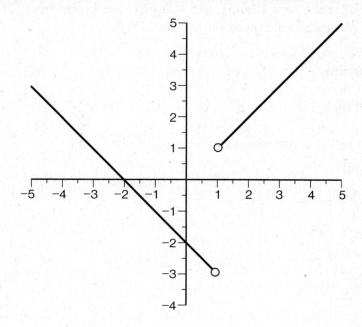

6. $\lim\limits_{x \to 1} f(x) =$

   (A) 1 and –3
   (B) Does not exist
   (C) 1 or –3
   (D) 1 and –3

7. $\lim\limits_{x \to 1^-} f(x) =$

   (A) –3
   (B) Does not exist
   (C) 1 or –3
   (D) 1 and –3

8. $\lim\limits_{x \to 1^+} f(x) =$

   (A) 1 and –3
   (B) Does not exist
   (C) 1 or –3
   (D) 1

9. During an 8-hour flight, a plane flew 350 mph for the first 3 hours, 500 mph for the next 4 hours, and 400 mph for the last hour. What was the plane's average speed for the entire flight?

   (A) 417 mph
   (B) 420 mph
   (C) 431 mph
   (D) 440 mph

10. $\log(9) - \log(5)$ is the same as

   (A) $\log(4)$

   (B) $\log\left(\dfrac{9}{5}\right)$

   (C) $\dfrac{\log(9)}{\log(5)}$

   (D) $\log(45)$

11. $\sqrt{18} + \sqrt{50} =$

   (A) $8\sqrt{2}$

   (B) $2\sqrt{17}$

   (C) $34\sqrt{2}$

   (D) $\sqrt{68}$

12. Mike can wash a car in 45 minutes. His brother takes twice as long to do the same job. Working together, how many cars can they wash in 6 hours?

   (A) 12
   (B) 10
   (C) 8
   (D) 14

13. If a coin is tossed four times, what is the probability of obtaining tails on the last toss?

   (A) $\dfrac{1}{2}$

   (B) $\dfrac{3}{5}$

   (C) $\dfrac{2}{5}$

   (D) $\dfrac{5}{8}$

14. A number is chosen at random from the set $\{1, 2, 3, 4, 5, 6, 7, 8, 9, 10\}$.
What is the probability that the chosen number is divisible by 2 or
divisible by 3?

   (A) 20%
   (B) 40%
   (C) 80%
   (D) 70%

15. $\left(\dfrac{1}{x}\right)^6 + \left(\dfrac{2}{x^2}\right)^3 =$

   (A) $3x^4$

   (B) $\dfrac{9}{x^6}$

   (C) $6x$

   (D) $\dfrac{1}{2x^4}$

16. $\log_5(125) =$

   (A) 3

   (B) $\dfrac{1}{3}$

   (C) 5

   (D) $\dfrac{1}{5}$

17. $-4 - 3\{2 + 1[3 - (2 + 3) + 2] + 2\} + 4 =$

   (A) -12
   (B) 0
   (C) 2
   (D) 8

18. 8 feet is approximately

   (A) 260 cm
   (B) 244 cm
   (C) 282 cm
   (D) 278 cm

For questions 19 and 20, consider the graph data shown below.

19. What is the mean value for miles per gallon?

    (A) 27.33
    (B) 26
    (C) 29
    (D) 25.24

20. What is the median value for miles per gallon?

    (A) 29
    (B) 24.89
    (C) 26
    (D) 25.24

21. $\int\limits_{1}^{\sqrt{e}} \left(\dfrac{10}{x} \right) dx =$

    (A) 5

    (B) $\dfrac{10}{\sqrt{e}} - 10$

    (C) 10

    (D) $\dfrac{10}{\sqrt{e}} + 10$

22. Event A has a probability of 7/10. What is the probability that event A does NOT occur?

    (A) 10/7
    (B) 3/10
    (C) 10/3
    (D) Not enough information

23. Parks leaves home for work and drives at 30 miles per hour. Twenty minutes later Susan, his wife, realizes he left his tool box at home. If Susan drives at 40 miles per hour, how far must she drive before she overtakes him?

    (A) 20 miles
    (B) 30 miles
    (C) 40 miles
    (D) 60 miles

For questions 24–27, consider the given graph of the function $y = f(x)$.

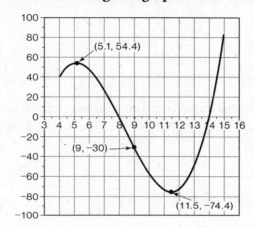

24. Identify the x value(s) at which the slope of the graph equals zero.

    (A) $x = 5.1$, $x = 11.5$
    (B) $x = 8$, $x = 14$
    (C) $x = 9$
    (D) $x = 54.4$, $y = -74.4$

25. Identify the x value(s) at which the graph has an inflection point.

    (A) $x = 5.1$, $x = 11.5$
    (B) $x = 8$, $x = 14$
    (C) $x = 9$
    (D) $x = -30$

26. Identify the interval(s) on which $f'(x) < 0$.

    (A) $(9, 15)$
    (B) $(8, 14)$
    (C) $(4, 9)$
    (D) $(5.1, 11.5)$

27. $\lim\limits_{x \to 5.1}\left(\dfrac{f(x) - f(5.1)}{x - 5.1} \right) =$

    (A) 11.4
    (B) 0
    (C) 5.1
    (D) Not enough information

28. A pair of fair six-sided dice is thrown. What is the probability that the sum of the numbers shown is equal to 7?

   (A) $\dfrac{1}{6}$

   (B) $\dfrac{1}{12}$

   (C) $\dfrac{1}{3}$

   (D) $\dfrac{2}{3}$

29. A computer password consists of four different characters chosen from the set {*A, B, C, D, E, F*, 1, 2, 3, 4, 5}. How many different passwords are possible?

   (A) $\dfrac{11!}{4!}$

   (B) $\dfrac{11!}{7!}$

   (C) $\dfrac{11!}{7!4!}$

   (D) $\dfrac{11!}{7! + 4!}$

30. A box contains apples and oranges in a ratio of 8:5. If the box contains 45 oranges, how many apples does the box contain?

   (A) 72
   (B) 48
   (C) 36
   (D) 63

31. In a student survey, 200 indicated that they would attend Summer Session I, and 150 indicated Summer Session II. If 75 students plan to attend both summer sessions and 275 indicated that they would attend neither session, how many students participated in the survey?

   (A) 550
   (B) 625
   (C) 700
   (D) Not enough information

32. Find the extreme value of the given function and state whether that value represents a maximum or a minimum value for the function.

$$P(x) = -100x^2 + 400x - 200$$

(A) 2, minimum
(B) 2, maximum
(C) 200, minimum
(D) 200, maximum

33. One hundred and forty pounds are equivalent to how many kilograms?

(A) 60.2
(B) 63.6
(C) 65.2
(D) 67.7

34. Find the vertex for the given function.

$$f(x) = 3x^2 - 12x + 5$$

(A) (2,0)
(B) (−2,41)
(C) (−2,0)
(D) (2,−7)

35. A truck is 60 miles from its destination at 4:00 P.M. At what speed must the truck travel to arrive by 4:45 P.M.?

(A) 80 mph
(B) 75 mph
(C) 70 mph
(D) 85 mph

36. Given the following equation:

$$°C = \frac{5}{9}(°F - 32)$$

Convert 50°F to °C.

(A) 10
(B) 14
(C) 12
(D) 16

37. Find all real solutions for the quadratic equation $3x^2 + 2x + 5 = 0$.

   (A) $x = \dfrac{-2 \pm \sqrt{56}}{6}$

   (B) No real solutions

   (C) $x = \dfrac{-2 \pm \sqrt{-56}}{6}$

   (D) $x = \dfrac{-2 \pm \sqrt{60}}{6}$

38. $6^2 \cdot 6^3 =$
   (A) 46,656
   (B) 7,776
   (C) 1,296
   (D) 248,832

39. $\dfrac{8}{9} - \dfrac{1}{2} =$

   (A) $\dfrac{6}{18}$

   (B) $\dfrac{7}{18}$

   (C) $\dfrac{5}{18}$

   (D) $\dfrac{3}{18}$

40. Given that 600 milligrams of drug A equals 800 milligrams of drug B, what is the equivalent dose of drug A for a patient taking 500 milligrams of drug B?

   (A) 350 mg
   (B) 325 mg
   (C) 375 mg
   (D) 450 mg

41. $3^2 + 3^4 =$
   (A) 729
   (B) 1,296
   (C) 90
   (D) 18

42. A number is chosen at random from the set $\{1, 2, 3, 4, 5, 6, 7, 8, 9, 10, 11, 12\}$. What is the probability that the chosen number is NOT divisible by 2 and NOT divisible by 3?

(A) $\dfrac{1}{3}$

(B) $\dfrac{3}{5}$

(C) $\dfrac{3}{4}$

(D) $\dfrac{2}{5}$

43. 250 milligrams of aminophylline injection is equivalent to 200 milligrams of theophylline. The strength of aminophylline injection is 25 milligrams per milliliter. How many milliliters of aminophylline injection are needed to provide a dose of 320 milligrams theophylline?

(A) 10.67
(B) 12.8
(C) 16
(D) 20

44. A patient's creatine clearance rate (CrCl) can be calculated by using the following formula:

$$CrCl = \frac{140 - \text{age in years}}{72 \cdot SCr} \cdot (\text{ideal body weight in kilograms}).$$

What is the CrCl for a 74-year-old patient who has a SCr of 3.2 and an ideal body weight of 84 kg?

(A) 34
(B) 24
(C) 28
(D) 38

45. The graph of a function $y = f(x)$ contains the point $(9, 6)$. Determine which point must be on the graph of $y = 7f(x - 3) + 1$.

(A) $(12, 43)$
(B) $(6, 43)$
(C) $(12, 85)$
(D) $(6, 85)$

46. Determine the derivative for the function $f(x) = e^{5x} \cdot \cos(x)$.

(A) $5e^{5x} \cdot \cos(x) + e^{5x} \cdot \sin(x)$

(B) $5e^{5x} \cdot \cos(x) - e^{5x} \cdot \sin(x)$

(C) $e^{5x} \cdot \cos(x) - e^{5x} \cdot \sin(x)$

(D) $e^{5x} \cdot \cos(x) + e^{5x} \cdot \sin(x)$

For questions 47 and 48, consider the graph below.

47. What is the maximum plasma concentration?

(A) 300 nmol/L
(B) 200 nmol/L
(C) 400 nmol/L
(D) 500 nmol/L

48. When does the maximum plasma concentration occur?

(A) Approximately 2 hours
(B) Approximately 4 hours
(C) Approximately 10 hours
(D) Approximately 3 hours

49. Determine the length of the line segment with endpoints (3, 6) and (–2, 5).

    (A) $\sqrt{24}$

    (B) $\sqrt{23}$

    (C) $\sqrt{26}$

    (D) $\sqrt{27}$

50. Larry's house is 12 miles from the park. Larry rode his bicycle from his house to the park at 12 miles per hour. He then walked the bicycle home from the park at 3 miles per hour. If he took the same route on both trips, what was his average speed?

    (A) 4.8 mph
    (B) 7.5 mph
    (C) 1.6 mph
    (D) 4.0 mph

51. Identify the graph that demonstrates a linear relationship between the variables x and y.

    (A)

    (B)

    (C)

    (D)

52. Determine the radius of the circle with equation $x^2 + y^2 + 12x - 14y - 1 = 0$.

    (A) $\sqrt{86}$

    (B) 86

    (C) 85

    (D) $\sqrt{85}$

53. What is the mean of this series of values: 12, 8, 17, 22, 5, 13?

    (A) 16.3
    (B) 12.8
    (C) 14.5
    (D) 14.1

54. Determine the slope of the tangent line to the graph of the function $f(x) = 5x^4 + 6x$ at the point whose x coordinate equals -1.

    (A) -14
    (B) 14
    (C) -1
    (D) 1

55. Given that $\ln(a) = 6$ and $\ln(b) = 2$, $\ln(a \cdot b) =$

    (A) 8
    (B) 12
    (C) $\ln(8)$
    (D) $\ln(12)$

56. Evaluate the integral $\int_{2}^{3} \left(4x^3\right) dx$.

    (A) -65
    (B) 60
    (C) -60
    (D) 65

For questions 57 and 58, consider the given graph of the function $y = f(x)$.

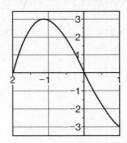

57. Identify the graph of the function $y = f(x - 2)$.

(A)

(B)

(C)

(D)

58. Identify the graph of the function $y = f(x) - 2$.

(A)

(B)

(C)

(D)

59. Lisa's gas tank is $\dfrac{2}{3}$ full. She completely filled the tank by putting in an additional 8 gallons. What is the capacity of the gas tank?

(A) 18 gallons
(B) 24 gallons
(C) 26 gallons
(D) 20 gallons

60. A walk-in clinic sees approximately 45% of its daily patients before noon. If the clinic sees a total of 40 patients on a given day, how many patients were seen **after** noon?

(A) 18
(B) 20
(C) 24
(D) 22

61. The height h of a projectile is given by $h(x) = -0.002x^2 + x$, where x is the horizontal distance the projectile travels. The projectile hits the ground after it has traveled a horizontal distance of

(A) 600 feet
(B) 400 feet
(C) 200 feet
(D) 500 feet

62. Express the distance from point P to point Q as a function of the x coordinate of point P.

(A) $\sqrt{x^2 - \left(6 - x^2\right)^2}$

(B) $x^2 + \left(6 - x^2\right)^2$

(C) $\sqrt{x^2 + \left(6 - x^2\right)^2}$

(D) $x^2 - \left(6 - x^2\right)^2$

63. If four red balls were placed in a bag with eight black balls, what is the probability of obtaining a red ball?

(A) $\dfrac{1}{3}$

(B) $\dfrac{8}{5}$

(C) 3

(D) 1

64. $\log(4) + \log(25) =$

(A) $\log(4)\log(25)$
(B) $\log(29)$
(C) 2
(D) 10

65. A jar contains 5 pennies, 4 nickels, and 6 dimes. What is the probability that a randomly chosen coin is NOT a dime?

   (A) 60%
   (B) 40%
   (C) 0.40%
   (D) 0.60%

For questions 66–71, consider the given graph of the function $y = f(x)$.

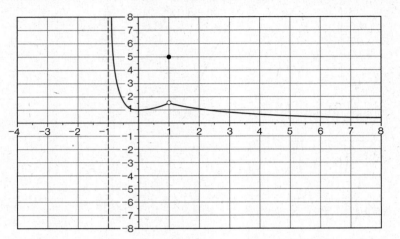

66. $\lim_{x \to -1^+} f(x) =$

   (A) 1.5
   (B) 5
   (C) Undefined
   (D) 0

67. $\lim_{x \to -1^-} f(x) =$

   (A) ∞
   (B) –1
   (C) $-\infty$
   (D) $\pm\infty$

68. $\lim_{x \to \infty} f(x) =$

   (A) ∞
   (B) Undefined
   (C) $-\infty$
   (D) 0

69. The equation of the vertical asymptote is

    (A) $x = -1$.
    (B) $x = \infty$.
    (C) $x = -\infty$.
    (D) $x = 0$.

70. The equation of the horizontal asymptote is

    (A) $y = -1$.
    (B) $y = 0$.
    (C) $y = \infty$.
    (D) $y = -\infty$.

71. $f'(1) =$

    (A) 0
    (B) 1.5
    (C) Undefined
    (D) 5

72. Determine the average rate of change of the function $f(x) = x^2$ on the interval $1 \leq x \leq 3$.

    (A) 4
    (B) 8
    (C) 3
    (D) 6

73. If 500 milligrams of drug A equal 400 milligrams of drug B, what is the equivalent dose of drug B for a patient taking 250 mg of drug A?

    (A) 200 mg
    (B) 240 mg
    (C) 250 mg
    (D) 300 mg

74. Determine the **domain** for the function $f(x) = \dfrac{x-1}{x^2 + 6x - 55}$.

    (A) $\{x : x = -11, x = 5\}$
    (B) $\{x : x = -11, x = -5\}$
    (C) $\{x : x \neq -11, x \neq -5\}$
    (D) $\{x : x \neq -11, x \neq 5\}$

75. $\dfrac{\sqrt{36} \cdot \sqrt{16}}{\sqrt{9}}$

   (A) $\dfrac{6 \cdot 4}{3} = 12$

   (B) $\dfrac{6 \cdot 4}{3} = 8$

   (C) $\dfrac{4 \cdot 4}{4} = 4$

   (D) $\dfrac{4 \cdot 3}{2} = 6$

76. The quadratic equation $ax^2 + bx + c = 0$ has solutions given by

   (A) $x = \dfrac{-b \pm \sqrt{b^2 - 4ac}}{2a}$.

   (B) $x = \dfrac{b \pm \sqrt{b^2 + 4ac}}{2a}$.

   (C) $x = -b \pm \dfrac{\sqrt{b^2 - 4ac}}{2a}$.

   (D) $x = -b \pm \dfrac{\sqrt{b^2 + 4ac}}{2a}$.

77. Given the function $f(x) = \begin{cases} 3x^2 & \text{for } x < 2 \\ 1 - 5x & \text{for } x > 2 \end{cases}$, evaluate the limit.

   $\lim\limits_{x \to 2} f(x) =$

   (A) Undefined
   (B) 12
   (C) –9
   (D) –9 and 12

78. The equation $5(x + 2)(x - 1) = 5x^2 + 6x$ has solution

   (A) $x = 10$.

   (B) $x = -10$.

   (C) $x = -\dfrac{2}{5}$.

   (D) $x = \dfrac{2}{5}$.

For questions 79 and 80, consider the survey data shown in the table below.

Seat Belt Worn	Probability
Never	0.0262
Rarely	0.0678
Sometimes	0.1156
Most of the time	0.2632
Always	0.5272

79. What is the probability that someone rarely or never wears a seat belt?

   (A) 5.32%
   (B) 2.62%
   (C) 6.78%
   (D) 9.40%

80. If 8,000 people participated in the survey, how many people sometimes wear a seat belt?

   (A) 1,156
   (B) 925
   (C) 116
   (D) 654

81. A pair of six-sided dice is thrown. What is the probability that the sum of the numbers shown is NOT equal to 7?

   (A) $\dfrac{2}{3}$

   (B) $\dfrac{1}{6}$

   (C) $\dfrac{1}{3}$

   (D) $\dfrac{11}{12}$

82. Find the exact value of the shaded area in the graph below.

$f(x) = \sin(2x)$

(A) 4

(B) 1

(C) 2

(D) $\dfrac{1}{2}$

83. Determine the inverse function for $f(x) = \dfrac{5x}{x-3}$.

(A) $f^{-1}(x) = \dfrac{x-3}{5x}$

(B) $f^{-1}(x) = \dfrac{-3}{5-x}$

(C) $f^{-1}(x) = \dfrac{5-x}{-3}$

(D) $f^{-1}(x) = \dfrac{3x}{x-5}$

84. If $x < 10$, then $\dfrac{x^2 - 11x + 10}{|x - 10|} =$

    (A) $-x + 1$
    (B) $-x - 1$
    (C) $x - 1$
    (D) $x + 1$

85. Event A has a probability of 0.26. Event B has a probability of 0.42. The probability that events A and B both occur is 0.12. What is the probability that either event A or event B occurs?

    (A) 0.68
    (B) 0.44
    (C) 0.56
    (D) 0.32

86. Set A contains 20 elements. Set B contains 11 elements. Set $A \cap B$ contains 5 elements. Determine the number of elements in the set $A \cup B$.

    (A) 26
    (B) 31
    (C) 36
    (D) Not enough information

87. Determine the slope of the line passing through the points $(5, 3)$ and $(2, -1)$.

    (A) $\dfrac{4}{3}$

    (B) $-\dfrac{4}{3}$

    (C) $\dfrac{3}{4}$

    (D) $-\dfrac{3}{4}$

88. If $\ln(w + 5x) = 3$, then

(A) $x = \dfrac{e^3 - w}{5}$

(B) $x = \dfrac{e^3 + w}{5}$

(C) $x = \dfrac{3e - w}{5}$

(D) $x = \dfrac{3e + w}{5}$

89. Write the equation of the **circle** with center point $C = (5, -6)$ and containing the point $P = (8, 3)$.

(A) $(x - 5)^2 + (y + 6)^2 = \sqrt{90}$

(B) $(x - 5)^2 + (y + 6)^2 = 90$

(C) $(x + 5)^2 + (y - 6)^2 = 90$

(D) $(x + 5)^2 + (y - 6)^2 = \sqrt{90}$

90. Find the equation of the horizontal asymptote, if any, for the given function.

$$f(x) = \dfrac{3x + 1}{5 - 4x}$$

(A) $y = -\dfrac{4}{5}$

(B) $y = \dfrac{3}{4}$

(C) $y = \dfrac{4}{5}$

(D) $y = -\dfrac{3}{4}$

91. Write the equation of the line passing through the point (5, –7) that is perpendicular to the line with equation $y = 4$.

    (A) $x = -\dfrac{1}{4}$

    (B) $x = -4$

    (C) $x = 5$

    (D) $x = -7$

92. How many different ways can a 5-person committee be chosen from a group of 12 people?

    (A) $\dfrac{12!}{7!}$

    (B) $\dfrac{12!}{5!}$

    (C) $\dfrac{12!}{5!7!}$

    (D) $\dfrac{12!}{5! + 7!}$

93. Convert 86°F to Kelvin.

    (A) 30
    (B) 243
    (C) 54
    (D) 303

94. Determine the domain of the function $f(x) = \ln(4x - 2)$.

    (A) $(-\infty, \infty)$
    (B) $[-\infty, \infty]$
    (C) $[0.5, \infty)$
    (D) $(0.5, \infty)$

95. A rental car company charges $25 per day, plus 12 cents per mile. Express the total rental cost of a 6-day rental as a function of the number of miles driven, x.

    (A) $C(x) = 25 + 12x$
    (B) $C(x) = 25 + 0.12x$
    (C) $C(x) = 150 + 12x$
    (D) $C(x) = 150 + 0.12x$

For questions 96–98, consider the given graph of the function $y = f(x)$.

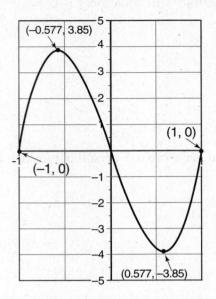

96. Choose the statement that best describes the function $y = f(x)$ with the given graph.

   (A) $y = f(x)$ is an even function.
   (B) $y = f(x)$ is a quadratic function.
   (C) $y = f(x)$ is an odd function.
   (D) $y = f(x)$ is a linear function.

97. Determine the domain of the function $y = f(x)$ with the given graph.

   (A) $(-1, 1)$
   (B) $[-1, 1]$
   (C) $(-3.85, 3.85)$
   (D) $[-3.85, 3.85]$

98. Determine the range of the function $y = f(x)$ with the given graph.

   (A) $(-1, 1)$
   (B) $[-1, 1]$
   (C) $(-3.85, 3.85)$
   (D) $[-3.85, 3.85]$

99. Kate had a box of red and blue crayons in a ratio of 5:9. If she had 20 red crayons, how many more blue crayons did she have than red?

(A) 9
(B) 16
(C) 4
(D) 11

100. $\dfrac{4}{11} - \dfrac{3}{8} =$

(A) $\dfrac{1}{3}$

(B) $\dfrac{1}{88}$

(C) $-\dfrac{1}{3}$

(D) $-\dfrac{1}{88}$

Answer Key
QUANTITATIVE ABILITY

1. **B**	26. **D**	51. **B**	76. **A**
2. **C**	27. **B**	52. **A**	77. **A**
3. **A**	28. **B**	53. **B**	78. **B**
4. **D**	29. **B**	54. **A**	79. **D**
5. **C**	30. **A**	55. **A**	80. **B**
6. **B**	31. **A**	56. **D**	81. **D**
7. **A**	32. **D**	57. **A**	82. **D**
8. **D**	33. **B**	58. **D**	83. **D**
9. **C**	34. **D**	59. **B**	84. **A**
10. **B**	35. **A**	60. **D**	85. **C**
11. **A**	36. **A**	61. **D**	86. **A**
12. **A**	37. **B**	62. **C**	87. **A**
13. **A**	38. **B**	63. **A**	88. **A**
14. **D**	39. **B**	64. **C**	89. **B**
15. **B**	40. **C**	65. **A**	90. **D**
16. **A**	41. **C**	66. **A**	91. **C**
17. **A**	42. **A**	67. **A**	92. **C**
18. **B**	43. **C**	68. **D**	93. **D**
19. **A**	44. **B**	69. **A**	94. **D**
20. **C**	45. **A**	70. **B**	95. **D**
21. **A**	46. **B**	71. **C**	96. **C**
22. **B**	47. **D**	72. **A**	97. **B**
23. **C**	48. **A**	73. **A**	98. **D**
24. **A**	49. **C**	74. **D**	99. **B**
25. **C**	50. **A**	75. **B**	100. **D**

EXPLANATORY ANSWERS

1. **(B)** We use the Quotient Rule for derivatives.

$$\frac{d}{dx}\left(\frac{f(x)}{g(x)}\right) = \frac{g(x) \cdot f'(x) - g'(x) \cdot f(x)}{\left(g(x)\right)^2}$$

2. **(C)** There were $142 + 115 = 257$ deaths due to suicide or congenital anomalies. There were 2,000 total deaths. Thus,

$$\text{probability} = \frac{257}{2000} = 0.1285 = 12.85\%.$$

3. **(A)** The percentage of deaths due to malignant neoplasms was

$$\frac{55}{2,000} = 0.0275 = 2.75\%.$$ Thus, the percentage of deaths NOT due to malignant neoplasms was $1 - 0.0275 = 0.9725 = 97.25\%$.

4. **(D)** Let $x =$ the number of quarters, and $2x =$ the number of dimes. This yields the equation $25 \cdot x + 10 \cdot 2x =$ money in cents. So we solve $25 \cdot x + 10 \cdot 2x = 900$

$$45x = 900 \Rightarrow x = \frac{900}{45} = 20.$$

5. **(C)** We simplify the expression as follows.

$$\frac{x^2 - 12x + 35}{x - 5} = \frac{\left(x - 5\right)\left(x - 7\right)}{x - 5} = x - 7$$

6. **(B)** The left- and right-hand limits are not equal.

7. **(A)** As x approaches 1 from the left-hand side, the values of $f(x)$ approach -3.

8. **(D)** As x approaches 1 from the right-hand side, the values of $f(x)$ approach 1.

9. **(C)** The plane travels $350 \cdot 3 = 1,050$ miles during the first 3 hours, $500 \cdot 4 = 2,000$ miles during the next 4 hours, and 400 miles during the last hour. So we have

$$\text{avg speed} = \frac{\text{total distance}}{\text{total time}} = \frac{3,450}{8 \text{ hrs}} = 431 \text{ mph.}$$

10. **(B)** The *Quotient Rule* for logarithms states that $\log(M) - \log(N) = \log\left(\dfrac{M}{N}\right)$.

11. **(A)** Note that $\sqrt{18} + \sqrt{50} = \sqrt{9 \cdot 2} + \sqrt{25 \cdot 2} = 3\sqrt{2} + 5\sqrt{2} = 8\sqrt{2}$.

12. **(A)** Mike can wash 1 car every 45 minutes = 0.75 hours. Thus, in 6 hours he can wash $\dfrac{6}{0.75} = 8$ cars. His brother can wash 1 car every 90 minutes = 1.5 hours. Thus, in 6 hours he can wash $\dfrac{6}{1.5} = 4$ cars. Working together, they can wash 12 cars (8 + 4 = 12 cars) in 6 hours.

13. **(A)** Each time a coin is tossed, there are two possible outcomes, heads and tails. The probability of heads is $\dfrac{1}{2}$. The outcome of the fourth coin toss is independent of the outcomes of the three earlier tosses.

14. **(D)** There are 7 numbers divisible by 2 or 3; that is, 2, 3, 4, 6, 8, 9, 10. We use the formula: probability $= \dfrac{7}{10} = 0.70 = 70\%$.

15. **(B)**

$$\left(\frac{1}{x}\right)^6 + \left(\frac{2}{x^2}\right)^3 = \frac{1^6}{x^6} + \frac{2^3}{\left(x^2\right)^3}$$

Rule: $\left(\dfrac{a}{b}\right)^n = \dfrac{a^n}{b^n}$

$$= \frac{1}{x^6} + \frac{8}{x^6}$$

Rule: $\left(a^n\right)^m = a^{n \bullet m}$

$$= \frac{9}{x^6}$$

16. **(A)** Note that $\log_5(125) = x$ is equivalent to the equation $5^x = 125$. This equation has solution $x = 3$.

17. **(A)** Begin with the innermost parentheses, and work outward.
$-4 - 3\{2 + 1\,[3 - (2 + 3) + 2] + 2\} + 4 =$
$-4 - 3\{2 + 1\,[\,3 - 5 + 2] + 2\} + 4 =$
$-4 - 3\{2 + 1 \cdot 0 + 2\} + 4 =$
$-4 - 3 \cdot 4 + 4 =$
$-4 - 12 + 4 =$
-12

18. **(B)** We use the conversion 1 foot = 30.5 cm; 1 inch = 2.54 cm; 12 inches = 1 foot, so 8 ft = 96 inches. Therefore, 96 inches = 96 · 2.54 = 244 cm.

19. **(A)** We compute

$$\frac{18 + 20 + 24 + 28 + 35 + 40 + 33 + 26 + 22}{9} = \frac{246}{9} = 27.33.$$

20. **(C)** We list the values in increasing order: 18, 20, 22, 24, 26, 28, 33, 35, 40. The median value occurs at the middle position in the list, that is, the median = 26.

21. **(A)** We use the Fundamental Theorem of Calculus to compute the definite integral. Note that

$$\int \frac{10}{x}\, dx = 10\ln(x).$$

$$\int_{1}^{\sqrt{e}} \left(\frac{10}{x}\right) dx = 10\ln(x)\big]_{1}^{\sqrt{e}} = 10\ln\left(\sqrt{e}\right) - 10\ln(1)$$

$$= 10\ln\left(e^{1/2}\right) - 10\ln(1) = 10\left(\frac{1}{2}\right) - 10(0) = 5.$$

22. **(B)** We use the formula $P(\overline{A}) = 1 - P(A) = 1 - \dfrac{7}{10} = \dfrac{3}{10}.$

23. **(C)** In 20 min. ($\frac{1}{3}$ hr.), Parks has gone 10 mi. In another hour, he will have covered a total of 40 mi. (10 + 30). Therefore, Susan must drive 40 mi. (for 1 hr.) to catch him.

24. **(A)** The graph has a horizontal tangent line at $x = 5.1$ and $x = 11.5$.

25. **(C)** The graph changes its concavity at $x = 9$. That is, the graph is concave down ("bends downward") for $x < 9$, and the graph is concave up ("bends upward") for $x > 9$.

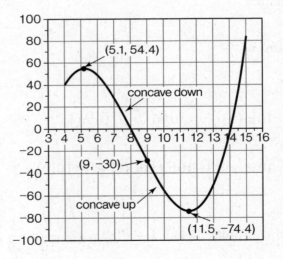

26. **(D)** The graph is decreasing on the interval (5.1, 11.5).

27. **(B)** Note that $\lim\limits_{x \to 5.1} \left(\dfrac{f(x) - f(5.1)}{x - 5.1} \right)$ gives the derivative of f at $x = 5.1$.

Recall that the derivative gives the slope of the tangent line to the graph at the point of the tangency. Note that the tangent line to the given graph is horizontal at the point where $x = 5.1$. Thus, the slope equals 0 there.

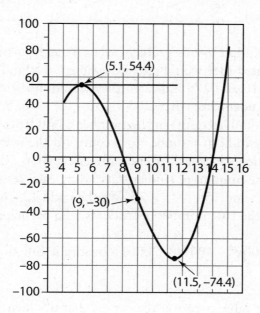

28. **(B)** There are 3 ways that the sum of the numbers shown can equal 7, that is, $1 + 6$, $2 + 5$, and $3 + 4$. Note that there are 6 possible outcomes for each die in the pair. Therefore, to calculate the possible combinations for the pair, we multiple $6 \cdot 6 = 36$.

Thus, probability $= \dfrac{3}{36} = \dfrac{1}{12}$.

29. **(B)** We are choosing 4 elements from an 11-element set, without repetition, such that order matters. Thus, we are counting permutations.

    We use the formula $_{11}P_4 = \dfrac{11!}{(11-4)!} = \dfrac{11!}{7!}$.

30. **(A)** Since the ratio of apples to oranges is 8:5, we solve the following proportion:

    $$\frac{8 \text{ apples}}{5 \text{ oranges}} = \frac{x \text{ apples}}{45 \text{ oranges}}$$

    Note that $5 \cdot 9 = 45$. Thus, $8 \cdot 9 = x$, i.e., $x = 72$.

31. **(A)** Consider the Venn diagram.

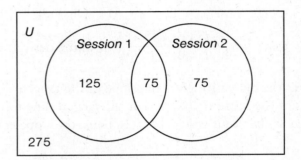

    Initially, the solution to this problem seems straightforward. Two hundred students indicated they would attend Session 1, 150 indicated they would attend Session II, and 275 indicated they would not attend either session. If we add these students together, $200 + 150 + 275 = 625$. However, there is an overlap (or double count) in the number of students, as 75 indicated they would attend both sessions. To account for the overlap and learn the number of students who will attend only one session, 75 should be subtracted from the number of students attending each session. In this case, $200 - 75 = 125$ and $150 - 75 = 75$. We then add $125 + 275 + 75 + 75 = 550$ to obtain the true number of students who participated in the survey.

32. **(D)** $P(x) = -100x^2 + 400x^2 - 200$ is a quadratic function whose graph opens down.

    The maximum value occurs at the vertex, that is, when $x = -\dfrac{400}{-200} = 2$.

    Thus, $P(2) = 200$.

33. **(B)** $\dfrac{1 \text{ kg}}{2.2 \text{ lb.}} \cdot 140 \text{ lb.} = 63.6$

34. **(D)** A quadratic function $f(x) = ax^2 + bx + c$ will have its vertex at the point

$$\left(-\frac{b}{2a}, f\left(-\frac{b}{2a}\right)\right)$$

$$f(x) = 3x^2 - 12x + 5 \Rightarrow x = -\frac{b}{2a} = -\frac{-12}{2(3)} = \frac{12}{6} = 2$$

$$f(2) = 3(2)^2 - 12(2) + 5 = 12 - 24 + 5 = -7$$

Thus, the vertex is (2,–7).

35. **(A)** The truck must travel 60 miles in 45 minutes = 0.75 hour. We have the formula

$$\text{speed} = \frac{\text{distance}}{\text{time}} = \frac{60 \text{ miles}}{0.75 \text{ hr}} = 80 \text{ mph.}$$

36. **(A)** $°C = \dfrac{5}{9}(50 - 32) = \dfrac{5}{9}(18) = 10.$

37. **(B)** We use the quadratic formula.

$$x = \frac{-b \pm \sqrt{b^2 - 4ac}}{2a} = \frac{-2 \pm \sqrt{2^2 - 4 \cdot 3 \cdot 5}}{2 \cdot 3} = \frac{-2 \pm \sqrt{-56}}{6}.$$

Since $\sqrt{-56}$ is not a real number, the equation has no real solutions.

38. **(B)** Note that $6^2 \cdot 6^3 = 6^{2+3} = 6^5 = 7{,}776.$

39. **(B)** The least common denominator for $\dfrac{8}{9}$ and $\dfrac{1}{2}$ is 18. Rewrite the fractions, using the least common denominator: $\dfrac{8 \cdot 2}{18} - \dfrac{1 \cdot 9}{18} = \dfrac{16}{18} - \dfrac{9}{18} = \dfrac{7}{18}.$

40. **(C)** We have the ratio $\dfrac{600 \text{ mg drug A}}{800 \text{ mg drug B}}$. Thus,

$$\frac{600 \text{ mg drug A}}{800 \text{ mg drug B}} \cdot \frac{x}{500 \text{ mg drug B}}$$

$800x = (600 \cdot 500)$

$800x = 300{,}000$

$$x = \frac{300{,}000}{800}$$

$x = 375$

41. **(C)** $3^2 + 3^4 = 9 + 81 = 90$.

42. **(A)** There are four numbers not divisible by either 2 or 3, that is 1, 5, 7, 11. Thus, probability $= \dfrac{4}{12} = \dfrac{1}{3}$.

43. **(C)** 250 milligrams of aminophylline injection is equivalent to 200 milligrams of theophylline. Thus, aminophylline is 80% theophylline $\left(\dfrac{200}{250} = 80\%\right)$; therefore, 25 mg (1 mL) of aminophylline will contain only 20 mg of theophylline. Divide 320 mg by 20 mg/mL to obtain 16 mL.

44. **(B)** We plug into the given formula

$$\text{CrCl} = \left(\frac{140 - 74}{72 \cdot 3.2}\right) \cdot (84) = \left(\frac{66}{72 \cdot 3.2}\right) \cdot (84) \approx 24 \, .$$

45. **(A)** Each point on the graph of $y = 7f(x - 3) + 1$ is obtained by transforming the points on the graph of $y = f(x)$ as follows. Add 3 to each x coordinate (in this case, $3 + 9 = 12$); multiply each y coordinate by 7 and then add 1 (in this case, $7 \cdot 6 = 42 + 1 = 43$). Therefore, the answer is (12, 43).

46. **(B)** We use the Product Rule for derivatives

$$\frac{d}{dx}\left(f(x) \cdot g(x)\right) = f'(x) \cdot g(x) + f(x) \cdot g'(x)$$

and the fact that $\dfrac{d}{dx}e^{5x} = 5e^{5x}$ and $\dfrac{d}{dx}\cos(x) = -\sin(x)$.

47. **(D)** The highest point on the graph has y coordinate equal to 500.

48. **(A)** The highest point on the graph occurs when the x coordinate equals 2.

49. **(C)** We calculate the distance using the formula

$$\sqrt{(x_2 - x_1)^2 + (y_2 - y_1)^2} = \sqrt{(-2 - 3)^2 + (5 - 6)^2} = \sqrt{25 + 1} = \sqrt{26} \, .$$

50. **(A)** If the house is 12 mi. from the park, at 12 mph Larry needed 1 hr. to make the trip. At only 3 mph, he needed 4 hr. to get back home. Thus, he traveled 24 mi. (2 · 12 mi.) in 5 hr. (1 + 4 hr.). Divide 24 by 5 to get an average speed of 4.8 mph.

51. **(B)** A linear relationship between two variables yields a graph that is a nonvertical line, which is represented in choice (B). The relationships represented in the answer choices are as follows: (A) quadratic, (B) linear, (C) polynomial, and (D) exponential.

52. **(A)** Note that an equation of the form $(x - h)^2 + (y - k)^2 = r^2$ represents a circle with radius equal to r. We can apply the technique of completing the square to the given equation as follows:

$$x^2 + y^2 + 12x - 14y - 1 = 0$$
$$x^2 + 12x + y^2 - 14y = 1$$
$$x^2 + 12x + 36 + y^2 - 14y + 49 = 1 + 36 + 49$$
$$(x + 6)^2 + (y - 7)^2 = 86$$
$$(x + 6)^2 + (y - 7)^2 = \left(\sqrt{86}\right)^2$$

Thus, $r = \sqrt{86}$.

53. **(B)** To find the mean, add all the values together ($12 + 8 + 17 + 22 + 5 + 13 = 77$), then divide the sum by the number of values in the series ($\frac{77}{6} = 12.8$).

54. **(A)** We compute the derivative $f'(x) = 20x^3 + 6$, and then evaluate $f'(-1) = 20(-1)^3 + 6 = -20 + 6 = -14$.

55. **(A)** We use the Product Rule for logarithms. $\ln(a \cdot b) = \ln(a) + \ln(b) = 6 + 2 = 8$

56. **(D)** We use the Fundamental theorem of calculus for integrals.

$$\int_2^3 \left(4x^3\right)dx = \frac{4x^4}{4}\bigg|_2^3 = x^4\bigg|_2^3 = 3^4 - 2^4 = 81 - 16 = 65$$

57. **(A)** The original graph is shifted 2 units to the right.

58. **(D)** The original graph is shifted 2 units down.

59. **(B)** Since the tank is already 2/3 full, the additional 8 gallons equals 1/3 of the tank's capacity. Thus, $8 = \frac{1}{3}x \Rightarrow x = 24$.

60. **(D)** The clinic sees 55% of its daily patients after noon. So we have $(0.55)(40) = 22$.

61. **(D)** The projectile hits the ground when the height equals zero. So we solve the equation $-0.002x^2 + x = 0$.

$$-0.002x^2 + x = 0$$
$$x(-0.002x + 1) = 0$$

$$x = 0, \quad -0.002x + 1 = 0 \Rightarrow x = \frac{-1}{-0.002} = 500$$

62. **(C)** We apply the distance formula to points P and Q.

$$\sqrt{(x-0)^2 + (y-2)^2} = \sqrt{x^2 + (8-x^2-2)^2} = \sqrt{x^2 + (6-x^2)^2}$$

63. **(A)** If four red balls were placed in a bag with eight black balls, the probability of obtaining a red ball would be 4 out of 12 (total number of balls in the bag). After being simplified, the answer is $\frac{1}{3}$.

64. **(C)** The *Product Rule* for logarithms states that

$$\log(M) + \log(N) = \log(M \cdot N).$$

Thus, we have $\log(4) + \log(25) = \log(4 \cdot 25) = \log(100)$.
Note that $\log(100)$ asks the question: Base 10 raised to what power will yield 100?

$$\log(100) = \log(10^2)$$
$$10^x = 10^2$$
$$x = 2$$

65. **(A)** There are 9 possible ways not to choose a dime from a total of 15 coins. We use the formula: probability $= \frac{9}{15} = 0.60 = 60\%$.

66. **(A)** As x approaches 1 from the right, y approaches 1.5.

67. **(A)** As x approaches -1 from the left, y approaches ∞.

68. **(D)** As x approaches ∞, y approaches 0.

69. **(A)** Since $\lim_{x \to -1} f(x) = \pm\infty$, $x = 1$ represents a vertical line at which the function values become infinite.

70. **(B)** Since $\lim_{x \to \infty} f(x) = 0$.

71. **(C)** There is no tangent line to the graph when $x = 1$, so the derivative does not exist there.

72. **(A)** We compute $\dfrac{f(3) - f(1)}{3 - 1} = \dfrac{9 - 1}{2} = 4$.

73. **(A)** Set up a proportion: $\dfrac{500 \text{ mg drug A}}{100 \text{ mg drug B}} = \dfrac{250 \text{ mg drug A}}{x \text{ mg}}$

    Cross multiply and divide: $500x = 250 \cdot 400$
    $$500x = 10,000$$
    $$x = 200 \text{ mg}$$

74. **(D)** We must exclude any values of x that cause $x^2 + 6x - 55 = 0$. Since $x^2 + 6x - 55 = 0 \Rightarrow (x + 11)(x - 5) = 0$, we must exclude $x = -11$, and $x = 5$.

75. **(B)** $\dfrac{\sqrt{36} \cdot \sqrt{16}}{9} = \dfrac{6 \cdot 4}{3} = 8$.

76. **(A)** This is the quadratic formula.

77. **(A)** Since the left-hand limit yields $\lim\limits_{x \to 2^-} f(x) = 3(2)^2 = 12$,

    but the right-hand limit yields $\lim\limits_{x \to 2^+} f(x) = 1 - 5(2) = -9$,

    the overall limit $\lim\limits_{x \to 2} f(x)$ is undefined.

78. **(B)** We solve the equation as follows.

    $$5(x + 2)(x - 1) = 5x^2 + 6x$$
    $$5(x^2 + x - 2) = 5x^2 + 6x$$
    $$5x^2 + 5x - 10 = 5x^2 + 6x$$
    $$5x - 10 = 6x \Rightarrow -10 = x$$

79. **(D)** Using data from the table, add together "Rarely" (0.0678) and "Never" (0.0262). We compute $0.0678 + 0.0262 = 0.094 = 9.4\%$.

80. **(B)** We compute $(0.1156)(8,000) = 924.8 \approx 925$.

81. **(D)** There are 3 ways that the sum of the numbers shown can equal 7, i.e., 1 + 6, 2 + 5, 3 + 4. Note that there are 6 possible outcomes for each die in the pair. Therefore, to calculate the possible combinations for the pair, we multiple 6 · 6 = 36. So, the probability that the sum of the numbers shown equals 7 is $\dfrac{3}{36} = \dfrac{1}{12}$. Thus, the probability that the sum of the numbers shown is NOT equal to 7 is $1 - \dfrac{1}{12} = \dfrac{11}{12}$.

82. **(D)** We use the Fundamental Theorem of Calculus to compute the definite integral. Note that $\int \sin(2x)\,dx = -\dfrac{1}{2}\cos(2x)$.

$$\int_{0}^{\pi/4} \sin(2x)\,dx = -\frac{1}{2}\cos(2x)\Big]_{0}^{\pi/4} = -\frac{1}{2}\cos\left(2\left(\frac{\pi}{4}\right)\right) + \frac{1}{2}\cos(2(0)) = 4$$

$$= -\frac{1}{2}\cos\left(\frac{\pi}{2}\right) + \frac{1}{2}\cos(0) = 0 + \frac{1}{2} = \frac{1}{2}$$

83. **(D)** Given the function $f(x) = \dfrac{5x}{x-3}$, we solve for y in the equation

$x = \dfrac{5y}{y-3}$, i.e.,

$$x = \frac{5y}{y-3}$$
$$xy - 3x = 5y$$
$$-3x = 5y - xy$$
$$-3x = y(5 - x) \Rightarrow y = \frac{-3x}{5-x} = \frac{3x}{x-5}$$

84. **(A)** Since $x < 10$, this means that $x - 10 < 0$. Thus, $|x - 10| = -(x - 10)$.

Therefore,

$$\frac{x^2 - 11x + 10}{|x-10|} = \frac{(x-10)(x-1)}{-(x-10)} = -(x-1) = -x+1$$

85. **(C)** With the understanding that the symbol $\cup$ means the set of elements either in A or B or in both, and $\cap$ means the set that contains all those elements that A and B have in common, we use the formula:

$$P(A \cup B) = P(A) + P(B) - P(A \cap B) = 0.26 + 0.42 - 0.12 = 0.56.$$

86. **(A)** We use the formula

$n(A \cup B) = n(A) + n(B) - n(A \cap B) = 20 + 11 - 5 = 26.$

87. **(A)** We calculate the slope using the formula $\dfrac{\Delta y}{\Delta x} = \dfrac{3 - (-1)}{5 - 2} = \dfrac{4}{3}$.

88. **(A)** We solve the equation as follows.

$\ln(w + 5x) = 3$

$e^{\ln(w + 5x)} = e^3$

$w + 5x = e^3$

$5x = e^3 - w \Rightarrow x = \dfrac{e^3 - w}{5}$

89. **(B)** We apply the distance formula to points C and P to determine

the radius of the circle $r = \sqrt{(5 - 8)^2 + (-6 - 3)^2} = \sqrt{9 + 81} = \sqrt{90}$.

Now use the fact that a circle with equation $(x - h)^2 + (y - k)^2 = r^2$ has center point (h, k) and radius equal to r.

90. **(D)** A rational function will have a horizontal asymptote of $y = L$, provided

$\lim\limits_{x \to \pm\infty} f(x) = L.$

$\lim\limits_{x \to \pm\infty} f(x) = \lim\limits_{x \to \pm\infty} \left(\dfrac{3x + 1}{5 - 4x} \right) \to \dfrac{3x}{-4x} \to -\dfrac{3}{4}$

91. **(C)** The line with equation $y = 4$ is horizontal. So we need the equation of the vertical line passing through the point $(5, -7)$. The answer is $x = 5$.

92. **(C)** We are choosing 5 elements from a 12-element set, without repetition, such that order does not matter. Thus, we are counting combinations.

We use the formula $_{12}C_5 = \dfrac{12!}{5!(12 - 5)!} = \dfrac{12!}{5!7!}$.

93. **(D)** To convert from °F to °K, you must first convert the temperature from °F to °C. Therefore, the first step is to use

$$T_C = (T_F - 32) \left(\dfrac{5}{9} \right)$$

to convert the temperature to Celsius. Then, to convert the Celsius temperature to Kelvin, add 273.15.

Step 1: $$T_C = (T_F - 32)\left(\frac{5}{9}\right)$$

$$= (86 - 32)\left(\frac{5}{9}\right)$$

$$= (54)\left(\frac{5}{9}\right)$$

$$= 30°C$$

Step 2: $$K = 30 + 273.15 \approx 303$$

94. **(D)** A logarithmic function is undefined unless the input value is strictly greater than zero. Thus, we solve $4x - 2 > 0$ and obtain $x > 0.5$.

95. **(D)** The total rental cost is given by the daily cost plus the mileage cost. Daily cost = ($25 per day)(6 days) = $150. Mileage cost = ($0.12 per mile)(x miles) = $0.12x$.

96. **(C)** The graph has symmetry with respect to the origin.

97. **(B)** The domain is given by the set of x coordinates of the points on the graph.

98. **(D)** The range is given by the set of y coordinates of the points on the graph.

99. **(B)** Since the red and blue crayons are in a 5:9 ratio, we can set up the proportion $\dfrac{5 \text{ red}}{9 \text{ blue}} = \dfrac{20 \text{ red}}{x \text{ blue}}$. Now solve for x and then calculate $20 - x$.

Step 1:
$$\frac{5}{9} = \frac{20}{x}$$
$$5x = (20)(9)$$
$$5x = 180$$
$$x = 36$$

Step 2:
$$20 - 36 = 16 \text{ more blue crayons than red crayons.}$$

100. **(D)** Note that $\dfrac{4}{11} - \dfrac{3}{8} = \dfrac{8 \cdot 4 - 3 \cdot 11}{11 \cdot 8} = \dfrac{32 - 33}{88} = -\dfrac{1}{88}$.

Reading Comprehension Review and Practice

CHAPTER 8

TIPS FOR THE READING COMPREHENSION SECTION

The reading comprehension section of the PCAT presents relatively short passages. You are asked to read each passage carefully and then answer questions related to it. For each passage, there are generally 4–8 questions, with a total of 48 questions for the entire section. Keep in mind that the correct answer may be a direct statement taken from the reading passage. You will have 50 minutes to complete the reading comprehension section. Be careful to pace yourself to prevent running out of time.

Practice the reading passages and sample questions in this book. Read the passage first, and then answer the questions. Do not be concerned with how many times you need to refer to the passage to answer questions; just complete the section as quickly as possible, making sure you find the correct answer to every question.

Try to determine where your general strengths and weaknesses as a reader lie. Do you tend to get a quick grasp of the overall sense of a passage but miss the details? Or do you as a reader sometimes fail to see the forest for the trees? In other words, do you remember only the details and find yourself unable to state the basic meaning of the passage as a whole? In either case, take some time to improve your "weak" areas. Be patient with yourself as you practice. With adequate review, you should be able to work at your normal pace when you take the actual PCAT.

Answer Sheet
READING COMPREHENSION

1 Ⓐ Ⓑ Ⓒ Ⓓ		26 Ⓐ Ⓑ Ⓒ Ⓓ	
2 Ⓐ Ⓑ Ⓒ Ⓓ		27 Ⓐ Ⓑ Ⓒ Ⓓ	
3 Ⓐ Ⓑ Ⓒ Ⓓ		28 Ⓐ Ⓑ Ⓒ Ⓓ	
4 Ⓐ Ⓑ Ⓒ Ⓓ		29 Ⓐ Ⓑ Ⓒ Ⓓ	
5 Ⓐ Ⓑ Ⓒ Ⓓ		30 Ⓐ Ⓑ Ⓒ Ⓓ	
6 Ⓐ Ⓑ Ⓒ Ⓓ		31 Ⓐ Ⓑ Ⓒ Ⓓ	
7 Ⓐ Ⓑ Ⓒ Ⓓ		32 Ⓐ Ⓑ Ⓒ Ⓓ	
8 Ⓐ Ⓑ Ⓒ Ⓓ		33 Ⓐ Ⓑ Ⓒ Ⓓ	
9 Ⓐ Ⓑ Ⓒ Ⓓ		34 Ⓐ Ⓑ Ⓒ Ⓓ	
10 Ⓐ Ⓑ Ⓒ Ⓓ		35 Ⓐ Ⓑ Ⓒ Ⓓ	
11 Ⓐ Ⓑ Ⓒ Ⓓ		36 Ⓐ Ⓑ Ⓒ Ⓓ	
12 Ⓐ Ⓑ Ⓒ Ⓓ		37 Ⓐ Ⓑ Ⓒ Ⓓ	
13 Ⓐ Ⓑ Ⓒ Ⓓ		38 Ⓐ Ⓑ Ⓒ Ⓓ	
14 Ⓐ Ⓑ Ⓒ Ⓓ		39 Ⓐ Ⓑ Ⓒ Ⓓ	
15 Ⓐ Ⓑ Ⓒ Ⓓ		40 Ⓐ Ⓑ Ⓒ Ⓓ	
16 Ⓐ Ⓑ Ⓒ Ⓓ		41 Ⓐ Ⓑ Ⓒ Ⓓ	
17 Ⓐ Ⓑ Ⓒ Ⓓ		42 Ⓐ Ⓑ Ⓒ Ⓓ	
18 Ⓐ Ⓑ Ⓒ Ⓓ		43 Ⓐ Ⓑ Ⓒ Ⓓ	
19 Ⓐ Ⓑ Ⓒ Ⓓ		44 Ⓐ Ⓑ Ⓒ Ⓓ	
20 Ⓐ Ⓑ Ⓒ Ⓓ		45 Ⓐ Ⓑ Ⓒ Ⓓ	
21 Ⓐ Ⓑ Ⓒ Ⓓ		46 Ⓐ Ⓑ Ⓒ Ⓓ	
22 Ⓐ Ⓑ Ⓒ Ⓓ		47 Ⓐ Ⓑ Ⓒ Ⓓ	
23 Ⓐ Ⓑ Ⓒ Ⓓ		48 Ⓐ Ⓑ Ⓒ Ⓓ	
24 Ⓐ Ⓑ Ⓒ Ⓓ		49 Ⓐ Ⓑ Ⓒ Ⓓ	
25 Ⓐ Ⓑ Ⓒ Ⓓ		50 Ⓐ Ⓑ Ⓒ Ⓓ	

Practice Questions

50 Questions

Passage 1

In the past two decades, people living in the northeastern, north-central, and western United States have unwittingly entered a dangerous enzootic cycle—a cycle of disease that typically is restricted to wildlife. Wild mammals and birds host a wide variety of disease agents, with effects ranging from mild symptoms to mortality, but in most cases the pathogen affects only one or a few host species and never causes disease in humans. However, as a result of a complicated sequence of events, people have become frequent accidental hosts for ticks and the disease agents they carry, including a corkscrew-shaped bacterium called *Borrelia burgdorferi*, the agent of Lyme disease. As of 1995, cases of Lyme disease had been reported in 48 of the 50 states and appear to be increasing, both in numbers of people affected and in geographic distribution.

Where does this disease come from, why has it emerged so rapidly, and what can people do to reduce their risk of exposure? It is possible to address these questions not from a medical point of view, but rather from an ecological one. All living organisms—from the *B. burgdorferi* bacterium and the ticks it infects to the mice and deer on which the ticks feed—form an ecological relationship with their habitats. Understanding the complex interactions between plant and animal species within those habitats may help people to predict the places where they are most likely to encounter disease-bearing ticks and become infected. Thus armed, individuals may ultimately be able to protect themselves from Lyme disease.

Currently, to prevent Lyme disease people wear protective clothing when they are in wooded areas and perform "tick checks" after leaving the woods. One underemphasized means to avoid exposure to Lyme disease, however, is avoiding the most heavily tick-infested habitats at the times of year when ticks are most abundant or dangerous. Recent research has suggested that such habitats can be predicted, often well in advance. Ultimately, it is the hope of ecologists studying this problem that we can use our expertise in pinpointing these habitats to warn the public away from areas that are likely to contain an abundance of disease-carrying ticks.

Excerpted from "The Ecology of Lyme-Disease Risk," by Richard S. Ostfeld, The American Scientist, Vol. 85, p. 338, reprinted by permission of *American Scientist*, magazine of Sigma Xi, The Scientific Research Society.

1. What is primary message or theme of the first paragraph of the passage?

   (A) Diseases found in mammals and birds are never found in humans.
   (B) Lyme disease has been diagnosed throughout almost all states in the United States and is expected to increase.
   (C) Humans living in the United States are immune to pathogens carried by ticks, and therefore are not contributors to the spread of Lyme disease.
   (D) Humans living in the United States have become hosts for ticks and disease agents, contributing to the spread of pathogens such as *Borrelia burgdorferi.*

2. The aim of understanding Lyme disease from an ecological as well as a medical point of view is

   (A) to help preserve the mice and deer on which the ticks feed.
   (B) to help people predict the places where they are most likely to encounter disease-bearing ticks and become infected.
   (C) to develop a vaccine against the disease.
   (D) to further our understanding of the relationship between ticks and their habitats.

3. Prevention of Lyme disease

   (A) is the purview of medical professionals and ecologists.
   (B) does not have an ecological component.
   (C) may be accomplished through the use of herbal remedies.
   (D) requires proactive consideration of factors both before and after exploring the woods.

4. As of 1995, Lyme disease had been reported in 48 of 50 states and

   (A) had been eradicated in the two remaining states.
   (B) appeared to be increasing in number of people affected and in geographic distribution.
   (C) appeared to be decreasing in number of people affected.
   (D) appeared to be increasing in geographic distribution within those 48 states.

5. One underemphasized means to avoid exposure to Lyme disease is

   (A) wearing protective clothing.
   (B) avoiding the most heavily tick-infested areas at certain times of the year.
   (C) using insect repellent.
   (D) remembering to get vaccinated before going into areas that are known to be heavily tick-infested.

Passage 2

To the average physician, Lyme disease is suspected when a patient arrives at a clinic or hospital complaining of a strange bull's-eye rash, known as erythema migrans, or EM, together with one or more flulike symptoms, such as fever, chills, muscle aches, or lethargy. The physician will take a blood sample for laboratory confirmation, but will feel quite confident to make a diagnosis of Lyme disease after noting the telltale combination of symptoms, as well as the circumstances surrounding the infection. The patient will undoubtedly have been bitten by the black-legged tick *Ixodes scaplaris*, formerly called the deer tick, or a close relative, which transferred to him or her the *B. burgdorferi* bacterium. Most likely, the physician will prescribe an oral course of antibiotics and will duly report the case to the county or state health department, which will include it in the morbidity statistics for Lyme disease.

Accurate diagnosis and effective treatment of Lyme disease are not always so straightforward, particularly in regions of the country newly invaded by the epidemic. In these regions, health care professionals and the public need to be educated about the confusing and generalized symptoms, the generally poor, but growing, accuracy of lab tests, and the efficacy of various antibiotic treatments. If Lyme disease is left untreated for some time, *B. burgdorferi* may persist in the patient's tissues and can migrate to the central and peripheral nervous systems or to joints and cause more severe late-stage symptoms, which include arthritis and neurological disorders, such as dizziness, memory loss, and disorientation. Vaccines that protect against Lyme disease are now being field tested by pharmaceutical companies, but none has yet been approved by the Food and Drug Administration for public use. Even if an effective vaccine were certified and marketed, the primary means that individuals have of protecting themselves against the disease is avoiding the tick in the first place.

Excerpted from "The Ecology of Lyme-Disease Risk," by Richard S. Ostfeld, The American Scientist, Vol. 85, p. 338, reprinted by permission of *American Scientist*, magazine of Sigma Xi, The Scientific Research Society.

6. When a patient reports to a clinic or hospital with symptoms of Lyme disease, he or she has undoubtedly been bitten by

   (A) the black-legged tick *Ixodes scaplaris.*
   (B) a tick-bearing wild mammal.
   (C) *B. burgdorferi.*
   (D) none of the above; Lyme disease is generally believed to be spread by an airborne pathogen.

7. An appropriate title for this passage would be

   (A) Diagnosis of Lyme Disease
   (B) Diagnosis, Treatment, and Challenges of Lyme Disease
   (C) Developing Vaccinations to Protect Against Lyme Disease
   (D) Complications of Lyme Disease

8. Lyme disease may affect the human body's

   (A) gastrointestinal system.
   (B) cardiovascular system.
   (C) reproductive system.
   (D) musculoskeletal system.

9. In addition to noting the telltale combination of symptoms in a patient with Lyme disease, a physician is likely to

   (A) seek laboratory confirmation of the diagnosis.
   (B) prescribe an analgesic to alleviate symptoms.
   (C) recommend bed rest for a brief duration.
   (D) hospitalize the patient for treatment.

10. If Lyme disease is left untreated for some time,

    (A) health care professionals and the public will not be educated about its confusing and generalized symptoms.
    (B) the accuracy of diagnostic lab tests may be poor.
    (C) the disease may progress, with symptoms increasing in severity.
    (D) antibiotic treatments will no longer be effective.

Passage 3

Rabies is a master dissembler. No other disease so completely manipulates its stricken host while barely leaving a trace of its presence. And rabies is preeminently adaptive: even if one host species is eliminated, the virus resurfaces in another. It bides its time, shadowing its victims, waiting for new hosts to emerge as people disrupt habitats and force animals to congregate more densely. Despite the war chest of vaccines designed to stop it and the near certain death of every organism infected by it, rabies persists.

In the United States, on average, fewer than two people a year die of rabies, about the same number as in Western Europe. Vaccination and animal control policies ensure that few, if any, of those cases come from dog bites. Worldwide, between 20,000 and 100,000 people die of rabies in a given year, most of them in developing countries, and some 10 million are treated annually for possible exposures, mostly from dog bites. Compared with the dangers of becoming infected with HIV, tuberculosis, or malaria, each of which strikes millions of people every year, the risk of contracting rabies is vanishingly small. But rabies has had far greater influence on culture and science than its current incidence might suggest. And its devastating effects assure that it is never far from people's minds. Rabies has the highest fatality rate of any known human infection.

Excerpted from "The Deadliest Virus," by Cynthia Mills, from the January/ February 1997 issue of THE SCIENCES, reprinted by permission of The Sciences, 2 East 63rd Street, New York, NY 10021.

11. Rabies persist

    (A) due to lack of vaccines designed to stop it.
    (B) because of its highly adaptive nature.
    (C) because of the stability of its hosts' habitats.
    (D) because of a lack of animal control policies.

12. In the United States, the number of people who die of rabies every year is

    (A) between 2,000 and 10,000.
    (B) comparable to the number who die of rabies in Western Europe.
    (C) increasing in spite of efforts to bring it under control.
    (D) approaching the number in danger of becoming infected with malaria.

13. Excluding the United States and Western Europe, worldwide transmission of rabies is most commonly through

    (A) transfusion of contaminated blood.
    (B) contaminated drinking water.
    (C) dog bites.
    (D) bat bites.

14. The passage describes rabies as a "master dissembler"; what does this mean?

    (A) Rabies has had a significant influence on science and culture.
    (B) Rabies has not been eradicated despite the numerous vaccinations developed.
    (C) Rabies is able to conceal or mask its appearance or presence.
    (D) Rabies has a high fatality rate.

Passage 4

Unlike an electron, a single red blood cell cannot go through two openings at once. Indeed, it is generally true that the physicist seeking to understand the circulation of the blood can ignore most of the perplexities of twentieth-century physics. Given the scale of the circulatory system and the speed of blood flow, neither quantum mechanics nor relativity applies. Instead the flow of blood through the heart and the vascular tree can be adequately described by the familiar mechanics of Newton and Galileo.

If the circulation of the blood obeys the laws of classical mechanics, however, this does not mean that it is simple. An early experimental model of the vascular tree was a system of glass tubes filled with water. But unlike water, blood is not an "ideal" fluid. Instead it is a suspension of cells that, under certain circumstances, can behave in non-Newtonian ways. Moreover, flow through the vascular tree is pulsatile rather than steady; blood vessels taper and are elastic rather than rigid; and flow in any part of the densely interconnected system is affected by flow in neighboring regions. When these factors and the fantastic geometrical complexity of the labyrinthine vascular system are taken into account, the equations of blood flow, while remaining classical in inspiration, quickly become too complex to be solved explicitly.

Confronted with a system of overwhelming complexity, scientists typically resort to the intelligent simplification, that is, to a model. The first mathematical model of the human circulation was the *windkessel*, or compression chamber, model developed by Otto Frank in 1899 to explain how pulsatile flow from the heart is converted into steadier flow in the peripheral circulation. Sophisticated analytical models, the descendants of the windkessel model, still provide insight into the functioning of the circulatory system. But they are increasingly supplemented by numerical models, which exploit the power of the computer to arrive at accurate approximations of values that satisfy systems of equations that would otherwise be unsolvable. The computer can also be used to produce stunning images that allow otherwise cryptic measurements or calculations to be grasped intuitively.

Excerpted from "The Biophysics of Stroke," by George J. Hademenos, The American Scientist, Vol. 85, p. 226, reprinted by permission of *American Scientist*, magazine of Sigma Xi, The Scientific Research Society.

15. Quantum physics and relativity may be ignored by the physicist seeking to understand the circulation of the blood because

    (A) electrons cannot go through two openings at once in the vascular tree.
    (B) the mechanics of Newton and Galileo do not apply.
    (C) the scale of the circulatory system and the speed of blood flow can be adequately described by the mechanics of Newton and Galileo.
    (D) blood is an "ideal" fluid.

16. An early experimental model of the vascular tree

    (A) revealed that blood cannot behave in non-Newtonian ways.
    (B) consisted of a system of glass tubes filled with water.
    (C) was developed by Galileo.
    (D) yielded equations that although complex, could be solved quickly and explicitly.

17. When scientists are confronted with a system of overwhelming complexity, they typically

    (A) give up.
    (B) resort to intelligent simplification, that is, to a model.
    (C) adjust their most arbitrary assumptions accordingly.
    (D) abandon the mechanics of Galileo and Newton.

18. Otto Frank developed the *windkessel* model in 1899 for the purpose of

    (A) explaining how pulsatile flow from the heart is converted into steadier flow in the peripheral circulation.
    (B) improving on previous mathematical models.
    (C) converting the flow of blood from the heart into steadier flow in the peripheral circulation of human subjects.
    (D) augmenting the mechanics of Galileo and Newton.

19. In the twentieth century

    (A) quantum physics and relativity have given us some useful insights into the functioning of the circulatory system.
    (B) the windkessel model is still in use.
    (C) computers have not proved as useful as physicists had hoped since many systems of equations remain unsolvable.
    (D) computers can be used to produce images that allow cryptic measurements or calculations to be grasped intuitively.

Passage 5

A taxonomist viewing insects or crustaceans tends to see tough, jointed exoskeletons and elaborate limbs as their salient features—so salient, in fact, that the taxonomists who named the phylum to which these animals belong called it Arthropoda, or "jointed foot." The same biologist will also notice that the arthropod body plan is that of a modified worm, where the worm's more-or-less uniform series of segmented units becomes well differentiated along the length of the arthropod body. This gives arthropods distinct head, middle, and tail regions.

As neurobiologists considering evolution from simple to more complex animals, we are interested in the changes in the neural circuits serving locomotion and sensory coding that accompanied the transition from worm to arthropod. Such evolution is crucial to the emergence of advanced mobile animals. Because brains and body plans must have evolved in step from their simpler antecedents, comparative studies of neural development and of the mature nervous systems of animals promise to reveal much about arthropod evolution. In arthropods almost every nerve cell grows in a particular pattern and makes specific synaptic connections to form the elaborate neural circuits that give an animal its mobility and control; these features make each cell a recognizable identity.

Just as vertebrae and ribs are serially repeated, sets of neurons are repeated in each segment of an insect's body, or beneath each facet of the compound eye. Using identified neurons, anatomists can compare the development and structure of nervous systems from different arthropods much as they can compare vertebrate skeletons. In addition, we can record the electrical activity from a single neuron, which allows us to compare physiological function in different lineages. So far, most work has been done on insects, but comparisons can also be made between insects and crustaceans. Such comparisons tell biologists how these arthropods, with their jointed exoskeletons and specialized limbs, evolved from simpler ancestors and how they have subsequently diversified during evolutionary history.

Excerpted from "The Evolution of Anthropod Nervous Systems," by Daniel Ororio, Jonathan P. Bacon, and Paul M. Whitington, *The American Scientist*, Vol. 85, p. 244, reprinted by permission of *American Scientist*, magazine of Sigma Xi, The Scientific Research Society.

20. The passage suggests that

    (A) neurobiologists do not agree with taxonomists about the evolution of arthropods from worms.
    (B) the arthropod body plan is that of a modified worm.
    (C) since arthropods evolved from worms, they have no distinct head, middle, and tail regions.
    (D) neurobiologists consider the salient features of insects and crustaceans to be more clearly differentiated than those of arthropods.

21. As worms evolved into arthropods

    (A) the neural circuits serving locomotion and sensory coding changed.
    (B) they maintained a uniform series of segmented units.
    (C) they did not become particularly mobile.
    (D) their neural circuits became more simplified.

22. The name Arthropoda means

    (A) "jointed foot."
    (B) "wormlike."
    (C) "well-differentiated."
    (D) "mobile."

23. The phylum Arthropoda is distinguished by

    (A) a lack of sets of repeated neurons.
    (B) simple neural circuits.
    (C) a tough, jointed exoskeleton.
    (D) opposable thumbs.

24. Using identified neurons, anatomists can compare the development and structure of the nervous systems of different arthropods just as they can compare

    (A) sets of nonrepeating neurons.
    (B) vertebrate skeletons.
    (C) exoskeletons and specialized limbs.
    (D) worms and arthropods.

25. The passage suggests that neurobiologists are seeking to discover more about

    (A) how arthropods evolved from more complex ancestors.
    (B) how arthropods have failed to diversify during their evolutionary history.
    (C) how the neural circuits of insects and crustaceans function.
    (D) how human behavior changes in proximity to arthropods.

Passage 6

Allergic drug reactions account for 5% to 20% of all observed adverse drug reactions. Adverse drug reactions have been reported to occur in as many as 30% of hospitalized patients, and 3% of all hospitalizations are a result of adverse drug reactions. In a computerized surveillance study of over 36,000 hospitalized patients, 731 adverse events were identified. Of those, 1% were categorized as severe, life threatening, and allergic in nature. The potential morbidity and mortality associated with allergic drug reactions is great even though these outcomes occur infrequently.

In order to appropriately diagnose and treat a patient experiencing an allergic reaction, it is necessary to be able to differentiate allergic reactions from other closely related adverse drug reactions. One method of classification divides adverse reactions into those that are "predictable, usually dose-dependent, and related to the pharmacologic actions of the drug," and those that are "unpredictable, often dose independent, and related to the individual's immunologic response or to genetic differences in susceptible patients." Under this classification scheme, drug allergy or drug hypersensitivity is an unpredictable adverse drug reaction that is immunologically mediated.

Excerpted with permission from "Chapter 6, Anaphylaxis and Drug Allergies," page 6-1, Applied Therapeutics: The Clinical Use of Drugs, Sixth Edition, edited by Lloyd Yee Young and Mary Anne Koda-Kimble, published by Applied Therapeutics, Inc., Vancouver, Washington, © 1995.

26. Which of the following is necessary in order to appropriately diagnose and treat a patient experiencing an allergic reaction to a drug?

   (A) A way to differentiate allergic reactions from other adverse drug reactions
   (B) Determination that the reaction is dose-dependent and related to the pharmacological actions of the drug
   (C) Access to appropriate statistics, such as computerized surveillance studies
   (D) Hospitalization

27. If an adverse reaction is not predictable, dose-independent, and related to the pharmacologic actions of the drug, then it is likely to be

   (A) adverse but not allergic.
   (B) unrelated to genetic differences in patients
   (C) related to the individual's immunologic response.
   (D) unrelated to the individual's immunologic response.

28. Allergic drug reactions account for as many as what percent of all observed adverse drug reactions?

   (A) 1% to 5%
   (B) 5% to 20%
   (C) 30%
   (D) 1%

29. Of 731 adverse drug events identified in a surveillance study of over 36,000 patients, 1% were characterized as

   (A) dose-dependent.
   (B) allergic but not severe or life-threatening.
   (C) severe, life-threatening, and allergic in nature.
   (D) adverse but not allergic.

Passage 7

You have seen the photographs, of course: An apple flaring on two sides as a bullet passes through it; tennis balls flattening themselves against rackets; jagged-edge balloons frozen in mid-pop; droplets in mid-drip; bubbles in mid-burst. They were the work of Harold E. Edgerton, an M.I.T. professor whose invention of the stroboscopic flash in the early 1930s made it possible, for the first time, to capture events as fleeting as a millionth of a second.

For decades chemists and solid-state physicists have yearned for a way of observing even more subtle alterations in matter: chemical reactions, or changes of state such as freezing or evaporation. Those changes depend on the breaking of bonds between atoms, a process that can take place in less than a picosecond—millions of times faster than anything Edgerton ever attempted. A fifth of a picosecond, for instance, is all the time it takes for photons entering your retina to trigger chemical changes in a pigment called rhodopsin—a reaction that makes it possible for you to read this article.

Lasers can flash that quickly. But laser light is too coarse a tool to give sharp closeup pictures of matter. Visible wavelengths are thousands of times longer than the space between the atoms in a solid material. Furthermore, visible light tends to interact with the fuzzy outer electron clouds of an atom—not with the tightly bound inner electrons that give a much better idea of where the atom is. For those reasons, physicists studying atomic structure have long relied on much shorter-wavelength radiation: X-rays. Stroboscopic X-ray crystallography, however, has been a long time coming. Now a team at Lawrence Berkeley National Laboratory in Berkeley, California, has taken a step in that direction by generating the shortest X-ray flash ever.

The main problem with X-rays is that their well known tendency to zip through materials makes them an optical nightmare. "You can't steer them the way you can light. It's difficult. You can't make a good mirror that operates at short wavelengths," says Robert W. Schoenlein, a staff scientist who coheaded the Lawrence Berkeley team. To point their X-rays in the right direction, Schoenlein and his colleagues generated them via Thomson scattering, an effect described early in this century by the English physicist J. J. Thomson. "Fast-moving particles such as electrons," Thomson said, "can transfer energy to photons, much as a Ping-Pong paddle energizes a ball." Thus, if you shoot a laser beam into a stream of high-velocity electrons, some of the photons in the beam may pick up enough energy to turn into X-rays. To produce X-ray flashes, some investigators fire a pulse of electrons head-on into a laser beam. The shorter the pulse, the shorter the flash. So far, however, the X-ray flashes have been too long to be useful.

Excerpted from "Flash Point," by Robert J. Coontz Jr., from the January/February 1997 issue of THE SCIENCES, reprinted by permission of The Sciences, 2 East 63rd Street, New York, NY 10021.

30. The passage identifies Harold E. Edgerton as

(A) head of the research team at Lawrence Berkeley National Laboratory.
(B) an English physicist.
(C) an M.I.T. professor who invented the stroboscopic flash.
(D) the discoverer of X-rays in the early 1930s.

31. The time it takes for photons entering your retina to trigger chemical changes in a pigment called rhodopsin is

(A) about a picosecond.
(B) a millionth of a second.
(C) a single pulse.
(D) a fifth of a picosecond.

32. According to Robert W. Schoenlein, the main problem with X-rays is that

(A) they cannot be steered the way light can.
(B) they cannot penetrate through materials.
(C) they make a mirror that operates at short wavelengths.
(D) their flashes are too short to be useful.

33. Physicists studying atomic structure have relied on X-rays rather than lasers because

(A) lasers cannot flash quickly enough.
(B) laser light is too coarse a tool to give good close-up pictures of matter.
(C) visible light tends to interact with the tightly bound inner electron clouds of an atom.
(D) laser wavelength radiation is too short.

34. The main point of this passage is best summarized by which of the following statements?

(A) Robert W. Schoenlein has invented a technique to transfer energy from electrons to photons, much as a Ping-Pong paddle energizes a ball.
(B) Lasers have proved to be the most efficient way to produce sharp close-up pictures of matter.
(C) Robert W. Schoenlein, a staff scientist at Lawrence Berkeley National Laboratory, and his team have succeeded in creating the shortest X-ray flashes ever.
(D) Robert W. Schoenlein and his research team have succeeded in disproving the Thomson effect.

Passage 8

Sulfasalazine, the most frequently prescribed drug for inflammatory bowel disease therapy, has been used commonly for 50 years for the induction of disease remission in patients with mild acute exacerbations of ulcerative colitis. Initial uncontrolled observations of its efficacy indicated that 80% to 90% of patients improved with the use of this agent. The first placebo-controlled trial using objective parameters of efficacy demonstrated that 80% of the treated group improved as compared to 35% receiving placebo. These data were confirmed subsequently, although improvement may not occur until after four weeks of therapy. Sulfasalazine, 250 to 500 mg four times a day, often is considered the drug of choice in ulcerative colitis exacerbation because its efficacy has been demonstrated and because it has less severe adverse effects than corticosteroids. However, controlled trials have shown that corticosteroids may be more prompt in onset of action than sulfasalazine, alone or in combination with corticosteroid, for the treatment of severe acute ulcerative colitis. While comparative efficacy trials are lacking, the combination of sulfasalazine and prednisone does not appear to be detrimental and often has been used in hope of alleviating patients' symptoms.

Excerpted with permission from "Chapter 24, Inflammatory Bowel Disease," page 24-3, Applied Therapeutics: The Clinical Use of Drugs, Sixth Edition, edited by Lloyd Yee Young and Mary Anne Koda-Kimble, published by Applied Therapeutics, Inc., Vancouver, Washington, © 1995.

35. The most frequently prescribed drug for inflammatory bowel disease therapy is

    (A) prednisone.
    (B) sulfasalazine.
    (C) estrogen.
    (D) aspirin.

36. What percentage of the patients in the uncontrolled observation did NOT improve with sulfasalazine therapy?

    (A) 35% to 50%
    (B) 5% to 10%
    (C) 10% to 20%
    (D) 80% to 90%

37. What percentage of the patients in the placebo group in the placebo-controlled trial did NOT improve?

    (A) 35%
    (B) 45%
    (C) 55%
    (D) 65%

38. According to the passage, how many times per day is sulfasalazine given?

    (A) Four
    (B) Five
    (C) Six
    (D) Eight

39. The combination of sulfasalazine and prednisone

    (A) appears to be dangerous.
    (B) offers hope.
    (C) shows no benefit.
    (D) is not recommended.

Passage 9

Angina pectoris can be defined as a sense of discomfort arising in the myocardium as a result of myocardial ischemia in the absence of infarction. Although angina usually implies severe chest pain or discomfort, its presentation is variable. At one extreme, angina may occur predictably with strenuous exercise; at the other, angina may develop unexpectedly with little or no exertion.

Patients who have a reproducible pattern of angina that is associated with a certain level of physical activity have chronic stable angina or exertional angina. In contrast, patients with unstable angina are experiencing new angina or a change in their angina intensity, frequency, or duration. Both chronic stable angina and unstable angina often reflect underlying atherosclerotic narrowing of coronary arteries. Classic Prinzmetal's variant angina, or vasospastic angina, occurs in patients without coronary heart disease and is due to a spasm of the coronary artery that decreases myocardial blood flow. When coronary vasospasm occurs at the site of a fixed atherosclerotic plaque, mixed angina can result.

Silent myocardial ischemia, which is a transient change in myocardial perfusion, function, or electrical activity, can be detected on an electrocardiogram (ECG) in most angina patients. The patient, however, does not experience chest pain or other signs of angina [e.g., jaw pain, shortness of breath] during these episodes. Silent myocardial ischemia also can occur in patients with no angina history.

Excerpted with permission from "Chapter 13, Ischematic Heart Disease: Anginal Syndromes," pages 13-1 to 13-2, Applied Therapeutics: The Clinical Use of Drugs, Sixth Edition, edited by Lloyd Yee Young and Mary Anne Koda-Kimble, published by Applied Therapeutics, Inc., Vancouver, Washington, © 1995.

40. The term angina usually refers to

   (A) headache.
   (B) chest pain.
   (C) athlete's foot.
   (D) sore throat.

41. Angina associated with physical activity is

   (A) Prinzmetal's angina.
   (B) variant angina.
   (C) vasocolonic angina.
   (D) stable angina.

42. Which type of angina occurs in patients without coronary heart disease?

   (A) Variant angina
   (B) Exertional angina
   (C) Prinzmetal's variant angina
   (D) Unstable angina

43. Silent myocardial ischemia

   (A) is atherosclerotic plaque.
   (B) has no consequences.
   (C) is a permanent change in myocardial perfusion, function, or electrical activity.
   (D) is a transient change in myocardial perfusion, function, or electrical activity.

44. Of the titles below, which would best describe the passage?

   (A) Angina—the Silent Killer
   (B) The Different Types of Angina
   (C) Chest Pain
   (D) Treating Chest Pain

Passage 10

Many scientists would agree that prions (pronounced PREE-ons) are the most bizarre pathogenic substances ever discovered. The late renowned physician and researcher Dr. Lewis Thomas called them one of the Seven Wonders of the World. Biologists are still arguing as to their composition. Prions had been an elusive, controversial, and well-kept secret in the medical community but this is no longer true.

A new book, *Deadly Feasts*, written by Pulitzer Prize-winning author Richard Rhodes, reveals much of the mystery surrounding these strange and deadly agents. Rhodes believes prions will be responsible for the next worldwide plague. His concern is plausible; prions have been responsible for the deaths of more than 100,000 cows in Great Britain and other countries. The cattle were suspected of carrying bovine spongiform encephalopathy or BSE (also known as "mad cow disease"). This epidemic in English cattle raises concerns about whether Creutzfeldt-Jakob disease, the human counterpart of BSE, will also increase in incidence.

The known prion diseases are sometimes referred to as transmissible spongiform encephalopathies. They are so named because they frequently cause the brain to become riddled with holes. The diseases are distinguished by long incubation periods and failure to produce an inflammatory response.

Dr. Thomas's decision to place these agents on the Seven Wonders list was based on the fact that no nucleic acid had yet been found among the infectious material. Prions have been found to consist of protein and nothing else. (The word *prion* is derived from the words *proteinaceous* and *infectious*. The letters *o* and *i* were transposed by poetic license.) It has been generally accepted that conveyers of transmissible diseases require genetic material, composed of nucleic acid (DNA or RNA), in order to establish an infection in a host. Even viruses, which are among the simplest microbes, rely on such material to direct the synthesis of the proteins needed for survival and replication.

Prions appear to convert normal protein molecules into dangerous ones simply by inducing the benign molecules to change shape. Much of the infectious nature of a prion appears to depend on the similarity of prion protein (PrP) between species. The degree of similarity between bovine and human PrP may therefore be an important determinant of the risk of infection.

45. The passage indicates that Creutzfeld-Jakob disease is

    (A) responsible for the deaths of 100,000 sheep.
    (B) a controversial and well-kept secret.
    (C) the human counterpart of BSE (bovine spongiform encephalopathy).
    (D) "mad cow disease."

46. Dr. Thomas decided to place prions on the Seven Wonders list because

    (A) prions have highly unusual DNA.
    (B) no nucleic acid was found among the infectious material.
    (C) prions have no proteins.
    (D) prions cause the brain to become riddled with holes.

47. Prions appear to convert normal protein molecules into dangerous ones by

    (A) inducing benign molecules to change shape.
    (B) using their DNA to direct the synthesis of dangerous proteins.
    (C) using their RNA to direct the synthesis of dangerous proteins.
    (D) inducing hostile molecules to change shape.

48. The word *prion* is derived from

    (A) proteinaceous and infectious.
    (B) the name of Pulitzer Prize-winning author Richard Prion.
    (C) peritoneal infection.
    (D) protein imbalance.

49. The new book *Deadly Feasts* warns that

    (A) prions will be responsible for the next worldwide plague.
    (B) prions will wipe out cattle herds worldwide.
    (C) prions will become our deadliest viruses.
    (D) prions cannot be defeated until their DNA is understood.

50. The known prion diseases are characterized by

    (A) short incubation periods.
    (B) failure to produce an inflammatory response.
    (C) frequently causing benign brain tumors.
    (D) production of an inflammatory response.

Answer Key
READING COMPREHENSION

1. D	11. B	21. A	31. D	41. D
2. B	12. B	22. A	32. A	42. C
3. D	13. C	23. C	33. B	43. D
4. B	14. C	24. B	34. C	44. B
5. B	15. C	25. C	35. B	45. C
6. A	16. B	26. A	36. C	46. B
7. B	17. B	27. C	37. D	47. A
8. D	18. A	28. B	38. A	48. A
9. A	19. D	29. C	39. B	49. A
10. C	20. B	30. C	40. B	50. B

EXPLANATORY ANSWERS

The numbers in the margins of the reprinted passages indicate the statements in which the answer to the questions can be found.

PASSAGE 1

In the past two decades, people living in the northeastern, north-central, and western United States have unwittingly entered a dangerous enzootic cycle—a cycle of disease that typically is restricted to wildlife. Wild mammals and birds host a wide variety of disease agents, with effects ranging from mild symptoms to mortality, but in most cases the pathogen affects only one or a few host species and never
1 causes disease in humans. However, as a result of a complicated sequence of events, people have become frequent accidental hosts for ticks and the disease agents they carry, including a corkscrew-shaped bacterium called *Borrelia burgdorferi,* the agent
4 of Lyme disease. As of 1995, cases of Lyme disease had been reported in 48 of the 50 states and appear to be increasing, both in numbers of people affected and in geographic distribution.

Where does this disease come from, why has it emerged so rapidly, and what can people do to reduce their risk of exposure? It is possible to address these questions not from a medical point of view, but rather from an ecological one. All living organisms—from the *B. burgdorferi* bacterium and the ticks it infects to the mice and deer on which the ticks feed—form an ecological relationship with their habi-
2 tats. Understanding the complex interactions between plant and animal species within those habitats may help people to predict the places where they are most likely to encounter disease-bearing ticks and become infected. Thus armed, individuals may ultimately be able to protect themselves from Lyme disease.

3 Currently, to prevent Lyme disease people wear protective clothing when they are in wooded areas and perform "tick checks" after leaving the woods. One underemphasized means to avoid exposure to Lyme disease, however, is avoiding the most heavily tick-infested habitats at the times of year when ticks are most abundant or dangerous. Recent research has suggested that such habitats can be predicted, often well in advance. Ultimately, it is the hope of ecologists studying this problem that we can use our expertise in pinpointing these habitats to warn the public away from areas that are likely to contain an abundance of disease-carrying ticks.

1. **(D)** The first paragraph clearly describes how humans have accidentally become hosts to ticks and pathogens such as *Borrelia burgdorferi.* While answer B is a true statement, it is not the primary focus of the paragraph. Answers A and C are not true.

2. **(B)** While A and D might well be sound ecological goals in other circumstances, when it comes to Lyme disease, ecologists are motivated by a desire to help people predict and avoid the places where they are likely to become infected (B). Although C is an important medical consideration, the development of a vaccine is not the province of ecologists.

3. **(D)** As stated in the last paragraph of the passage, preventative steps in remaining Lyme disease–free include wearing protective clothing (a step taken prior to exploring the woods) and performing physical "tick checks" after leaving the woods. The remaining answer choices are not true.

4. **(B)** Answer B is a true statement, taken directly from the passage. Answer A states the opposite of the truth, and C and D each combine a false statement with a true one.

5. **(B)** Answer B states the main point of the passage. Answer A is mentioned as an often-used, rather than an underemployed protective measure. Answers C and D are irrelevant.

PASSAGE 2

To the average physician, Lyme disease is suspected when a patient arrives at a clinic or hospital complaining of a strange bull's-eye rash, known as erythema migrans, or EM, together with one or more flulike symptoms, such as fever, chills, muscle aches, or lethargy. The doctor will take a blood sample for laboratory confirmation, but will feel quite confident to make a diagnosis of Lyme disease after noting the telltale combination of symptoms, as well as the circumstances surrounding the infection. The patient will undoubtedly have been bitten by the black-legged tick *Ixodes scaplaris*, formerly called the deer tick, or a close relative, which transferred to him or her the *B. burgdorferi* bacterium. Most likely, the doctor will prescribe an oral course of antibiotics and will duly report the case to the county or state health department, which will include it in the morbidity statistics for Lyme disease.

Accurate diagnosis and effective treatment of Lyme disease are not always so straightforward, particularly in regions of the country newly invaded by the epidemic. In these regions, health care professionals and the public need to be educated about the confusing and generalized symptoms, the generally poor, but growing, accuracy of lab tests, and the efficacy of various antibiotic treatments. If Lyme disease is left untreated for some time, *B. burgdorferi* may persist in the patient's tissues and can migrate to the central and peripheral nervous system or to joints and cause more severe late-stage symptoms, which include arthritis and neurological disorders, such as dizziness, memory loss and disorientation. Vaccines that protect against Lyme disease are now being field tested by pharmaceutical companies, but none has yet been approved by the Food and Drug Administration for public use. Even if an effective vaccine were certified and marketed, the primary means that individuals have of protecting themselves against the disease is avoiding the tick in the first place.

6. **(A)** In order for the pathogen *B. burgdorferi* to pass from tick to human, the human must be bitten by the tick—in this case, the black-legged tick, *Ixodes scaplaris*. A tick-bearing mammal (B) might provide the tick, but not the bite. The microbe *B. burgdorferi* is not capable of biting, so C cannot be correct. Answer D is irrelevant (Lyme disease is not airborne).

7. **(B)** Because the passage discusses both diagnosis of and strategies to treat Lyme disease, as well as challenges in addressing Lyme disease such as lack of public awareness, answer B represents the most appropriate title. Answer A addresses only one part of the passage, a similar problem with answers C and D.

8. **(D)** As noted in the second paragraph of the passage, Lyme disease can migrate to joints, which belong to the musculoskeletal system.

9. **(A)** As stated in the passage, the physician will take a blood sample to get laboratory confirmation of the diagnosis. Answers B, C, and D are not true.

10. **(C)** Answer A is not addressed in the paragraph. Answer B is false since leaving the disease untreated is not mentioned in the passage as having any effect on lab tests; D is neither stated nor implied in the passage. The result of leaving Lyme disease untreated is clearly described in C.

PASSAGE 3

14   Rabies is a master dissembler. No other disease so completely manipulates its stricken host while barely leaving a trace of its presence. And rabies is preeminently
11   adaptive: even if one host species is eliminated, the virus resurfaces in another. It bides its time, shadowing its victims, waiting for new hosts to emerge as people disrupt habitats and force animals to congregate more densely. Despite the war chest of vaccines designed to stop it and the near-certain death of every organism infected by it, rabies persists.

12   In the United States, on average, fewer than two people a year die of rabies, about the same number as in Western Europe. Vaccination and animal control policies
13   ensure that few, if any, of those cases come from dog bites. Worldwide, between 20,000 and 100,000 people die of rabies in a given year, most of them in develop-
13   ing countries, and some 10 million are treated annually for possible exposures, mostly from dog bites. Compared with the dangers of becoming infected with HIV, tuberculosis or malaria, each of which strikes millions of people every year, the risk of contracting rabies is vanishingly small. But rabies has had far greater influence on culture and science than its current incidence might suggest. And its devastating effects assure that it is never far from people's minds. Rabies has the highest fatality rate of any known human infection.

11. **(B)** Answer B states a fact taken directly from the passage. Answers A, C, and D are not true.

12. **(B)** Although you might be tempted to complete the statement with an incorrect figure (A), B is actually stated in the passage. Both C and D are false.

13. **(C)** C is true. Answers A, B, and D are false.

14. **(C)** Although statements A, B, and D are factually true, they do not address the question regarding the meaning of the description of rabies as a "master dissembler." "Dissembler" means to give a false or misleading appearance or conceal one's true nature. It is a fitting descriptor for rabies, as the presence of the disease is barely detectable in an infected individual despite its insidious impact.

PASSAGE 4

Unlike an electron, a single red blood cell cannot go through two openings at once. <u>Indeed, it is generally true that the physicist seeking to understand the circulation of the blood can ignore most of the perplexities of twentieth century physics. Given the scale of the circulatory system and the speed of blood flow, neither quantum mechanics nor relativity applies. Instead the flow of blood through the heart and the vascular tree can be adequately described by the familiar mechanics of Newton and Galileo.</u> 15

If the circulation of the blood obeys the laws of classical mechanics, however, this does not mean that it is simple. <u>An early experimental model of the vascular tree was a system of glass tubes filled with water.</u> But unlike water, blood is not an "ideal" fluid. Instead it is a suspension of cells that, under certain circumstances, can behave in non-Newtonian ways. Moreover, flow through the vascular tree is pulsatile rather than steady; blood vessels taper and are elastic rather than rigid; and flow in any part of the densely interconnected system is affected by flow in neighboring regions. When these factors and the fantastic geometrical complexity of the labyrinthine vascular system are taken into account, the equations of blood flow, while remaining classical in inspiration, quickly become too complex to be solved explicitly. 16

<u>Confronted with a system of overwhelming complexity, scientists typically resort to the intelligent simplification, that is, to a model.</u> <u>The first mathematical model of the human circulation was the *windkessel*, or compression chamber, model developed by Otto Frank in 1899 to explain how pulsatile flow from the heart is converted into steadier flow in the peripheral circulation.</u> Sophisticated analytical models, the descendants of the *windkessel* model, still provide insight into the functioning of the circulatory system. But they are increasingly supplemented by numerical models, which exploit the power of the computer to arrive at accurate approximations of values that satisfy systems of equations that would otherwise be unsolvable. <u>The computer can also be used to produce stunning images that allow otherwise cryptic measurements or calculations to be grasped intuitively.</u> 17 18 19

15. **(C)** The passage states that the mechanics of Newton and Galileo are adequate for describing the circulatory system and blood flow. Answer A is irrelevant; B and D contradict information given in the passage.

16. **(B)** As described in the passage, an early experimental model was a system of glass tubes filled with water. Answer A is irrelevant; C is false; and D is both false and absurd.

17. **(B)** According to the passage, scientists are likely to turn to a model when confronted with a system of overwhelming complexity. Answers A and D are decidedly untrue; in fact, D contradicts information given in the passage.

18. **(A)** As stated in the passage, Frank developed his *windkessel* model of the circulatory system to explain how pulsatile flow from the heart is converted into steadier flow in the peripheral circulation. Since he made use of the model, not human subjects, the answer cannot be C (which is a nonsense statement anyway). His was the first mathematical model, so B cannot be

correct, and Frank was not attempting to augment the mechanics of Galileo and Newton (D).

19. **(D)** As the passage indicates, quantum physics and relativity are not relevant to the study of the circulatory system, so A cannot be the correct answer. Nor is B correct, since the windkessel dates back to 1899 and is no longer in use. Answer C contradicts information stated in the passage. Only D actually occurs as a statement in the passage.

PASSAGE 5

23   A taxonomist viewing insects or crustaceans tends to see tough, jointed exoskeletons and elaborate limbs as their salient features—so salient, in fact, that the tax-

22   onomists who named the phylum to which these animals belong called it Arthropoda, or "jointed foot." The same biologist will also notice that the arthro-

20   pod body plan is that of a modified worm, where the worm's more-or-less uniform series of segmented units becomes well differentiated along the length of the arthropod body. This gives arthropods distinct head, middle and tail regions.

21   As neurobiologists considering evolution from simple to more complex animals, we are interested in the changes in the neural circuits serving locomotion and sensory coding that accompanied the transition from worm to arthropod. Such evolution is crucial to the emergence of advanced mobile animals. Because brains and body plans must have evolved in step from their simpler antecedents, comparative studies of neural development and of the mature nervous systems of animals promise to reveal much about arthropod evolution. In arthropods almost every nerve cell grows in a particular pattern and makes specific synaptic connections to form the elaborate neural circuits that give an animal its mobility and control; these features make each cell a recognizable identity.

Just as vertebrae and ribs are serially repeated, sets of neurons are repeated in each segment of an insect's body, or beneath each facet of the compound eye. Using iden-

24   tified neurons, anatomists can compare the development and structure of nervous systems from different arthropods much as they can compare vertebrate skeletons.

25   In addition, we can record the electrical activity from a single neuron, which allows us to compare physiological function in different lineages. So far, most work has been done on insects, but comparisons can also be made between insects and crustaceans. Such comparisons tell biologists how these arthropods, with their jointed exoskeletons and specialized limbs, evolved from simpler ancestors and how they have subsequently diversified during evolutionary history.

20. **(B)** The passage states that the arthropod body plan is that of a modified worm (B). A contradicts information given in the passage, as does C; D is a nonsense statement since insects and crustaceans are arthropods.

21. **(A)** The passage states A as a change that took place as worms evolved into arthropods. Answers B, C, and D are false.

22. **(A)** As the passage states, arthropod means "jointed foot." Answers B, C, and D are false.

23. **(C)** Answers A and B contradict information given in the passage, but answer C is accurate. Answer D is not true.

24. **(B)** The passage draws an analogy between the work done by anatomists who compare neurons to learn more about the development and structure of the nervous systems of different arthropods and the work done by anatomists who compare the skeletons of different vertebrates. Answers A, C, and D do not make sense in the context of the passage.

25. **(C)** The passage directly mentions answer C as a subject that neurobiologists are seeking to discover more about. Answers A and B contradict information in the passage. Answer D is not discussed in the passage.

PASSAGE 6

Allergic drug reactions account for 5% to 20% of all observed adverse drug reactions. Adverse drug reactions have been reported to occur in as many as 30% of hospitalized patients, and 3% of all hospitalizations are a result of adverse drug reactions. In a computerized surveillance study of over 36,000 hospitalized patients, 731 adverse events were identified. Of those, 1% were categorized as severe, life threatening, and allergic in nature. The potential morbidity and mortality associated with allergic drug reactions is great even though these outcomes occur infrequently.

In order to appropriately diagnose and treat a patient experiencing an allergic reaction, it is necessary to be able to differentiate allergic reactions from other closely related adverse drug reactions. One method of classification divides adverse reactions into those that are "predictable, usually dose-dependent, and related to the pharmacologic actions of the drug," and those that are "unpredictable, often dose independent, and are related to the individual's immunologic response or to genetic differences in susceptible patients." Under this classification scheme, drug allergy or drug hypersensitivity is an unpredictable adverse drug reaction that is immunologically mediated.

26. **(A)** As the passage states, allergic reactions must be differentiated from other closely related adverse drug reactions. Answer B describes reactions that are typically adverse but not allergic, and C is irrelevant to diagnosing and treating allergic drug reactions appropriately. While some allergic reactions may require hospitalization (D), this is not necessary to diagnose appropriately and treat all allergic reactions to drugs.

27. **(C)** C appears in the passage. A, B, and D are not true.

28. **(B)** According to the passage, 5% to 20% of all observed drug reactions represent allergic drug reactions.

29. **(C)** That 1% of the 731 adverse drug events were characterized as severe, life-threatening, and allergic in nature is stated in the passage (C). Answer B is only partially true, since the allergic reactions identified were of a severe and life-threatening nature. Both A and D refer to adverse reactions that are not classified as allergic.

PASSAGE 7

You have seen the photographs, of course: An apple flaring on two sides as a bullet passes through it; tennis balls flattening themselves against rackets; jagged-edge balloons frozen in mid-pop; droplets in mid-drip; bubbles in mid-burst. <u>They</u>
30 <u>were the work of Harold E. Edgerton, an M.I.T. professor whose invention of the</u> <u>stroboscopic flash in the early 1930s made it possible, for the first time, to capture</u> <u>events as fleeting as a millionth of a second.</u>

For decades chemists and solid-state physicists have yearned for a way of observing even more subtle alterations in matter: chemical reactions, or changes of state such as freezing or evaporation. Those changes depend on the breaking or forging of bonds between atoms, a process that can take place in less than a picosecond—millions of times faster than anything Edgerton ever attempted. <u>A fifth of a picosec-</u>
31 <u>ond, for instance, is all the time it takes for photons entering your retina to trigger</u> <u>chemical changes in a pigment called rhodopsin—a reaction that makes it possible</u> <u>for you to read this article.</u>

33 <u>Lasers can flash that quickly. But laser light is too coarse a tool to give sharp</u> <u>closeup pictures of matter. Visible wavelengths are thousands of times longer than</u> <u>the space between the atoms in a solid material. Furthermore, visible light tends to</u> <u>interact with the fuzzy outer electron clouds of an atom—not with the tightly</u> <u>bound inner electrons that give a much better idea of where the atom is. For those</u> <u>reasons, physicists studying atomic structure have long relied on much shorter-</u> <u>wavelength radiation: X rays.</u> Stroboscopic X-ray crystallography, however, has been
34 a long time coming. <u>Now a team at Lawrence Berkeley National Laboratory in</u> <u>Berkeley, California, has taken a step in that direction by generating the shortest</u> <u>X-ray flash ever.</u>

The main problem with X rays is that their well known tendency to zip through
32 materials makes them an optical nightmare. <u>"You can't steer them the way you can</u> <u>light. It's difficult. You can't make a good mirror that operates at short wavelengths,"</u>
34 <u>says Robert W. Schoenlein, a staff scientist who coheaded the Lawrence Berkeley</u> <u>team.</u> To point their X rays in the right direction, Schoenlein and his colleagues generated them via Thomson scattering, an effect described early in this century by the English physicist J. J. Thomson. "Fast-moving particles such as electrons," Thomson said, "can transfer energy to photons, much as a Ping-Pong paddle energizes a ball." Thus, if you shoot a laser beam into a stream of high-velocity electrons, some of the photons in the beam may pick up enough energy to turn into X rays. To produce X-ray flashes, some investigators fire a pulse of electrons head-on into a laser beam. The shorter the pulse, the shorter the flash. So far, however, the X-ray flashes have been too long to be useful.

30. **(C)** The passage identifies Harold E. Edgerton as an M.I.T. professor who invented the stroboscopic flash.

31. **(D)** A precise figure is required here. According to the passage, the correct answer is a fifth of a picosecond.

32. **(A)** Schoenlein is quoted in the passage as complaining about A. Answers B, C, and D are contradicted in the passage.

33. **(B)** The passage reports that physicists have had problems with B, but not A, since lasers do flash quickly enough. C and D are not true.

34. **(C)** The main thrust of the passage is that Shoenlein and his team have created the shortest X-ray flashes ever (even if they are still not short enough to be truly useful). Answer A is false, since this technique was described in the early 1900s by the English physicist J. J. Thomson. Answer B contradicts information given in the passage, and D is untrue because Schoenlein's research depends on the Thomson effect.

PASSAGE 8

Sulfasalazine, the most frequently prescribed drug for inflammatory bowel 35
disease therapy, has been used commonly for 50 years for the induction of disease remission in patients with mild acute exacerbations of ulcerative colitis. Initial uncontrolled observations of its efficacy indicated that 80% to 90% of patients 36 improved with the use of this agent. The first placebo-controlled trial using objective parameters of efficacy demonstrated that 80% of the treated group improved as 37 compared to 35% receiving placebo. These data were confirmed subsequently, although improvement may not occur until after four weeks of therapy. Sulfasalazine, 250 to 500 mg four times a day, often is considered the drug of choice 38 in ulcerative colitis exacerbation because its efficacy has been demonstrated and because it has less severe adverse effects than corticosteroids. However, controlled trials have shown that corticosteroids may be more prompt in onset of action than sulfasalazine, alone or in combination with corticosteroid, for the treatment of severe acute ulcerative colitis. While comparative efficacy trials are lacking, the combination of sulfasalazine and prednisone does not appear to be detrimental and 39 often has been used in hope of alleviating patients' symptoms.

35. **(B)** Although prednisone (A) is used to treat inflammatory bowel disease, the first sentence of the passage states clearly that the most frequently prescribed drug for inflammatory bowel disease therapy is sulfasalazine. Ulcerative colitis (C) is a type of inflammatory bowel disease. Answer D is not true.

36. **(C)** The passage states that 80% to 90% of patients improved during the initial uncontrolled observations, leaving 10% to 20% who did not improve.

37. **(D)** The passage states 35% of patients in the placebo group improved, leaving 65% who did not improve.

38. **(A)** Sulfasalazine is given four times per day at doses of 250–500 mg.

39. **(B)** The passage clearly states that the combination of sulfasalazine and prednisone does not appear to be detrimental (dangerous, A) and often has been used in hope of alleviating patients' symptoms.

PASSAGE 9

Angina pectoris can be defined as a sense of discomfort arising in the myocardium as a result of myocardial ischemia in the absence of infarction. Although angina 40 usually implies severe chest pain or discomfort, its presentation is variable. At one extreme, angina may occur predictably with strenuous exercise; at the other, angina may develop unexpectedly with little or no exertion.

41 Patients who have a reproducible pattern of angina that is associated with a certain level of physical activity have chronic stable angina or exertional angina. In contrast, patients with unstable angina are experiencing new angina or a change in their angina intensity, frequency, or duration. Both chronic stable angina and unstable angina often reflect underlying atherosclerotic narrowing of coronary arteries.

42 Classic Prinzmetal's variant angina, or vasospastic angina, occurs in patients without coronary heart disease and is due to a spasm of the coronary artery that decreases myocardial blood flow. When coronary vasospasm occurs at the site of a fixed atherosclerotic plaque, mixed angina can result.

43 Silent myocardial ischemia, which is a transient change in myocardial perfusion, function, or electrical activity, can be detected on an electrocardiogram (ECG) in most angina patients. The patient, however, does not experience chest pain or other signs of angina [e.g., jaw pain, shortness of breath] during these episodes. Silent myocardial ischemia also can occur in patients with no angina history.

40. **(B)** Although a headache (A) may accompany chest pain (B), angina usually implies severe chest pain. Answer C is absurd in the context of the passage. Answer D is not true.

41. **(D)** Prinzmetal's and variant angina (A and B) are due to a spasm of the coronary artery. There is no such disorder as vasocolonic angina. Angina that is associated with a certain level of physical activity is called stable angina or exertional angina.

42. **(C)** The passage states that Prinzmetal's variant angina occurs in patients without coronary heart disease. Answers A, B, and D are untrue.

43. **(D)** The passage states that silent myocardial ischemia is a transient change in myocardial perfusion, function, or electrical activity, therefore answer D is correct, while C is incorrect. Silent myocardial ischemia is not atherosclerotic plaque (A), although atherosclerotic plaque may cause ischemia. Myocardial ischemia can cause serious damage (consequences, B).

44. **(B)** Since the passage does not discuss the mortality rates associated with angina or the treatment of chest pain, answers A and D are incorrect. Chest pain (C) is too broad a title for this passage. Answer B, The Different Types of Angina, best describes the focus of this passage.

PASSAGE 10

Many scientists would agree that prions (pronounced PREE-ons) are the most bizarre pathogenic substances ever discovered. The late, renowned physician and researcher Dr. Lewis Thomas called them one of the Seven Wonders of the World. Biologists are still arguing as to their composition. Prions had been an elusive, controversial, and well-kept secret in the medical community but this is no longer true.

A new book, *Deadly Feasts*, written by Pulitzer Prize-winning author Richard   49
Rhodes, reveals much of the mystery surrounding these strange and deadly agents. Rhodes believes prions will be responsible for the next worldwide plague. His concern is plausible; prions have been responsible for the deaths of more than 100,000 cows in Great Britain and other countries. The cattle were suspected of carrying bovine spongiform encephalopathy or BSE (also known as "mad cow disease"). This epidemic in English cattle raises concerns about whether Creutzfeldt-Jakob   45
disease, the human counterpart of BSE, will also increase in incidence.

The known prion diseases are sometimes referred to as transmissible spongiform encephalopathies. They are so named because they frequently cause the brain to become riddled with holes. The diseases are distinguished by long incubation   50
periods and failure to produce an inflammatory response.

Dr. Thomas's decision to place these agents on the Seven Wonders list was based   46
on the fact that no nucleic acid had yet been found among the infectious material. Prions have been found to consist of protein and nothing else. (The word *prion* is   48
derived from the words *proteinaceous* and *infectious*. The letters *o* and *i* were transposed by poetic license.) It has been generally accepted that conveyers of transmissible diseases require genetic material, composed of nucleic acid (DNA or RNA), in order to establish an infection in a host. Even viruses, which are among the simplest microbes, rely on such material to direct the synthesis of the proteins needed for survival and replication.

Prions appear to convert normal protein molecules into dangerous ones simply   47
by inducing the benign molecules to change shape. Much of the infectious nature of a prion appears to depend on the similarity of prion protein (PrP) between species. The degree of similarity between bovine and human PrP may therefore be an important determinant of the risk of infection.

45. **(C)** Creutzfeldt-Jakob disease is the human counterpart of BSE, according to the passage. Answer A is false (prions killed more than 100,000 cows, not sheep, according to the passage). Answer B refers to prions in general rather than to Creutzfeld-Jakob disease; D is BSE, a disease of animals.

46. **(B)** Prions are regarded as an oddity because they have no nucleic acid and consist only of protein. Both A and C, therefore, are false. D is definitely a result of diseases caused by prions but is not the reason that Thomas placed them on the Seven Wonders list.

47. **(A)** That prions appear to induce benign molecules to change shape is the only true statement. Since prions have no nucleic acid, they have neither RNA nor DNA, thereby ruling out B and C. Answer D is incorrect.

48. **(A)** The word *prion* is formed from two adjectives, proteinaceous and infectious. "Richard Prion" (B) is not mentioned in the passage although the passage states that Richard Rhodes is the Pulitzer Prize-winning author of *Deadly Feasts*. Answers C and D are incorrect.

49. **(A)** The passage warns that prions will be responsible for the next worldwide plague. While theoretically possible, B is not mentioned in the passage; C is clearly false (prions are not viruses), and D is false as well (prions have no DNA).

50. **(B)** Prion diseases are characterized by B. Answers A, C, and D are incorrect.

The PCAT Essay

CHAPTER 9

PCAT WRITING TEST

The writing section of the PCAT presents a topic that requires you to write a short literary composition as a "problem-solving" essay. The problem-solving essay topic is presented in the form of a statement that poses a problem to be solved. The essay should present and coherently explain your suggested solution to the problem presented in the statement, as well as possible alternatives to the primary solution being presented. The writing sections are scored according to two writing rubrics: "Conventions of Language" and "Problem Solving."

You will not be able to use a dictionary or any other reference material(s). You will have 30 minutes to complete the essay. You should allow yourself enough time to determine what your response to the topic will be (brainstorm), to organize and write your essay (you may find that writing a quick outline may help with this), and to edit and proofread your response. The greatest portion of the 30-minute time allotment should be spent writing the essay; remember to pace yourself and to keep track of time. As with the other sections of the PCAT, the essay will be written on the computer using the computer-based platform provided at the testing center.

TIP

Be sure to present and coherently explain your suggested solution to the problem.

PCAT WRITING SECTION SCORES

On the PCAT score report, you will receive a score for the writing test as well as the mean of all writing scores for the same test administration period. The score on the writing test will utilize a six-point scale, ranging from 1 = "Inadequate" to 6 = "Superior." The six score possibilities for each rubric are characterized on the next page, as outlined on the PCAT website (*www.pcatweb.info*).

The writing score will be included on the score report received by the candidate and sent to those institutions chosen by the candidate. However, the score is not incorporated into the composite scaled or percentile scores of the PCAT. Some schools do not use the PCAT writing score at all in their admission processes. Please confirm with the school you are interested in as to what they do with the PCAT writing score as it relates to your candidacy evaluation.

Writing Section Score	Conventions of Language Description
One—"Inadequate"	Application of the conventions of language is limited.
Two–"Marginal"	Several mistakes distract from the essay response that is being presented, and the ability to fully understand the points of the essay may be diminished.
Three–"Satisfactory"	There are several mistakes in structure that may interfere with the ease of the essay's interpretation, but the basic structural pattern (beginning, middle, end) is intact.
Four–"Effective"	While there are several mistakes in structure that may interfere with the essay's flow, the general meaning is not compromised.
Five–"Proficient"	Overall, the writer correctly applies the conventions of language. There may be slight errors, but they do not interfere with understanding of the points intended or the flow of the essay.
Six–"Superior"	Few, if any, errors are made and the writer exhibits good technique in presentation of the essay components.

Writing Section Score	Problem-Solving Description
One—"Inadequate"	The relationship between the problem and the solution is not clear, support is unconvincing, and the organization is problematic.
Two—"Marginal"	Although the solution is related to the problem, the structure of the essay detracts from the flow of ideas, the essay lacks a logical argument, and the solution is not clear.
Three—"Satisfactory"	The essay's solution is adequately related to the problem, but too general in presentation to be persuasive, and organization may be weak.
Four—"Effective"	The essay's solution is clear, but too general in presentation, and organization may be weak so as to lessen the effectiveness of the argument.
Five—"Proficient"	The essay shows a clear relationship between problem and solution. However, while support is appropriate and logical, it lacks depth.
Six—"Superior"	The essay presents a clear, well-reasoned relationship between problem and solution with convincing support and a powerful argument. Organization has logical flow.

PCAT ESSAY WRITING TIPS

There are many existing guides and tutorials that discuss the construction of an effective essay. For additional guidance on how to write a persuasive essay, refer to *www.hamilton.edu/writing/writing-resources/persuasive-essays* (please note that this website is not specific to the PCAT). You must keep in mind the 30-minute time limit for the PCAT writing section. Below are several tips you can use to help compose an essay.

- The introduction paragraph is the first paragraph of your essay. In your introduction, include some background information and the problem to be solved based on the topic. Use a clear thesis statement to present the topic and inform the reader as to what the essay will be about.
- Follow your introduction with one or more supporting paragraphs to make up the main body of your essay. It is important to develop each point in your essay in a properly structured paragraph. Make sure there is a link between your thesis and the supporting paragraphs. Present applicable and appropriate references based on academic studies or personal experiences.
- Use clear and simple structure to your sentences. Avoid the use of clichés, slang, jargon, and abstract terms that tend to fill space but provide no specific points in your essay. Elaborate on your ideas, leading the reader to your conclusions. You are to present a solution or build a case in support of your viewpoint.
- Use a clear writing style. Avoid redundant words, long sentences, and vague information. Do not use 35 words when five words will efficiently and effectively present your information. Write concisely and cover the topic presented.
- Use appropriate grammar, punctuation, usage, and style. Avoid abbreviations and acronyms when possible.
- Finish with a conclusion, either as a statement or a closing paragraph after the main body of your essay. It is important that your conclusion logically follow the points you have developed in the supporting paragraphs of the essay.
- Always proofread your essay. Glaring or frequent spelling or grammatical errors could be construed as poor writing.

Practice Essay Questions

(Please note, in 2014 the actual PCAT exam will have only one question/writing section.)

Directions: Write a well-constructed essay addressing the statement below.

According to the Centers for Disease Control and Prevention, obesity has doubled in children and tripled in adolescents over the past three decades, resulting in increased risk for cardiovascular disease and diabetes, among other disease states. Discuss a solution to the problem of childhood obesity and its associated health risks.

Directions: Write a well-constructed essay addressing the statement below.

Although controversial, some research has suggested that graphic and violent television programming may negatively impact the behavior of children. Discuss a solution to the problem that may be posed by graphic and violent television programming regarding its influence on children.

PRACTICE TESTS
AND ANSWERS

Practice Test 1

This sample PCAT is not a copy of an actual PCAT, but it has been designed to closely represent the types of questions that may be included in an actual exam. As in the actual PCAT, this test has six separate sections—Verbal Ability, Biology, Chemistry, Quantitative Ability, Reading Comprehension, and a Writing section. The actual PCAT may have additional experimental questions that are being tested for use on future exams. Because the experimental questions do not count toward your actual PCAT score, there are no equivalent questions included in this sample PCAT. It is important to do your best on every question since you will not be able to distinguish the experimental questions.

You may find it best to proceed with this practice exam as if you were taking the actual PCAT by adhering to the time allowed for each section in the table below. Your overall strategy should be to answer every question in the time allotted, while getting as many correct answers as possible. Do not leave any questions unanswered, as there will be no penalty for guessing on the actual PCAT. Your score on this sample PCAT will give you a good idea of the subject areas you need to study further. By timing yourself on the sample PCAT, you will also learn whether you need to increase your speed or slow down when you take the actual PCAT.

After completing the sample PCAT, you may grade your exam by using the answer key. Regardless of your score on the sample PCAT, it will benefit you to review all the explanatory answers at the end of the sample PCAT. If your answer to a question was incorrect, the explanation may help you understand where you went wrong. If your answer was correct, the explanation may broaden your understanding of the topic area being tested.

Before starting the exam, please refresh your memory on the test-taking strategies discussed earlier in this book. Good luck on the examination.

Section	Time Allowed*
1. Verbal Ability	25 minutes
2. Biology	35 minutes
3. Chemistry	35 minutes
4. Quantitative Ability	45 minutes
5. Reading Comprehension	50 minutes
6. Writing (Essay)	30 minutes

*Please note: The order of the subjects (test sections) may vary from test to test.

Answer Sheet
PRACTICE TEST 1

Verbal Ability (1–40)

1 Ⓐ Ⓑ Ⓒ Ⓓ	11 Ⓐ Ⓑ Ⓒ Ⓓ	21 Ⓐ Ⓑ Ⓒ Ⓓ	31 Ⓐ Ⓑ Ⓒ Ⓓ
2 Ⓐ Ⓑ Ⓒ Ⓓ	12 Ⓐ Ⓑ Ⓒ Ⓓ	22 Ⓐ Ⓑ Ⓒ Ⓓ	32 Ⓐ Ⓑ Ⓒ Ⓓ
3 Ⓐ Ⓑ Ⓒ Ⓓ	13 Ⓐ Ⓑ Ⓒ Ⓓ	23 Ⓐ Ⓑ Ⓒ Ⓓ	33 Ⓐ Ⓑ Ⓒ Ⓓ
4 Ⓐ Ⓑ Ⓒ Ⓓ	14 Ⓐ Ⓑ Ⓒ Ⓓ	24 Ⓐ Ⓑ Ⓒ Ⓓ	34 Ⓐ Ⓑ Ⓒ Ⓓ
5 Ⓐ Ⓑ Ⓒ Ⓓ	15 Ⓐ Ⓑ Ⓒ Ⓓ	25 Ⓐ Ⓑ Ⓒ Ⓓ	35 Ⓐ Ⓑ Ⓒ Ⓓ
6 Ⓐ Ⓑ Ⓒ Ⓓ	16 Ⓐ Ⓑ Ⓒ Ⓓ	26 Ⓐ Ⓑ Ⓒ Ⓓ	36 Ⓐ Ⓑ Ⓒ Ⓓ
7 Ⓐ Ⓑ Ⓒ Ⓓ	17 Ⓐ Ⓑ Ⓒ Ⓓ	27 Ⓐ Ⓑ Ⓒ Ⓓ	37 Ⓐ Ⓑ Ⓒ Ⓓ
8 Ⓐ Ⓑ Ⓒ Ⓓ	18 Ⓐ Ⓑ Ⓒ Ⓓ	28 Ⓐ Ⓑ Ⓒ Ⓓ	38 Ⓐ Ⓑ Ⓒ Ⓓ
9 Ⓐ Ⓑ Ⓒ Ⓓ	19 Ⓐ Ⓑ Ⓒ Ⓓ	29 Ⓐ Ⓑ Ⓒ Ⓓ	39 Ⓐ Ⓑ Ⓒ Ⓓ
10 Ⓐ Ⓑ Ⓒ Ⓓ	20 Ⓐ Ⓑ Ⓒ Ⓓ	30 Ⓐ Ⓑ Ⓒ Ⓓ	40 Ⓐ Ⓑ Ⓒ Ⓓ

Biology (41–88)

41 Ⓐ Ⓑ Ⓒ Ⓓ	53 Ⓐ Ⓑ Ⓒ Ⓓ	65 Ⓐ Ⓑ Ⓒ Ⓓ	77 Ⓐ Ⓑ Ⓒ Ⓓ
42 Ⓐ Ⓑ Ⓒ Ⓓ	54 Ⓐ Ⓑ Ⓒ Ⓓ	66 Ⓐ Ⓑ Ⓒ Ⓓ	78 Ⓐ Ⓑ Ⓒ Ⓓ
43 Ⓐ Ⓑ Ⓒ Ⓓ	55 Ⓐ Ⓑ Ⓒ Ⓓ	67 Ⓐ Ⓑ Ⓒ Ⓓ	79 Ⓐ Ⓑ Ⓒ Ⓓ
44 Ⓐ Ⓑ Ⓒ Ⓓ	56 Ⓐ Ⓑ Ⓒ Ⓓ	68 Ⓐ Ⓑ Ⓒ Ⓓ	80 Ⓐ Ⓑ Ⓒ Ⓓ
45 Ⓐ Ⓑ Ⓒ Ⓓ	57 Ⓐ Ⓑ Ⓒ Ⓓ	69 Ⓐ Ⓑ Ⓒ Ⓓ	81 Ⓐ Ⓑ Ⓒ Ⓓ
46 Ⓐ Ⓑ Ⓒ Ⓓ	58 Ⓐ Ⓑ Ⓒ Ⓓ	70 Ⓐ Ⓑ Ⓒ Ⓓ	82 Ⓐ Ⓑ Ⓒ Ⓓ
47 Ⓐ Ⓑ Ⓒ Ⓓ	59 Ⓐ Ⓑ Ⓒ Ⓓ	71 Ⓐ Ⓑ Ⓒ Ⓓ	83 Ⓐ Ⓑ Ⓒ Ⓓ
48 Ⓐ Ⓑ Ⓒ Ⓓ	60 Ⓐ Ⓑ Ⓒ Ⓓ	72 Ⓐ Ⓑ Ⓒ Ⓓ	84 Ⓐ Ⓑ Ⓒ Ⓓ
49 Ⓐ Ⓑ Ⓒ Ⓓ	61 Ⓐ Ⓑ Ⓒ Ⓓ	73 Ⓐ Ⓑ Ⓒ Ⓓ	85 Ⓐ Ⓑ Ⓒ Ⓓ
50 Ⓐ Ⓑ Ⓒ Ⓓ	62 Ⓐ Ⓑ Ⓒ Ⓓ	74 Ⓐ Ⓑ Ⓒ Ⓓ	86 Ⓐ Ⓑ Ⓒ Ⓓ
51 Ⓐ Ⓑ Ⓒ Ⓓ	63 Ⓐ Ⓑ Ⓒ Ⓓ	75 Ⓐ Ⓑ Ⓒ Ⓓ	87 Ⓐ Ⓑ Ⓒ Ⓓ
52 Ⓐ Ⓑ Ⓒ Ⓓ	64 Ⓐ Ⓑ Ⓒ Ⓓ	76 Ⓐ Ⓑ Ⓒ Ⓓ	88 Ⓐ Ⓑ Ⓒ Ⓓ

Answer Sheet

PRACTICE TEST 1

Chemistry (89–136)

89 Ⓐ Ⓑ Ⓒ Ⓓ	101 Ⓐ Ⓑ Ⓒ Ⓓ	113 Ⓐ Ⓑ Ⓒ Ⓓ	125 Ⓐ Ⓑ Ⓒ Ⓓ
90 Ⓐ Ⓑ Ⓒ Ⓓ	102 Ⓐ Ⓑ Ⓒ Ⓓ	114 Ⓐ Ⓑ Ⓒ Ⓓ	126 Ⓐ Ⓑ Ⓒ Ⓓ
91 Ⓐ Ⓑ Ⓒ Ⓓ	103 Ⓐ Ⓑ Ⓒ Ⓓ	115 Ⓐ Ⓑ Ⓒ Ⓓ	127 Ⓐ Ⓑ Ⓒ Ⓓ
92 Ⓐ Ⓑ Ⓒ Ⓓ	104 Ⓐ Ⓑ Ⓒ Ⓓ	116 Ⓐ Ⓑ Ⓒ Ⓓ	128 Ⓐ Ⓑ Ⓒ Ⓓ
93 Ⓐ Ⓑ Ⓒ Ⓓ	105 Ⓐ Ⓑ Ⓒ Ⓓ	117 Ⓐ Ⓑ Ⓒ Ⓓ	129 Ⓐ Ⓑ Ⓒ Ⓓ
94 Ⓐ Ⓑ Ⓒ Ⓓ	106 Ⓐ Ⓑ Ⓒ Ⓓ	118 Ⓐ Ⓑ Ⓒ Ⓓ	130 Ⓐ Ⓑ Ⓒ Ⓓ
95 Ⓐ Ⓑ Ⓒ Ⓓ	107 Ⓐ Ⓑ Ⓒ Ⓓ	119 Ⓐ Ⓑ Ⓒ Ⓓ	131 Ⓐ Ⓑ Ⓒ Ⓓ
96 Ⓐ Ⓑ Ⓒ Ⓓ	108 Ⓐ Ⓑ Ⓒ Ⓓ	120 Ⓐ Ⓑ Ⓒ Ⓓ	132 Ⓐ Ⓑ Ⓒ Ⓓ
97 Ⓐ Ⓑ Ⓒ Ⓓ	109 Ⓐ Ⓑ Ⓒ Ⓓ	121 Ⓐ Ⓑ Ⓒ Ⓓ	133 Ⓐ Ⓑ Ⓒ Ⓓ
98 Ⓐ Ⓑ Ⓒ Ⓓ	110 Ⓐ Ⓑ Ⓒ Ⓓ	122 Ⓐ Ⓑ Ⓒ Ⓓ	134 Ⓐ Ⓑ Ⓒ Ⓓ
99 Ⓐ Ⓑ Ⓒ Ⓓ	111 Ⓐ Ⓑ Ⓒ Ⓓ	123 Ⓐ Ⓑ Ⓒ Ⓓ	135 Ⓐ Ⓑ Ⓒ Ⓓ
100 Ⓐ Ⓑ Ⓒ Ⓓ	112 Ⓐ Ⓑ Ⓒ Ⓓ	124 Ⓐ Ⓑ Ⓒ Ⓓ	136 Ⓐ Ⓑ Ⓒ Ⓓ

Quantitative Ability (137–184)

137 Ⓐ Ⓑ Ⓒ Ⓓ	149 Ⓐ Ⓑ Ⓒ Ⓓ	161 Ⓐ Ⓑ Ⓒ Ⓓ	173 Ⓐ Ⓑ Ⓒ Ⓓ
138 Ⓐ Ⓑ Ⓒ Ⓓ	150 Ⓐ Ⓑ Ⓒ Ⓓ	162 Ⓐ Ⓑ Ⓒ Ⓓ	174 Ⓐ Ⓑ Ⓒ Ⓓ
139 Ⓐ Ⓑ Ⓒ Ⓓ	151 Ⓐ Ⓑ Ⓒ Ⓓ	163 Ⓐ Ⓑ Ⓒ Ⓓ	175 Ⓐ Ⓑ Ⓒ Ⓓ
140 Ⓐ Ⓑ Ⓒ Ⓓ	152 Ⓐ Ⓑ Ⓒ Ⓓ	164 Ⓐ Ⓑ Ⓒ Ⓓ	176 Ⓐ Ⓑ Ⓒ Ⓓ
141 Ⓐ Ⓑ Ⓒ Ⓓ	153 Ⓐ Ⓑ Ⓒ Ⓓ	165 Ⓐ Ⓑ Ⓒ Ⓓ	177 Ⓐ Ⓑ Ⓒ Ⓓ
142 Ⓐ Ⓑ Ⓒ Ⓓ	154 Ⓐ Ⓑ Ⓒ Ⓓ	166 Ⓐ Ⓑ Ⓒ Ⓓ	178 Ⓐ Ⓑ Ⓒ Ⓓ
143 Ⓐ Ⓑ Ⓒ Ⓓ	155 Ⓐ Ⓑ Ⓒ Ⓓ	167 Ⓐ Ⓑ Ⓒ Ⓓ	179 Ⓐ Ⓑ Ⓒ Ⓓ
144 Ⓐ Ⓑ Ⓒ Ⓓ	156 Ⓐ Ⓑ Ⓒ Ⓓ	168 Ⓐ Ⓑ Ⓒ Ⓓ	180 Ⓐ Ⓑ Ⓒ Ⓓ
145 Ⓐ Ⓑ Ⓒ Ⓓ	157 Ⓐ Ⓑ Ⓒ Ⓓ	169 Ⓐ Ⓑ Ⓒ Ⓓ	181 Ⓐ Ⓑ Ⓒ Ⓓ
146 Ⓐ Ⓑ Ⓒ Ⓓ	158 Ⓐ Ⓑ Ⓒ Ⓓ	170 Ⓐ Ⓑ Ⓒ Ⓓ	182 Ⓐ Ⓑ Ⓒ Ⓓ
147 Ⓐ Ⓑ Ⓒ Ⓓ	159 Ⓐ Ⓑ Ⓒ Ⓓ	171 Ⓐ Ⓑ Ⓒ Ⓓ	183 Ⓐ Ⓑ Ⓒ Ⓓ
148 Ⓐ Ⓑ Ⓒ Ⓓ	160 Ⓐ Ⓑ Ⓒ Ⓓ	172 Ⓐ Ⓑ Ⓒ Ⓓ	184 Ⓐ Ⓑ Ⓒ Ⓓ

Answer Sheet
PRACTICE TEST 1

Reading Comprehension (185–232)

185 Ⓐ Ⓑ Ⓒ Ⓓ	197 Ⓐ Ⓑ Ⓒ Ⓓ	209 Ⓐ Ⓑ Ⓒ Ⓓ	221 Ⓐ Ⓑ Ⓒ Ⓓ
186 Ⓐ Ⓑ Ⓒ Ⓓ	198 Ⓐ Ⓑ Ⓒ Ⓓ	210 Ⓐ Ⓑ Ⓒ Ⓓ	222 Ⓐ Ⓑ Ⓒ Ⓓ
187 Ⓐ Ⓑ Ⓒ Ⓓ	199 Ⓐ Ⓑ Ⓒ Ⓓ	211 Ⓐ Ⓑ Ⓒ Ⓓ	223 Ⓐ Ⓑ Ⓒ Ⓓ
188 Ⓐ Ⓑ Ⓒ Ⓓ	200 Ⓐ Ⓑ Ⓒ Ⓓ	212 Ⓐ Ⓑ Ⓒ Ⓓ	224 Ⓐ Ⓑ Ⓒ Ⓓ
189 Ⓐ Ⓑ Ⓒ Ⓓ	201 Ⓐ Ⓑ Ⓒ Ⓓ	213 Ⓐ Ⓑ Ⓒ Ⓓ	225 Ⓐ Ⓑ Ⓒ Ⓓ
190 Ⓐ Ⓑ Ⓒ Ⓓ	202 Ⓐ Ⓑ Ⓒ Ⓓ	214 Ⓐ Ⓑ Ⓒ Ⓓ	226 Ⓐ Ⓑ Ⓒ Ⓓ
191 Ⓐ Ⓑ Ⓒ Ⓓ	203 Ⓐ Ⓑ Ⓒ Ⓓ	215 Ⓐ Ⓑ Ⓒ Ⓓ	227 Ⓐ Ⓑ Ⓒ Ⓓ
192 Ⓐ Ⓑ Ⓒ Ⓓ	204 Ⓐ Ⓑ Ⓒ Ⓓ	216 Ⓐ Ⓑ Ⓒ Ⓓ	228 Ⓐ Ⓑ Ⓒ Ⓓ
193 Ⓐ Ⓑ Ⓒ Ⓓ	205 Ⓐ Ⓑ Ⓒ Ⓓ	217 Ⓐ Ⓑ Ⓒ Ⓓ	229 Ⓐ Ⓑ Ⓒ Ⓓ
194 Ⓐ Ⓑ Ⓒ Ⓓ	206 Ⓐ Ⓑ Ⓒ Ⓓ	218 Ⓐ Ⓑ Ⓒ Ⓓ	230 Ⓐ Ⓑ Ⓒ Ⓓ
195 Ⓐ Ⓑ Ⓒ Ⓓ	207 Ⓐ Ⓑ Ⓒ Ⓓ	219 Ⓐ Ⓑ Ⓒ Ⓓ	231 Ⓐ Ⓑ Ⓒ Ⓓ
196 Ⓐ Ⓑ Ⓒ Ⓓ	208 Ⓐ Ⓑ Ⓒ Ⓓ	220 Ⓐ Ⓑ Ⓒ Ⓓ	232 Ⓐ Ⓑ Ⓒ Ⓓ

Writing

For the essay portion of the test, please compose your response on a separate sheet of paper.

VERBAL ABILITY

40 QUESTIONS (#1–#40)

TIME: 25 MINUTES

Directions: Choose the word that **best** completes the analogy.

1. AUSTERE : DOUR :: AUSPICIOUS :

   (A) Sovereign
   (B) Suspect
   (C) Hopeful
   (D) Avarice

2. PLACATE : PACIFY :: CONFIRM :

   (A) Ratify
   (B) Invalidate
   (C) Comply
   (D) Reply

3. BUSTLE : REPOSE :: CALLOW :

   (A) Jejune
   (B) Sophomore
   (C) Sophisticated
   (D) Guileless

4. VIRUS : COLD :: DEITY :

   (A) Miracle
   (B) Transcendent
   (C) Ubiquitous
   (D) Prayer

5. RIM : VOLCANO :: MARGIN :

   (A) Wound
   (B) Edge
   (C) Probability
   (D) Erupt

6. BOOK : CHAPTER :: CONCERTO :

   (A) Oboe
   (B) Movement
   (C) Applause
   (D) Strings

7. SMALL INTESTINE : DUODENUM :: HAND :

   (A) Finger
   (B) Echidna
   (C) Knee
   (D) Elbow

8. NEEDLE : SEW :: HOSE :

   (A) Lawn
   (B) Down
   (C) Garter
   (D) Siphon

9. BARN : HORSE :: AVIARY :

   (A) Bird
   (B) Monkey
   (C) Spider
   (D) Fish

10. RECYCLE : PAPER :: INCUBATE :

    (A) Hatch
    (B) Egg
    (C) Sit on
    (D) Return

11. THEORY : REFUTE :: PRESIDENT :

    (A) Impeach
    (B) Congress
    (C) Veto
    (D) Obscure

12. EAR : CORN :: BOLL :

    (A) Weevil
    (B) Stem
    (C) Pod
    (D) Cotton

13. DEBRIS : COMPOST :: RESIN :

    (A) Tar
    (B) Amber
    (C) Industry
    (D) Pitchblende

14. SEAL : ROTUND :: CHEETAH :

(A) Fast
(B) Mammal
(C) Protected
(D) Sleek

15. COLD : FLU :: RECESSION :

(A) Temperature
(B) Danger
(C) Depression
(D) Glacier

16. ON : COMMENT :: OUT :

(A) Direction
(B) Pool
(C) Eke
(D) Down

17. PAINTER : PALETTE :: COOK :

(A) Spices
(B) Chef
(C) Spatula
(D) Bake

18. SENTENCE : ELLIPSIS :: SPEECH :

(A) Applause
(B) Pause
(C) Finale
(D) Silence

19. HAT : PANAMA :: SHARK :

(A) Predator
(B) Skin
(C) Cichlid
(D) Mako

20. DRUMS : BAND :: GOALIE :

(A) Position
(B) Team
(C) Puck
(D) Fans

21. DESPOT : DICTATOR :: AGITATOR :

(A) Cherub
(B) Narcissist
(C) Demagogue
(D) Epicure

22. HAIKU : SONNET :: CONCERTO :

(A) Madrigal
(B) Bauhaus
(C) Fable
(D) Parable

23. CANONIZE : EXALT :: MOURNFUL :

(A) Litigious
(B) Lugubrious
(C) Suspicious
(D) Contumacious

24. TELESCOPE : FOCUSER :: MICROSCOPE :

(A) Cathode
(B) Condenser
(C) Microprocessor
(D) Alternator

25. SEEMINGLY : OSTENSIBLY :: THOROUGHLY :

(A) Completely
(B) Openly
(C) Divisively
(D) Ruinously

Directions: Select the word or set of words that makes the most sense when inserted into the sentence and that best fits the meaning of the sentence as a whole.

26. In evolution, when a _____ is introduced into a population, it allows for genetic _____ within the population.

    (A) vernacular; utopia
    (B) compilation; concurrence
    (C) mutilation; displacement
    (D) mutation; variation

27. He was a _____ old gentleman who was always complaining and rude. His twin brother, on the other hand, was more _____, always laughing and joking.

    (A) mediocre; inordinate
    (B) cantankerous; mirthful
    (C) formal; militant
    (D) terrific; fastidious

28. Henry did not rely on his _____ to solve the problem; he used _____ data collected throughout the study.

    (A) curiosity; enigmatic
    (B) influence; cursory
    (C) intuition; empirical
    (D) callousness; compensatory

29. The ghost story he told around the campfire was _____, with several twists and turns before reaching the thrilling conclusion.

    (A) convoluted
    (B) dispassionate
    (C) insipid
    (D) placid

30. Ongoing interaction with the _____ and discourteous senior partner in her law firm left the young lawyer feeling _____ and longing to pursue another profession.

    (A) imperious; jaded
    (B) sanguine; tranquil
    (C) sincere; bucolic
    (D) humorous; chimerical

31. The _____ remarks made during the ceremony offended many audience members, and it seemed that _____ damage had been done to the sacred and dignified occasion.

    (A) jovial; reputable
    (B) transitory; unassuming
    (C) irreverent; irreparable
    (D) discrete; figurative

32. The man was _____ concerning his opinions, and everyone thought it would be better if he kept his ample thoughts to himself.

    (A) profuse
    (B) impassive
    (C) conservative
    (D) sparse

33. Karen thought the advertisements for the new clothing store were _____, filled with clashing colors and design patterns; however, her friends believed the opposite and were very positive about the style choices expressed in the ads.

    (A) opulent
    (B) ephemeral
    (C) alluring
    (D) meretricious

34. Without a doubt, it is _____ that we wait until the solution has completely stabilized. Until _____ is reached, we risk causing a violent chemical reaction.

    (A) immense; illumination
    (B) unfortunate; equivalence
    (C) imperative; equilibrium
    (D) insignificant; consensus

35. In contrast to the other _____ paintings, one painting stood out because of its _____.

    (A) flamboyant; simplicity
    (B) divergent; fortuitousness
    (C) rudimentary; coincidence
    (D) anecdotal; catharsis

36. It is essential that we do not act too hastily; it may be in our best interest to _____ the meeting until next week.

    (A) devour
    (B) shuffle
    (C) modernize
    (D) defer

37. After studying for several years and conducting numerous, well-received research projects, Dr. Smith was considered quite _____ on the subject of global economics.

    (A) foppish
    (B) inveterate
    (C) erudite
    (D) mawkish

38. Although multiple sclerosis was first described over 100 years ago, the cause remains a _____ and a cure is still _____.

    (A) problem; berated
    (B) coercion; obvious
    (C) mystery; undiscovered
    (D) possibility; changed

39. During the early _____ period of an individual's lifespan, many of the major organ systems appear and begin to develop.

    (A) enigmatic
    (B) asymmetric
    (C) audacious
    (D) embryonic

40. We must stir the solution for the experiment with a sterile rod to make sure that we do not _____ it.

    (A) impugn
    (B) contaminate
    (C) denounce
    (D) confound

STOP

End of Verbal Ability section. If you have any time left, you may go over your work in this section only.

BIOLOGY

48 QUESTIONS (#41–#88)

TIME: 35 MINUTES

Directions: Choose the **best** answer to each of the following questions.

41. A woman visits an emergency clinic complaining of a nagging cough. An X-ray of her lungs shows dark objects obstructing her alveoli. She is given a medicine to treat the infection. The medicine does not work. After two additional medications are tried, the fourth medicine clears up the infection. Below is a table of her four medications.

	Name	**Mode of Action**	**Effective (Yes/No)**
1st	Penicillin	Targets peptidoglycan production	No
2nd	Ciprofloxacin	Targets prokaryote DNA replication	No
3rd	Lincomycin	Targets 50S ribosome subunit	No
4th	Amphotericin B	Targets ergosterol in plasma membrane	Yes

Based on the mode of action of each drug tried, what type of organism likely caused her infection?

(A) Archaea
(B) Bacterium
(C) Plant
(D) Fungus

Use Figure 1 to answer question 42.

Figure 1.

42. In Figure 1, number 1 is pointing to what part of the cell?

(A) Nucleolus
(B) Nuclear envelope
(C) Ribosomes
(D) Nucleus

43. How do ions like Na$^+$ enter a cell?

(A) Ions pass directly through the cell plasma membrane.
(B) Ions pass through the cell plasma membrane via a transporter protein.
(C) Ions pass through the cell plasma membrane via a channel protein.
(D) Ions are never allowed to enter a cell.

44. The respiratory system has many ways to protect itself from unwanted materials. For example, epithelial cells that line the respiratory system possess cilia. These cilia are extensions of the cells that capture debris such as pollen, dust, and microorganisms. The cilia then bend in waves to move the debris back up the respiratory track to be removed.

    Which of the following cellular components, if absent, would prevent ciliated epithelial cells from ridding the respiratory system of unwanted debris?

    (A) Cell plasma membrane
    (B) Cytoskeleton
    (C) Endomembrane system
    (D) Cell wall

45. Which of the following organelles is a site of protein translation?

    (A) Lysosome
    (B) Golgi apparatus
    (C) Rough endoplasmic reticulum
    (D) Smooth endoplasmic reticulum

46. By which of the following mechanisms can a cell transport a substance from a lower to a higher concentration:

    (A) Simple diffusion
    (B) Active transport
    (C) Facilitated diffusion
    (D) Extracellular enzymes

47. Which of the following organelles are thought to have arisen from primitive prokaryotes?

    (A) The endoplasmic reticulum and Golgi complex
    (B) Mitochondria and chloroplasts
    (C) Vacuoles and transport vesicles
    (D) Lyposomes and peroxisomes

48. DNA replication results in

    (A) two DNA molecules, one with two newly synthesized strands and one with two parental strands.
    (B) two DNA molecules, each with two newly synthesized strands.
    (C) two DNA molecules, each of which has one parental strand and one newly synthesized strand.
    (D) two DNA molecules, each of which has strands of unknown origins.

49. Some genetic disorders can lead to an abnormal number of chromosomes. For example, Klinefelter's syndrome is the possession of three sex chromosomes, two 'X' chromosomes and one 'Y' chromosome. Individuals with Klinefelter's syndrome are often sterile and can have a variety of morphological and physiological abnormalities.

    The abnormal number of sex chromosomes is caused by the incorrect separation of chromosomes during the production of sex cells. This abnormal process is called non-disjunction. Based on this information, which of the following does *not* describe how Klinefelter's syndrome can occur?

    (A) A non-disjunction event in Meiosis I occurred during the production of sperm in the father of an individual with Klinefelter's syndrome.
    (B) A non-disjunction event occurred in Meiosis I during the production of an egg in the mother of an individual with Klinefelter's syndrome.
    (C) A non-disjunction event occurred in Meiosis II during the production of an egg in the mother of an individual with Klinefelter's syndrome.
    (D) A non-disjunction event occurred during the first round of mitosis in a fertilized egg resulting in an individual with Klinefelter's syndrome.

50. A microorganism that obtains its carbon, as well as its energy, from organic compounds is called

    (A) an autotroph.
    (B) a heterotroph.
    (C) a heterozygote.
    (D) a homozygote.

51. If A represents blue (dominant color) and a represents red (recessive color), which of the following crosses would be expected to result in 25% red offspring?

    (A) Aa × aa
    (B) AA × aa
    (C) Aa × Aa
    (D) Aa × AA

52. Which of the following structures respond(s) to dim light for black and white vision?

    (A) Cones
    (B) Rods
    (C) Iris
    (D) Cornea

53. Normal red blood cells have an average life span of

    (A) 30 days.
    (B) 60 days.
    (C) 120 days.
    (D) 180 days.

54. Which is a sign of infection?

    (A) An increase in white blood cell count
    (B) An increase in red blood cell count
    (C) A decrease in body temperature
    (D) A decrease in leukocytes

55. Which of the following is a monomer?

    (A) Starch
    (B) Peptidoglycan
    (C) Glucose
    (D) Chitin

56. Which of the following modifies materials synthesized in the rough and smooth endoplasmic reticulum?

    (A) Plastids
    (B) Golgi apparatus
    (C) Ribosomes
    (D) Mitochondria

57. In the cell cycle, what phase occurs just prior to cytokinesis?

    (A) Telophase
    (B) Metaphase
    (C) Prophase
    (D) Anaphase

58. Genes that are capable of relocating from one part of the genome to another are called:

    (A) Mesosomes
    (B) Transposons
    (C) Plasmids
    (D) Fimbriae

59. _____ are gram-positive, spore-forming bacilli. The major diseases associated with these bacteria are caused by exotoxins.

    (A) Acinomyces
    (B) Eubacterium
    (C) Clostridium
    (D) Lactobacillus

60. What organ filters blood from the digestive tract and returns the blood to the heart via hepatic veins?

    (A) The pancreas
    (B) The gallbladder
    (C) The kidneys
    (D) The liver

61. ATP is a molecule that stores energy in the form of a

    (A) hydrogen bond.
    (B) phosphate bond.
    (C) nitrogen bond.
    (D) carbon bond.

62. The medulla oblongata controls which of the following functions?

    (A) Respiration and heartbeat
    (B) Verbal communication and heartbeat
    (C) Vision and breathing
    (D) Verbal communication and vision

63. Which of the following enzymes connects Okazaki fragments on the lagging strand during DNA replication in eukaryotic cells?

    (A) DNA ligase
    (B) DNA helicase
    (C) DNA polymerase I
    (D) DNA polymerase III

64. What structure connects the middle ear to the throat?

    (A) Auricle
    (B) Eustachian tube
    (C) Tympanic membrane
    (D) Cochlea

65. A resistance to which hormone causes type 2 diabetes?

    (A) Glucose
    (B) Cortisol
    (C) Insulin
    (D) Testosterone

66. The heart wall is composed of three distinct layers. The outermost layer is

    (A) epicardium.
    (B) asocardium.
    (C) myocardium.
    (D) endocardium.

67. Microorganisms that lack cell walls are known as _____; they do not synthesize the precursors of peptidoglycan.

    (A) phototrophic
    (B) archaeobacteria
    (C) mycoplasmas
    (D) plasmids

68. In the cardiac cycle, the relaxation of the heart is referred to as

    (A) systole.
    (B) diastole.
    (C) cardiac rate.
    (D) systemic relaxation.

69. The superficial protective layer of the skin is the

    (A) dermis.
    (B) hypodermis.
    (C) epidermis.
    (D) exodermis.

70. What does the term *evolution* mean?

    (A) The characteristics of a population change through time.
    (B) The characteristics of a species become more complex over time.
    (C) The characteristics of an individual change through the course of its life in response to natural selection.
    (D) The strongest individuals produce the most offspring.

71. The adrenal glands produce which two hormones?

    (A) Melatonin and serotonin
    (B) Adrenalin and noradrenaline
    (C) Insulin and glucagon
    (D) Estrogen and testosterone

72. What part of the kidney first filters the blood?

    (A) The ureter
    (B) The renal vein
    (C) The glomerulus
    (D) The Loop of Henle

73. The process of endocytosis allows a cell to bring in a large volume of material from the environment via the formation of vesicles. Each vesicle enters the cell and fuses with the lysosome. Inside the lysosome, enzymes break down the material into a form that may be utilized by the cell. In the case of phagocytes, these cells engulf bacteria and kill them in lysosomes, helping rid the body of a potential pathogen attack.

    A study was done to show the importance of the function of four different subunits of the proton (H^+) pump protein complex found in the membrane of lysosomes. A series of four mutant phagocytes, A–D, were created, each with a mutation in a different subunit of the proton pump protein complex. The pH of the interior of the lysosome of each mutant strain was recorded. The results are shown in the table below. Based on this data, which mutant has the most functional lysosome?

	Resulting pH
Mutant A	4.5
Mutant B	2.0
Mutant C	10
Mutant D	8.5

    (A) Mutant A
    (B) Mutant B
    (C) Mutant C
    (D) Mutant D

74. In humans, gas exchange takes place in the

    (A) alveoli.
    (B) bronchi.
    (C) trachea.
    (D) bronchioles.

75. High-density lipoproteins (HDLs) and low-density lipoproteins (LDLs) are associated with which of the following?

    (A) Insulin
    (B) Cholesterol
    (C) Myelin sheaths
    (D) Neurotransmitters

76. In aerobic cellular respiration, most of the ATP is synthesized during

    (A) the Krebs cycle.
    (B) electron transport.
    (C) electron oxidation.
    (D) the citric acid cycle.

77. A normal cell spends approximately 90% of its time in

    (A) prophase.
    (B) metaphase.
    (C) interphase.
    (D) anaphase.

78. In the human respiratory system, there is a net diffusion of carbon dioxide from

    (A) hemoglobin to mitochondria.
    (B) alveoli to blood.
    (C) blood to air in the alveoli.
    (D) air to blood in bronchi.

79. Which of the following is a water-soluble vitamin?

    (A) Vitamin A
    (B) Vitamin E
    (C) Vitamin C
    (D) Vitamin D

80. Which of the following would detect the position of your head?

    (A) The cochlea
    (B) The vestibular apparatus
    (C) The pinna
    (D) The organ of Corte

81. Non-Hodgkin's lymphoma is a type of cancer in which blood cells do not develop correctly. The presence of abnormal white blood cells, such as T and B cells, are often a diagnosis for this disease. Additional symptoms include fever, swollen lymph nodes, and sudden weight loss.

    A person with non-Hodgkin's lymphoma symptoms can be treated. Which of the following would be the most effective, long-term treatment of this disease?

    (A) An injection of T and B cells
    (B) An injection of cytokines
    (C) A bone marrow transplant
    (D) Removal of the pancreas

82. Which of the following blood cells is a leukocyte?

    (A) Platelet
    (B) Red blood cell
    (C) Neutrophil
    (D) Megakaryocyte

83. In the thyroid hormone control network, the source of negative feedback is the

    (A) hypothalamus.
    (B) cerebrum.
    (C) pituitary gland.
    (D) thyroid gland.

84. Why is it difficult to develop a vaccine against viruses with high mutation rates like HIV?

    (A) The vaccines tend to be unstable and deteriorate over time.
    (B) The virus proteins are only recognized by killer T cells.
    (C) New viral mutations constantly change the viral proteins.
    (D) The virions contain so many different proteins that the immune system is overwhelmed.

85. Which of the following cell types would engulf and digest bacteria?

    (A) Killer T cells
    (B) B cells
    (C) Natural killer cells
    (D) Macrophages

86. The genomes of viruses may contain

    (A) double-stranded DNA only.
    (B) single-stranded RNA only.
    (C) double-stranded DNA or double-stranded RNA.
    (D) double-stranded DNA, single-stranded DNA, single-stranded RNA, or double-stranded RNA.

87. A bacteriophage

    (A) is a virus that infects bacteria.
    (B) is a fungus.
    (C) does not contain DNA or RNA.
    (D) is a bacterium that infects fungi.

88. In general, enzyme activity is influenced by temperature, enzyme concentration, substrate concentration, and

    (A) water.
    (B) pH.
    (C) oxygen concentration.
    (D) carbon dioxide concentration.

STOP

End of Biology section. If you have any time left, you may go over your work in this section only.

CHEMISTRY

48 QUESTIONS (#89–#136)

TIME: 35 MINUTES

Directions: Choose the **best** answer to each of the following questions.

89. The quantity of which subatomic particle is unique for each element?

    (A) Protons
    (B) Neutrons
    (C) Electrons
    (D) Nucleons

90. What is the molarity (M) of a solution prepared by dissolving 18.0 grams of sugar, $C_6H_{12}O_6$, in 500 milliliters of solution? (O = 16 amu, C = 12 amu, H = 1 amu)

    (A) 0.130
    (B) 0.230
    (C) 0.200
    (D) 0.910

91. In the following reaction:

    $$CS_2 + 2O_2 \rightarrow CO_2 + 2SO_2$$

    38.0 grams of CS_2 (carbon disufide) are reacted with excess O_2 to produce 32.0 grams of SO_2. What is the percent yield of this reaction? (S = 32 amu, O = 16 amu, C = 12 amu, H = 1 amu)

    (A) 50
    (B) 25
    (C) 38
    (D) 13

92. The functions of RNA molecules include all of the following EXCEPT

    (A) permanent storage of nucleotide sequence information.
    (B) transporting amino acids to the protein synthesis machinery in the cell.
    (C) providing the information from which proteins are synthesized.
    (D) participating in the construction and function of the ribosomes.

93. Prior to cell division (mitosis), the genetic material must be duplicated such that the DNA in each daughter cell is identical to that of the mother cell. Mitosis is part of the cell cycle and is called the M stage. Other parts of the cell cycle are two gaps (G1 and G2) and the S phase during which the cell's DNA is synthesized. During DNA synthesis, the polymerization of nucleotides is catalyzed by DNA polymerases. Details on the enzymes' requirements and functions are known, and in addition to the polymerization activity, they have an exonuclease or proofreading activity. Thus, errors in DNA synthesis are largely avoided. Since DNA is the permanent copy of genetic material in the cell and is used as a pattern for protein synthesis throughout the cell's life, fidelity in the process is required.

    What is the name of the process by which new DNA molecules are synthesized?

    (A) Transcription
    (B) Translation
    (C) Replication
    (D) Translocation

94. How many milliliters of 4.0 M NaOH solution must be used to prepare 100 milliliters of 2.0 M solution?

    (A) 50
    (B) 13
    (C) 800
    (D) 200

95. What is the density, in grams per liter, of oxygen gas, O_2, if the pressure is 1.00 atmosphere and the temperature is 15°C? (O = 16 amu, R = 0.082 L-atm/K-mole)

    (A) 1.35
    (B) 0.74
    (C) 8.74×10^{-3}
    (D) 1.43

96. A sample of gas contains approximately 56 grams nitrogen, N_2, and 64 grams oxygen, O_2. What is the partial pressure, in atmospheres, of nitrogen if the total pressure of the air is 1.6 atmospheres? (O = 16 amu, N = 14 amu)

    (A) 0.5
    (B) 3.2
    (C) 0.8
    (D) 2.0

97. The specific heat of copper, Cu, is 0.385 joule per gram °C. If 10.0 joules of heat is absorbed by a 5 g sample of Cu at 25°C, what will be the new temperature?

    (A) 20
    (B) 75
    (C) 30
    (D) 44

98. The amino acid sequence of proteins is determined by the

    (A) nucleotide sequence of the respective rRNA.
    (B) nucleotide sequence of the respective gene.
    (C) codon and anticodon base pairing in transcription.
    (D) cellular levels of amino acids.

99. Which of the following wavelengths of light will have the highest frequency?

    (A) 0.300 m
    (B) 2.75 mm
    (C) 630 nm
    (D) 0.69 km

100. A chloride ion and a sulfide ion

    (A) have the same charge.
    (B) have the same number of valence electrons.
    (C) have the same number of protons.
    (D) are diatomic ions.

101. Which of the following is a basic oxide?

    (A) CO_2
    (B) K_2O
    (C) SO_2
    (D) P_2O_5

102. Hydrogen bonding can exist between molecules of all the following EXCEPT

    (A) H_2O
    (B) CH_4
    (C) CH_3OH
    (D) NH_3

103. Which of the following is NOT true concerning triglycerides and phospholipids?

    (A) They are esters of glycerol and short-chain carboxylic acids.
    (B) They are found in adipose tissue and cell membranes.
    (C) They contain long-chain fatty acids.
    (D) They contain hydrophilic and hydrophobic regions.

104. The conversion of a gas into a liquid is called _____ and it is usually _____ at room temperature.

    (A) evaporation; endothermic
    (B) evaporation; exothermic
    (C) condensation; endothermic
    (D) condensation; exothermic

105. Gases are usually most soluble in liquids with

    (A) low temperature.
    (B) high temperature.
    (C) low pressure.
    (D) high agitation.

106. The statins are a class of drugs used in patients with high blood cholesterol (hypercholesterolemia). For many years, atorvastatin (Lipitor) was the number one selling drug in the United States. Hypercholesterolemia has been associated with an increased risk of myocardial infarction, stroke, and atherosclerosis. Appropriate dietary choices and increased exercise can lower serum cholesterol (a steroid) and is usually the first recommendation to patients diagnosed with hypercholesterolemia. If the target value for serum cholesterol is not achieved, a statin may be prescribed. Statins inhibit the first committed step in steroid biosynthesis, and thus decrease the amount of cholesterol found in the blood. This class of drugs, like all drugs, is not without side effects. Since the primary site of biosynthesis is the liver, liver function tests are recommended while taking a statin.

    Cholesterol is biosynthesized as well as absorbed from dietary fats and is necessary for

    (A) hormone production.
    (B) hemoglobin production.
    (C) DNA synthesis.
    (D) the prevention of cardiovascular disease.

107. The following reactions have equilibrium constants as indicated below:

$$A + B \leftrightarrow C + D \quad K^1$$
$$E + F \leftrightarrow G + H \quad K^2$$

    The reactions are added to give the following overall reaction. What will be the overall equilibrium constant for the new equation?

$$A + B + E + F \leftrightarrow C + D + G + H$$

    (A) $K^1 + K^2$
    (B) $(K^1)(K^2)$
    (C) K^1/K^2
    (D) K^2/K^1

108. The element having an atomic number of 21 and an atomic mass of 35 contains

    (A) 21 neutrons.
    (B) 14 neutrons.
    (C) 24 electrons.
    (D) 14 protons.

109. Beta sheets and alpha helices are examples of what level of protein structure?

    (A) Primary
    (B) Secondary
    (C) Tertiary
    (D) Quarternary

110. In which of the following are the acids listed correctly in decreasing order of strength (i.e., the strongest acid is first and the weakest acid last)?

    (A) HF > HCl > HBr > HI
    (B) HI > HBr > HCl > HF
    (C) HBr > HCl > HI > HF
    (D) HCl > HBr > HI > HF

111. Which of the following can be a buffer solution?

    (A) H_2SO_4, Na_2SO_4
    (B) H_2SO_4
    (C) CH_3COOH
    (D) CH_3COOH, CH_3COONa

112. The three-dimensional shape of proteins is intimately linked to their biological activity. Extreme changes in temperature or pH can disrupt the protein's secondary and tertiary structure and result in a loss of biological activity. Normal physiologic pH is 7.4, and the side chains of several amino acids are essentially 100% ionized at that pH. If the pKa of the functional group in the side chain is more than two units above or below 7.4, the side chain is assumed to be completely ionized. The ionization of side chains is important in forming "salt bridges" in proteins. Salt bridges are the attraction between oppositely charged functional groups on proteins. Changes in the pH can thus affect the percent of ionization, and thus destroy salt bridges necessary for biological function. Ionized side chains of proteins are also often involved in the active site binding of substrates and the mechanism of catalysis for enzymes.

The side chain of which of the following amino acids would be completely ionized at physiological pH?

(A) Alanine
(B) Glycine
(C) Lysine
(D) Valine

113. The following reaction:
$$^{90}_{38}\text{Sr} \rightarrow {}^{90}_{39}\text{Y} + {}^{0}_{-1}\text{e}$$
represents

(A) nuclear fission.
(B) gamma emission.
(C) beta decay.
(D) alpha decay.

114. Which of the following is a statement of the first law of thermodynamics?

(A) Entropy for a crystalline substance is zero at absolute zero temperature.
(B) Energy can be converted from one form to another but is neither created nor destroyed.
(C) Entropy increases in spontaneous reactions and remains the same in equilibrium systems.
(D) The Gibbs free energy is a measure of the spontaneity of a reaction.

115. If the Gibbs free energy for a certain reaction has a negative value, the

(A) reaction does not take place.
(B) reaction system is at equilibrium.
(C) reaction is non-spontaneous.
(D) reaction is spontaneous.

116. Which statement is true concerning aqueous solutions of Acid A ($Ka = 6 \times 10^{-8}$) and Acid B ($Ka = 3 \times 10^{-5}$)?

(A) Acid A is stronger than Acid B.
(B) The pH of the Acid B solution is less than that of Acid A.
(C) Both solutions are neutral.
(D) The pKa of Acid B is greater than the pKa of Acid A.

117. What reagents should be used to accomplish the following conversion?

(A) CH_3COCl, $AlCl_3$
(B) CH_3Cl, $AlCl_3$
(C) CH_3CH_3, CH_3MgCl
(D) CH_3MgCl, $AlCl_3$

118. What is a product of the following reaction?

$$\begin{array}{c} 1.\ \text{LiAlH}_4 \\ 2.\ \text{H}^+ \end{array}$$

$$\text{CH}_3\text{CO}_2\text{CH}_3 \xrightarrow{\hspace{3cm}}$$

   (A) $\text{CH}_3\text{CH}_2\text{OH}$
   (B) CH_4
   (C) $\text{CH}_3\text{CO}_2\text{H}$
   (D) $\text{H}_2\text{C}=\text{CH}_2$

119. Which statement describes the entry of molecules and ions into the cell?

   (A) Some enter via passive diffusion that requires ATP.
   (B) Those that enter via passive diffusion are usually polar or charged.
   (C) Some enter via transmembrane channels.
   (D) Molecules and ions indiscriminately move into and out of cells.

120. The reaction of Br_2 with C_2H_6 to produce $\text{C}_2\text{H}_5\text{Br}$ and HBr in the presence of ultraviolet light or heat is an example of

   (A) a nucleophilic substitution reaction.
   (B) a free radical substitution reaction.
   (C) an electrophilic addition reaction.
   (D) an elimination reaction.

121. The reaction of Br_2 with C_2H_4 to produce $\text{C}_2\text{H}_4\text{Br}_2$ is an example of

   (A) a nucleophilic substitution reaction.
   (B) a free radical reaction.
   (C) an electrophilic addition reaction.
   (D) an elimination reaction.

122. Many drug molecules contain chiral centers. A chiral center is most often a tetrahedral carbon to which four different groups are attached. Each chiral center has two possible configurations and these are designated, according to the Cahn-Ingold-Prelog system, as R or S. The R form is the nonsuperimposable mirror image of the S form. When molecules with a chiral center are synthesized in a laboratory using ordinary reagents, both forms (R and S) are synthesized and the resultant product is 50% R and 50% S (called a racemic mixture). It is well known that when drugs contain a chiral center, usually only one form (either R or S) is biologically active, but it is usually unnecessary and cost-prohibitive to isolate and market only the active form. For example, the laboratory synthesis of the nonsteroidal anti-inflammatory drug ibuprofen results in a racemic mixture. This mixture is found in the over-the-counter products containing ibuprofen.

Two molecules that are nonsuperimposable mirror images of each other are called

   (A) diastereomers.
   (B) enantiomers.
   (C) the same compound.
   (D) geometric isomers.

123. What is the organic starting material for the reaction given below performed under basic conditions?

   (A) ⌃⌄CHO
   (B) HCHO
   (C) $\text{CH}_2=\text{CH}_2$
   (D) CH_3CHO

124. For butanone, where would the most significant band be found in the infrared spectrum?

    (A) 3,300 cm^{-1}
    (B) 1,700 cm^{-1}
    (C) 2,100 cm^{-1}
    (D) 1,100 cm^{-1}

125. People are always trying to find a way to lose weight while still eating foods they enjoy. Low carb diets are advertised on the Internet and in grocery stores. Low carb diets limit the amount of carbohydrate consumed in an effort to cause the mobilization and oxidation of fat stores. The term "carbohydrate" describes monosaccharides like glucose, disaccharides like sucrose or table sugar, and polysaccharides like starch and cellulose. All carbohydrates structurally contain many alcohol functional groups and either an aldehyde/ketone (as in the monosaccharides) or a hemiacetal/acetal resulting from the reaction of an alcohol with an aldehyde/ketone (as in the disaccharides and polysaccharides). Even on low carb diets, however, lettuce (cellulose) is not prohibited. This is curious since cellulose is a carbohydrate but our bodies cannot hydrolyze the acetal linkages in this polysaccharide, meaning it leaves the body in the same form as it entered.

    Which statement describes carbohydrates?

    (A) They are used as monomers in protein synthesis.
    (B) They are oxidized to produce usable chemical energy.
    (C) They are composed of polymers of phosphates.
    (D) They are not commonly found inside cells.

126. Which of the following would NOT produce an ester?

    (A) The reaction of a carboxylic acid with an alcohol.
    (B) The reaction of a carboxylic acid halide with an alcohol.
    (C) The reaction of a carboxylic acid anhydride with an alcohol.
    (D) The reaction of an amide with an alcohol.

127. What functional group is most commonly present in proteins?

    (A) Alcohol
    (B) Amide
    (C) Ester
    (D) Ketone

128. Which of the following statements about benzene is INCORRECT?

    (A) The benzene molecule has 120° bond angles.
    (B) All bonds in benzene are equivalent in length.
    (C) Hybridization of the carbon atoms is sp^2.
    (D) The benzene molecule is planar.

129. The name of the following compound:

$$CH_3CH_2CHCH_2COOH$$
$$|$$
$$CH_3$$

is

    (A) 3-methylpentanoic acid.
    (B) 2-methylpentanoic acid.
    (C) 2-methylbutanoic acid.
    (D) 3-methylbutanoic acid.

130. What is the name of the following molecule?

   (A) (S)-isopentanol
   (B) (S)-3-methyl-2-butanol
   (C) (R)-3-methyl-2-butanol
   (D) (R)-2-methyl-3-butanol

131. What is the percentage of hydrogen, H, present in ammonium sulfate, $(NH_4)_2SO_4$? (S = 32 amu, O = 16 amu, N = 14 amu, H = 1 amu)

   (A) 11
   (B) 6
   (C) 3
   (D) 4

132. Oxidation of an aldehyde produces

   (A) a ketone.
   (B) an alcohol.
   (C) a carboxylic acid.
   (D) an amide.

133. How many grams of sodium hydroxide (FW 40) are needed to neutralize 2.2 mL of pentanoic acid (FW 102, density = 0.93 g/mL) by the equation

$$CH_3(CH_2)_3COOH + NaOH \rightarrow$$
$$H_2O + CH_3(CH_2)_3COONa$$

   (A) 0.80 g
   (B) 2.04 g
   (C) 0.02 g
   (D) 0.051 g

134. What is the final volume in milliliters of a solution prepared by dissolving 18 grams of sugar, $C_6H_{12}O_6$, in sufficient water to produce a 0.5 M solution? (O = 16 amu, C = 12 amu, H = 1 amu)

   (A) 36
   (B) 100
   (C) 200
   (D) 52

135. The reaction of a neutron with a uranium-235 nucleus to generate a strontium atom, a xenon atom, and three neutrons as shown in the equation below is known as

$$^{235}_{92}U + ^{1}_{0}n \rightarrow ^{90}_{38}Sr + ^{143}_{54}Xe + 3^{1}_{0}n$$

   (A) radioactive decay
   (B) nuclear fusion
   (C) carbon dating
   (D) nuclear fission

136. If two moles of acetic acid are generated from the cleavage of an organic molecule by ozonolysis followed by reductive work up, what is the name of the organic molecule?

   (A) 1-butyne
   (B) 2-butyne
   (C) 2-butene
   (D) cyclobutyne

STOP

End of Chemistry section. If you have any time left, you may go over your work in this section only.

QUANTITATIVE ABILITY

48 QUESTIONS (#137–#184)

TIME: 45 MINUTES

Directions: Choose the **best** answer to each of the following questions.

137. $\sqrt{32} + \sqrt{18} =$

    (A) $6\sqrt{2}$

    (B) $8\sqrt{2}$

    (C) $7\sqrt{2}$

    (D) $9\sqrt{2}$

138. Lisa's gas tank is 4/5 full. She completely filled the tank by putting in an additional 7 gallons. What is the capacity of the gas tank?

    (A) 30 gallons
    (B) 35 gallons
    (C) 25 gallons
    (D) 40 gallons

139. $\lim\limits_{x \to \infty} \left(\dfrac{8x^6 + 5x^4 - x + 1000}{3x^6 + 21x^3 - 4} \right)$

    (A) ∞

    (B) $\dfrac{8}{3}$

    (C) 1

    (D) $\dfrac{13}{24}$

140. Determine the inverse function for

    $f(x) = \dfrac{x+1}{10x}$.

    (A) $f^{-1}(x) = \dfrac{10x}{x+1}$

    (B) $f^{-1}(x) = \dfrac{1}{10x - 1}$

    (C) $f^{-1}(x) = \dfrac{1}{10x + 1}$

    (D) $f^{-1}(x) = \dfrac{x-1}{10x}$

141. $5^2 + 5^3$

    (A) 3,125
    (B) 1,000
    (C) 150
    (D) 25

142. A crate of fruit contains 11 limes, 10 oranges, and 4 lemons. What is the probability that a randomly chosen piece of fruit is NOT a lemon?

    (A) 16%
    (B) 84%
    (C) 0.84%
    (D) 0.16%

143. The quadratic equation $2x^2 + 5x + 1 = 0$ has

    (A) two real roots.
    (B) no real root.
    (C) one real root.
    (D) one real root and one complex root.

144. Find the **radius** of the circle with equation $x^2 + y^2 - 12x + 14y + 9 = 0$.

(A) $\sqrt{76}$

(B) 76

(C) 85

(D) $\sqrt{85}$

145. Find the exact value of the shaded area.

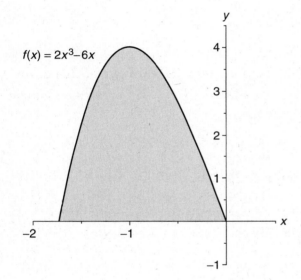

$f(x) = 2x^3 - 6x$

(A) −4.5

(B) 9

(C) 4.5

(D) −9

146. A number is chosen at random from the set $\{1, 2, 3, 4, 5, 6, 7, 8, 9, 10, 11, 12\}$. What is the probability that the chosen number is divisible by 3 or divisible by 4?

(A) 55%

(B) 45%

(C) 60%

(D) 50%

147. Evaluate the integral $\int_{1}^{2} (5x^4)\, dx$.

(A) 32

(B) 140

(C) 180

(D) 31

148. If $x < 6$, then $\dfrac{x^2 - 7x + 6}{|x - 6|} =$

(A) $x + 1$

(B) $-x - 1$

(C) $x - 1$

(D) $-x + 1$

149. Simplify the expression $\dfrac{x^2 - 11x + 24}{x - 8}$.

(A) $x + 3$

(B) $x - 14$

(C) $x - 3$

(D) $x + 14$

150. Find all real solutions for the quadratic equation $6x^2 + x + 2 = 0$.

(A) $x = \dfrac{-1 \pm \sqrt{23}}{12}$

(B) No real solutions

(C) $x = \dfrac{-1 \pm \sqrt{-23}}{12}$

(D) $x = \dfrac{1 \pm \sqrt{23}}{12}$

151. The graph of a function $y = f(x)$ contains the point $(3, 1)$. Determine which point must be on the graph of $y = 5f(x + 2) - 3$.

(A) $(1, 2)$

(B) $(5, 2)$

(C) $(1, -10)$

(D) $(5, -10)$

152. $\log_7 (49) =$

(A) 2

(B) $\dfrac{1}{2}$

(C) 7

(D) $\dfrac{1}{7}$

153. $\lim\limits_{x \to 4} \left(\dfrac{x^2 - 10x + 24}{4 - x} \right) =$

(A) Undefined
(B) 2
(C) –2
(D) 1

154. What is the mean of the following numbers: 8, 35, 8, 9, 5, 10, 7, 3, 12?

(A) 8
(B) 10.77
(C) 15.24
(D) 9

155. A rental car company charges $30 per day, plus 14 cents per mile. Express the total rental cost of a 7-day rental as a function of the number of miles driven, x.

(A) $C(x) = 30 + 14x$
(B) $C(x) = 30 + 0.14x$
(C) $C(x) = 210 + 14x$
(D) $C(x) = 210 + 0.14x$

156. If a coin is tossed four times, what is the probability that the outcome will be all heads?

(A) $\dfrac{1}{16}$

(B) $\dfrac{1}{4}$

(C) $\dfrac{1}{2}$

(D) $\dfrac{1}{8}$

157. Find the instantaneous rate of change for the function $f(t) = 4e^{t^2 - 9}$ at the moment when $t = 3$.

(A) 4
(B) $4e$
(C) $24e$
(D) 24

158. Given $f(x) = x^2 + 2x - 1$, and $g(x) = 2x + 1$, what is $(f + g)(x)$?

(A) $2x^2 + 4x$
(B) $x^2 - 4x$
(C) $x^2 + 4x$
(D) $2x^2 - 4x$

159. The equation $4(x + 3)(x - 2) = 4x^2 + x$ has solution

(A) $x = -8$
(B) $x = 8$
(C) $x = -2$
(D) $x = 2$

160. If a die is rolled, what is the probability that the number will be odd?

    (A) 50%
    (B) 100%
    (C) 25%
    (D) 0%

161. $\dfrac{5}{9} - \dfrac{3}{10} =$

    (A) $\dfrac{77}{90}$

    (B) $-\dfrac{23}{90}$

    (C) $-\dfrac{77}{90}$

    (D) $\dfrac{23}{90}$

162. Find the mode of the following data set: 3, 6, 29, 8, 6, 4, 2, 6, 8, 6, 9, 3.

    (A) 3
    (B) 6
    (C) 9
    (D) 29

163. A pair of fair six-sided dice is thrown. What is the probability that the sum of the numbers shown is NOT equal to 5?

    (A) $\dfrac{1}{6}$

    (B) $\dfrac{1}{18}$

    (C) $\dfrac{1}{3}$

    (D) $\dfrac{17}{18}$

164. Evaluate $\int (x + 2)\, dx$.

    (A) $\dfrac{1}{2}x^2 + 2x + C$

    (B) $\dfrac{1}{x^2} + C$

    (C) $x + C$

    (D) $\dfrac{x}{C}$

For questions 165 and 166, consider the given graph.

165. What is the maximum plasma concentration?

    (A) 100 nmol/L
    (B) 150 nmol/L
    (C) 200 nmol/L
    (D) 300 nmol/L

166. When does the maximum plasma concentration occur?

    (A) At 3 hours
    (B) At 1 hour
    (C) At 4 hours
    (D) At 2 hours

167. Determine the value(s) of q, if any, for which $10x^2 + \pi x - q = 0$ has a double root.

(A) $q = \dfrac{\pi^2}{40}$

(B) $q = \dfrac{40}{\pi^2}$

(C) $q > \dfrac{\pi^2}{40}$

(D) $q > \dfrac{40}{\pi^2}$

168. Find the domain of the given function.
$$f(x) = \frac{x-4}{x^2 + 9x + 18}$$

(A) $\{x \mid x \neq -6,\ x \neq -3\}$
(B) $\{x \mid x = -6,\ x = -3\}$
(C) $\{x \mid x \neq -6,\ x \neq -3,\ x \neq 4\}$
(D) $\{x \mid x = -6,\ x = -3,\ x = 4\}$

169. $9^3 \cdot 9^{-1} =$

(A) $\dfrac{1}{729}$

(B) 81
(C) -81

(D) $\dfrac{1}{81}$

170. Five people are chosen at random from a group of 3 boys and 5 girls. What is the probability that 3 girls and 1 boy are chosen?

(A) $\dfrac{4}{7}$

(B) $\dfrac{1}{2}$

(C) $\dfrac{3}{4}$

(D) $\dfrac{3}{7}$

171. Find the vertex for the given function.
$$f(x) = 9x^2 + 18x - 7$$

(A) $(-1,0)$
(B) $(-1,-16)$
(C) $(1,20)$
(D) $(1,0)$

172. Determine the slope of the tangent line to the graph of the function $f(x) = 4x^3 + 7x$ at the point whose x coordinate equals -1.

(A) 19
(B) -19
(C) -11
(D) 11

173. If $\ln(2w + 9x) = 4$, then

(A) $x = \dfrac{e^4 - 2w}{9}$

(B) $x = \dfrac{e^4 + 2w}{9}$

(C) $x = \dfrac{4e - 2w}{9}$

(D) $x = \dfrac{4e + 2w}{9}$

174. A box contains apples and oranges in a ratio of 3:7. If the box contains 9 apples, how many oranges does the box contain?

    (A) 13
    (B) 21
    (C) 10
    (D) 18

175. $\dfrac{2+\sqrt{3}}{2-\sqrt{3}}$ =

    (A) $7-4\sqrt{3}$

    (B) $-7+4\sqrt{3}$

    (C) $7+4\sqrt{3}$

    (D) $-7-4\sqrt{3}$

176. In an employee survey, 300 indicated they would attend Workshop I, and 120 indicated Workshop II. If 65 employees plan to attend both workshops and 260 indicated they could not attend either workshop, how many employees participated in the survey?

    (A) 615
    (B) 745
    (C) 550
    (D) Not enough information

177. Given the graph of the function $y = f(x)$, evaluate the limit.

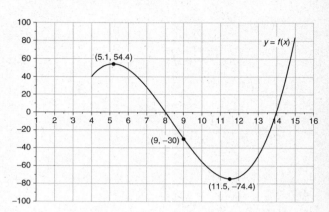

$$\lim_{x \to 5.1}\left(\frac{f(x)-f(5.1)}{x-5.1}\right) =$$

    (A) 54.4
    (B) 5.1
    (C) 0
    (D) Not enough information

178. Determine the domain of the function $f(x) = \ln(2x - 7)$.

    (A) $(-\infty, \infty)$
    (B) $[-\infty, \infty]$
    (C) $[3.5, \infty)$
    (D) $(3.5, \infty)$

179. Find the extreme value of the given function and state whether that value represents a maximum or a minimum value for the function.

$$P(x) = 35x^2 + 420x - 50$$

    (A) −1,310, maximum
    (B) −1,310, minimum
    (C) −6, maximum
    (D) −6, minimum

180. Simplify the expression $\dfrac{\sqrt{x-h}-\sqrt{x}}{h}$.

    (A) $-\dfrac{1}{\sqrt{x-h}+\sqrt{x}}$

    (B)   1

    (C) $\dfrac{1}{\sqrt{x-h}+\sqrt{x}}$

    (D)   –1

181. $\log(75) - \log(3) =$

    (A) $\dfrac{1}{25}$

    (B) $\log(25)$

    (C) $\dfrac{\log(75)}{3}$

    (D) $\log(72)$

182. A truck is 48 miles from its destination at 5:00 P.M. At what speed must the truck travel to arrive by 5:45 P.M.?

    (A)   64 mph
    (B)   60 mph
    (C)   70 mph
    (D)   74 mph

183. Determine the radius of the circle with equation $(x-4)^2 + (y+3)^2 = 36$.

    (A)   36
    (B)   6
    (C)   ±6
    (D)   ±36

184. Solve the equation $\dfrac{x}{x+3} + \dfrac{x}{x+2} = 2$.

    (A) $x = \dfrac{12}{5}$

    (B) $x = -\dfrac{5}{12}$

    (C) $x = \dfrac{5}{12}$

    (D) $x = -\dfrac{12}{5}$

STOP

End of Quantitative Ability section. If you have any time left, you may go over your work in this section only.

READING COMPREHENSION

48 QUESTIONS (#185–#232)

TIME: 50 MINUTES

Directions: Read each of the following passages, and choose the one **best** answer to each of the questions that follow each passage.

Passage 1

Bronchial asthma is a common disease of children and adults. Although the clinical manifestations of asthma have been known since antiquity, it is a disease that still defies precise definition. The word *asthma* is of Greek origin and means "panting." More than 2000 years ago, Hippocrates used the word *asthma* to describe episodic shortness of breath; however, the first detailed clinical description of the asthmatic patient was made by Aretaeus in the second century. Since that time *asthma* has been used to describe any disorder with episodic shortness of breath or dyspnea; thus, the terms *cardiac asthma* and *bronchial asthma* have been used to delineate the etiologies of the dyspnea. These terms are now obsolete and *asthma* refers to a disorder of the respiratory system characterized by episodes of difficulty in breathing. An Expert Panel of the National Institutes of Health National Asthma Education Program (NAEP) has defined asthma as a lung disease characterized by (1) airway obstruction that is reversible (but not completely so in some patients) either spontaneously or with treatment; (2) airway inflammation; and (3) increased airway responsiveness to a variety of stimuli. This descriptive definition for asthma is attributed to our lack of knowledge of the precise pathogenic defect that results in the clinical syndrome we recognize as asthma. The current definition does allow for the important heterogeneity of the clinical presentation of asthma. New technologies have added substantially to our understanding of the interrelationships of immunology, biochemistry, and physiology to the clinical presentation of asthma, and further research may yet uncover a specific genetic defect associated with asthma. Until such time, asthma will continue to defy exact definition.

An estimated 10 million persons in the United States have asthma (about 5% of the population). The reported prevalence increased 29% from 1980 to 1987 to 40.1 per 1000 population. African-Americans have a 19% higher incidence of asthma than whites and are twice as likely to be hospitalized. The estimated cost of asthma in the United States in 1990 was $6.2 billion. The largest single direct medical expenditure was for inpatient hospital services (emergency care), reaching almost $1.5 billion, followed by prescription medications ($1.1 billion). The costs of medication increased 54% between 1985 and 1990. In total, 43% of the economic impact was associated with emergency room use, hospitalization, and death. Asthma accounted for 1% of all ambulatory care visits according to the National Ambulatory Medical Care Survey and results in more than 450,000 hospitalizations per year.

Excerpted with permission from *Pharmacotherapy, A Pathophysiological Approach*, Third Edition, by Joseph T. DiPiro, et al., page 553. Stamford, CT: Appleton & Lange, 1996.

185. Bronchial asthma is best described as a

    (A) precisely defined disease commonly occurring in both children and adults.
    (B) common disease in children and adults that defies precise definition.
    (C) common disease found only in children that defies precise description.
    (D) precisely defined disease rarely occurring in children and adults.

186. The etiologies of the episodic shortness of breath were once divided into two terms:

    (A) antiquity and panting.
    (B) reversible and spontaneous.
    (C) inpatient and outpatient.
    (D) bronchial asthma and cardiac asthma.

187. According to the NAEP, one way to characterize asthma is by

    (A) the homogeneity of its clinical presentation.
    (B) inflamed airways.
    (C) a decrease in airway responsiveness.
    (D) airway obstruction that is always completely reversible.

188. What was the cost of asthma in the United States in 1990, not including the cost of prescription medications?

    (A) $1.5 billion
    (B) $6.2 billion
    (C) $5.1 billion
    (D) $1.1 billion

189. The passage suggests that in the future researchers are likely to understand more about

    (A) new technologies to treat asthma.
    (B) wheezing and episodes of shortness of breath.
    (C) a specific genetic defect associated with asthma.
    (D) the interrelationship of immunology, biochemistry, and physiology.

190. Asthma results in more than _____ hospitalizations per year.

    (A) 6.2 billion
    (B) 29% of
    (C) 10 million
    (D) 450,000

191. The estimated number of persons in the United States who have asthma is

    (A) 100 million.
    (B) 2.5 million.
    (C) fewer than 2%.
    (D) 10 million.

192. Today, the term *asthma* refers to

    (A) panting.
    (B) dyspnea of cardiac etiology.
    (C) dyspnea of bronchial etiology.
    (D) a disorder of the respiratory system characterized by episodes of difficulty in breathing.

193. The word *asthma* has a Greek origin and was used by

    (A) Aretaeus.
    (B) an Expert Panel of the National Institutes of Health.
    (C) Hippocrates.
    (D) the National Ambulatory Medical Care Survey.

194. The passage contains which of the following?

    (A) A description of pharmacists' role in asthma treatment
    (B) Facts about the prevalence of asthma in the United States
    (C) An explanation of the worldwide increase in prevalence of asthma
    (D) An in-depth treatment plan for asthma

Passage 2

Hypercalcemia, increased serum calcium concentrations, occurs in approximately 15% of individuals with cancer. Occurrences of this condition have been reported in most types of malignancies. The most effective management of this life-threatening disease is successful treatment of the malignancy. Unfortunately, successful treatment of the cancer may not be possible. In these cases, treatment goals should include correcting intravascular depletion, enhancing renal excretion of calcium, and inhibiting bone resorption. First line treatment of acute hypercalcemia includes the administration of normal saline and furosemide. Since many patients suffering from acute hypercalcemia are dehydrated, the administration of normal saline is warranted. In addition to treating dehydration, normal saline helps to increase renal excretion of calcium. The optimal administration of normal saline is dependent on the severity of hypercalcemia, the degree of dehydration, and the clinical status of the patient. An infusion rate of 400 mL per hour of normal saline is typical. Furosemide, a diuretic, is useful in the treatment of hypercalcemia due to its ability to enhance urinary excretion and more importantly calcium excretion. Additionally, furosemide protects patients from becoming volume overloaded due to the administration of the normal saline. It is very important that patients be adequately hydrated prior to the administration of furosemide in order to get maximum benefits. Intravenous doses of 100 mg of furosemide every 2 hours may be used. Although normal saline and furosemide are the most commonly used agents to treat acute cancer hypercalcemia, only a modest decrease in calcium levels are achieved from this regimen. The use of normal saline and furosemide may be sufficient for the management of mild to moderate hypercalcemia, but it is commonly insufficient for treating severe hypercalcemia.

195. Hypercalcemia may occur in

    (A) breast cancer only.
    (B) most types of cancer.
    (C) bone cancer only.
    (D) lung cancer only.

196. Which of the following is the most appropriate title for this passage?

    (A) The Pathogenesis of Cancer-Related Hypercalcemia
    (B) The Uses of Normal Saline and Furosemide
    (C) Hypercalcemia—a Life-Threatening Disorder
    (D) First Line Agents Used to Treat Acute Cancer-Related Hypercalcemia

197. In treating hypercalcemia with a diuretic, it is important to

    (A) use the diuretic every hour.
    (B) administer the diuretic by mouth.
    (C) hydrate the patient before administrating the diuretic.
    (D) give the diuretic before the normal saline.

198. Which of the following is the most effective method of treating cancer-related hypercalcemia?

    (A) The use of normal saline
    (B) The use of furosemide
    (C) The use of dialysis
    (D) Treatment of the malignancy

199. Which of the following is NOT a goal in the treatment of acute hypercalcemia?

    (A) Administration of calcium carbonate
    (B) Enhancing renal excretion of calcium
    (C) Inhibiting bone resorption
    (D) Correcting intravascular depletion

200. In patients who are being treated for acute hypercalcemia, the administration of normal saline is warranted because

    (A) the patients have cancer.
    (B) the patients are dehydrated.
    (C) the patients are seen in the clinic.
    (D) the patients are volume overloaded.

201. The use of normal saline and furosemide is NOT typically sufficient for which type of hypercalcemia?

    (A) Mild cancer-related hypercalcemia
    (B) Mild hypercalcemia
    (C) Moderate hypercalcemia
    (D) Severe hypercalcemia

Passage 3

Gastroesophageal reflux disease (GERD) is a common medical disorder seen by health care practitioners of all specialties. It is generally chronic in nature, and long-term therapy may be required. While the mortality associated with GERD is very low (1 death per 100,000 patients), the quality of life experienced by the patient can be greatly diminished.

GERD refers to any symptomatic clinical condition or histologic alteration that results from episodes of gastroesophageal reflux. Gastroesophageal reflux refers to the retrograde movement of gastric contents from the stomach into the esophagus. Many people experience some degree of reflux, especially after eating, which may be considered a benign physiologic process. When the esophagus is repeatedly exposed to refluxed material for prolonged periods of time, inflammation of the esophagus (i.e., reflux esophagitis) can occur. It is important to realize that gastroesophageal reflux must precede the development of GERD or reflux esophagitis. In severe cases, reflux may lead to a multitude of serious complications including esophageal strictures, esophageal ulcers, motility disorders, perforation, hemorrhage, aspiration, and Barrett's esophagus. While mild disease is often managed with life-style changes and antacids, more intensive therapeutic intervention with histamine (H_2) antagonists, sucralfate, prokinetic agents, or proton pump inhibitors is generally required for patients with more severe disease. In general, response to pharmacologic intervention is dependent on the efficacy of the agent, dosage regimen employed, duration of therapy, and severity of the disease. Following discontinuation of therapy, relapse is common and long-term maintenance therapy may be required. Historically, surgical intervention has been reserved for patients in whom conventional treatment modalities fail. However, the recent development of laparoscopic antireflux surgical procedures has led to a reevaluation of the role of surgery in the long-term management of GERD. Some clinicians have suggested that laparoscopic antireflux surgery may be a cost-effective alternative to long-term maintenance therapy in young patients. However, long-term comparative trials evaluating the cost effectiveness of the various treatment modalities are warranted.

The pathogenesis of gastroesophageal reflux is related to the complex balance between defense mechanisms and aggressive factors. Understanding both the normal protective mechanisms and the aggressive factors that may contribute to or promote gastroesophageal reflux helps one to design rational therapeutic treatment regimens. Gastric acid, pepsin, bile acids, and pancreatic enzymes are considered aggressive factors and may promote esophageal damage upon reflux into the esophagus. Thus, the composition (potency) and volume of the refluxate are aggressive factors that may lead to esophageal injury. Conversely, normal protective mechanisms include anatomic factors, the lower esophageal sphincter pressure, esophageal clearing, mucosal resistance, and gastric emptying. Rational therapeutic regimens in the treatment of gastroesophageal reflux are designed to maximize normal defense mechanisms and/or attenuate the aggressive factors.

Excerpted with permission from *Pharmacotherapy, A Pathophysiological Approach*, Third Edition, by Joseph T. DiPiro, et al., page 675. Stamford, CT: Appleton & Lange, 1996.

202. The mortality rate associated with GERD is

    (A) 1 death in 1,000 patients
    (B) 1 death in 10,000 patients
    (C) 1 death in 100,000 patients
    (D) 1 death in 1,000,000 patients

203. One possible complication of reflux is

    (A) perforation.
    (B) mucosal resistance.
    (C) gastric emptying.
    (D) lower esophageal sphincter pressure.

204. Reflux esophagitis is

   (A) a rational therapeutic treatment regimen.
   (B) a surgical intervention.
   (C) the inflammation of the esophagus due to repeated exposure to refluxed gastric contents for prolonged periods of time.
   (D) a normal defense mechanism.

205. After therapy is discontinued

   (A) no further intervention is needed.
   (B) brief periods of medication therapy will be needed periodically throughout the patient's life.
   (C) long-term maintenance may be required to prevent relapse following the discontinuation of therapy.
   (D) GERD is considered cured and no relapses are expected.

206. In GERD patients, response to pharmacologic intervention is dependent on

   (A) physical exercise.
   (B) efficacy of the agent.
   (C) intramuscular administration of drugs.
   (D) limiting duration of therapy.

207. Long-term comparative trials evaluating the cost effectiveness of various treatment modalities for GERD are

   (A) warranted.
   (B) not feasible.
   (C) premature.
   (D) aggressive.

208. Some clinicians have suggested that a cost-effective alternative therapy for GERD may be

   (A) histamine antagonists.
   (B) prokinetic agents.
   (C) laparoscopic antireflux surgery.
   (D) proton pump inhibitors.

209. Aggressive factors that may promote esophageal damage upon reflux into the esophagus are

   (A) gastric acid and pancreatic enzymes.
   (B) bile acids and esophageal clearing.
   (C) lower esophageal sphincter pressure and gastric emptying.
   (D) lipids and plaques.

Passage 4

Many people in the United States are diagnosed with diabetes mellitus. Type 2 diabetes is the most common type of diabetes and it is associated with a significant amount of morbidities and mortalities. Type 2 diabetes is classified as an endocrine disorder characterized by defects in insulin secretion as well as in insulin action. In type 2 diabetes patients, a defect also exists in insulin receptor binding. These defects lead to increased serum glucose concentrations or hyperglycemia.

Sulfonylureas are one of the most popular classes of agents used to treat type 2 diabetes. One of the newest agents to treat type 2 diabetes is acarbose, an oral alpha-glucosidase inhibitor. Acarbose interferes with the hydrolysis of dietary disaccharides and complex carbohydrates, thereby delaying absorption of glucose and other monosaccharides. Acarbose is available for oral administration only. To be most effective, it should be taken at the beginning of a meal. The recommended starting dose is 25 mg three times daily and doses as high as 200 mg three times a day have been safely used. The most common adverse experiences associated with the use of acarbose are abdominal cramps, flatulence, diarrhea, and abdominal distension. Most of the adverse effects are due to the unabsorbed carbohydrates undergoing fermentation in the colon. Acarbose has also been associated with decreased intestinal absorption of iron, thereby possibly leading to anemia. The occurrence of hypoglycemia when using acarbose in combination with other agents used to lower serum glucose is great. Glucose should be administered to treat hypoglycemia in patients taking acarbose because sucrose may not be adequately hydrolyzed and absorbed. The effectiveness of this agent to lower serum glucose concentrations in patients with type 2 diabetes has been clearly demonstrated in clinical trials. Acarbose provides another option for treating type 2 diabetes.

210. Which of the following does NOT describe the term *type 2 diabetes*?

(A) Endocrine in nature
(B) Hyperglycemia
(C) May be due to a defect in insulin receptor binding
(D) Results in iron deficiencies

211. Which of the following is the most common type of agent used to treat type 2 diabetes?

(A) A sulfonylurea agent
(B) Glucose
(C) Sucrose
(D) Fructose

212. To be most effective, when should acarbose be taken?

(A) At the beginning of a meal
(B) At bedtime
(C) At the end of a meal
(D) At noon

213. According to the passage, which of the following is the most common side effect associated with the use of acarbose?

(A) Hyperglycemia
(B) Anemia
(C) Gastrointestinal discomfort
(D) Rash

214. Which of the following is the best agent to treat hypoglycemia in patients taking acarbose?

(A) A sulfonylurea agent
(B) Glucose
(C) Sucrose
(D) Fructose

215. According to the passage, which of the following has NOT been associated with the use of acarbose?

(A) Low serum glucose concentrations
(B) Gastrointestinal discomfort
(C) Decreased iron absorption
(D) Obstruction of the urinary tract

216. Which of the following used in combination with acarbose increases the risk of experiencing hypoglycemia?

(A) A sulfonylurea agent
(B) Glucose
(C) Iron
(D) Increased caloric intake

217. Which of the following is the best title for this passage?

(A) Diabetes in the United States
(B) Agents Used to Treat Type 2 Diabetes
(C) The Use of Acarbose in the Treatment of Type 2 Diabetes
(D) Adverse Effects of Acarbose

Passage 5

Osteoporosis, the most common skeletal disorder associated with aging, is a significant cause of mortality and morbidity among the elderly. The two most common types of osteoporosis are type I (postmenopausal) osteoporosis and type II (senile) osteoporosis. Type I osteoporosis is due to a drastic decline in bone mass during the first five years of menopause and a slower rate of bone loss in subsequent years. Type II osteoporosis is characterized by a gradual, age-related loss of bone in females and males over the age of 65 years. By far, osteoporosis is most prevalent in the postmenopausal population. In addition to menopausal-associated hormonal changes, other risk factors for osteoporosis in women include low calcium intake, medical factors such as oophorectomy, and life-style factors such as inactivity and cigarette smoking. In osteoporosis, osteoclasts excavate areas in bone that the bone-forming cells, the osteoblasts, are unable to fully reconstitute. Often this defective bone loses compressive strength, thereby leading to an increased risk of fracture. Osteoporosis evolves as a silent disease with no obvious early warning signs. Many patients suffering from osteoporosis are not aware of their condition until a fracture occurs. This disease is responsible for at least 1.5 million fractures in Americans each year, with annual costs to the United States health care system of approximately $10 billion. Other consequences of osteoporosis include pain and spinal deformities such as dorsal kyphosis and dowager's or widow's hump. In addition, a decrease in appetite, fatigue, and weakness may be present. As the population continues to age, the cost of treating osteoporosis and its associated complications is predicted to double over the next 30 years.

218. Osteoporosis is most common in which population?

   (A) Postmenopausal women
   (B) Young males
   (C) Infants
   (D) Teenagers

219. Which of the following is NOT a risk factor for osteoporosis?

   (A) Age
   (B) Low calcium intake
   (C) Weight-bearing exercise
   (D) Cigarette smoking

220. Which of the following is a direct consequence of osteoporosis?

   (A) Height gain
   (B) Hypertension
   (C) Oophorectomy
   (D) Dowager's hump

221. Early warning signs of osteoporosis are

   (A) easily detectable.
   (B) not obvious.
   (C) evident by age 45.
   (D) common in women but not men.

222. What is the predicted U.S. cost of treating osteoporosis and its associated complications over the next 30 years?

   (A) $5 billion
   (B) $7 billion
   (C) $10 billion
   (D) $20 billion

223. Which cells are responsible for removing bone?

   (A) Osteoclasts
   (B) Osteoblasts
   (C) Osteomasts
   (D) Osteotrasts

224. Which cells are responsible for forming bone?

   (A) Osteoclasts
   (B) Osteoblasts
   (C) Osteomasts
   (D) Osteotrasts

Passage 6

Although phenytoin may be used to treat cardiac arrhythmias, migraines, and trigeminal neuralgia, the primary use of phenytoin is to treat seizure disorders. Phenytoin, one of the most important agents used to manage seizures, works similarly to other hydantoin-derivative anticonvulsants. It decreases seizure activity by stabilizing neuronal membranes and by increasing efflux or decreasing influx of sodium ions across cell membranes in the motor cortex during generation of nerve impulses. Phenytoin is commercially available as oral suspension, tablets, and capsules. It is also available as an injection. The dosage of phenytoin varies according to the frequency of seizures, the type of seizures, and the patient's tolerance for phenytoin. Therefore, it is extremely important to monitor the patient for seizure activity as well as to monitor phenytoin serum concentrations. Phenytoin has a narrow therapeutic window and monitoring of serum concentrations is necessary. Therapeutic serum concentrations of phenytoin are usually 10–20 mcg per mL (millimeter) and depend on the assay method used. Serum concentrations above 20 mcg per mL often result in toxicity. Adverse reactions associated with dose-related toxicities include blurred vision, lethargy, rash, fever, slurred speech, nystagmus, and confusion. In some patients, seizure control is not achieved when plasma concentrations are within the therapeutic concentration range and therefore clinical response of the patient is more meaningful than plasma concentrations. Generally, therapeutic steady state serum concentrations are achieved within 30 days of therapy with an oral dosage of 300 mg daily in adults. Following an intravenous administration of 1000–1500 mg, at a rate not exceeding 50 mg per minute, therapeutic concentrations can be attained within 2 hours. Rapid administration of intravenous phenytoin may result in adverse effects such as decreased blood pressure and other cardiac complications. The use of phenytoin has been associated with osteomalacia, thrombocytopenia, and gastrointestinal upset.

225. According to the passage, which of the following is treated with phenytoin?

(A) Trigeminal neuralgia
(B) Arthritis
(C) Osteomalacia
(D) Nystagmus

226. The primary use of phenytoin is to treat

(A) cardiac arrhythmias.
(B) migraines.
(C) seizure disorders.
(D) arthritis.

227. Which of the following best represents the mechanism of action of phenytoin in treating seizures?

(A) Increases neuronal activity
(B) Excites peripheral impulses to excite neuronal activity
(C) Stabilizes neuronal membranes and decreases seizure activity by decreasing the entrance of sodium ions across the cell membranes in the motor cortex during generation of nerve impulses
(D) Stabilizes neuronal membranes and decreases seizure activity by increasing the entrance of sodium ions across the cell membranes in the motor cortex during generation of nerve impulses

228. Which of the following does NOT affect the dosage of phenytoin?

(A) Phenytoin serum concentration
(B) Number of seizures experienced
(C) Adverse events experienced
(D) Puncture sites available

229. Which of the following best explains the meaning of the sentence "Phenytoin has a narrow therapeutic window and monitoring of serum concentrations is necessary"?

    (A) There is a small difference in the serum concentrations known to produce seizures and the serum concentrations known to produce adverse experiences. Therefore, serum concentrations should be monitored.
    (B) There is no difference in the serum concentrations known to produce desirable effects and the serum concentrations known to produce undesirable effects. Therefore, serum concentrations should be monitored.
    (C) There is a small difference in the serum concentrations known to control migraines and the serum concentrations known to produce migraines. Therefore, serum concentrations should be monitored.
    (D) There is a small difference in the serum concentrations known to control seizures and the serum concentrations known to produce toxicities and adverse effects. Therefore, serum concentrations should be monitored.

230. Which of the following statements describe why phenytoin should NOT be administered at a rate greater than 50 mg per minute?

    (A) A higher rate takes longer to achieve adequate plasma concentrations.
    (B) A higher rate may lower blood pressure.
    (C) A higher rate increases arthritis pain.
    (D) A higher rate may cause a rash.

231. According to the passage, which of the following is NOT a common adverse reaction associated with phenytoin toxicity?

    (A) Blurred vision
    (B) Lethargy
    (C) Dysuria
    (D) Mental confusion

232. When is the therapeutic steady-state serum concentration generally achieved with an oral dosage of 300 mg daily of phenytoin?

    (A) Within 5 days
    (B) Within 24 hours
    (C) Within 6 days
    (D) Within 30 days

STOP

End of Reading Comprehension section. If you have any time left, you may go over your work in this section only.

ESSAY

TIME: 30 MINUTES

Directions: Write a well-constructed essay addressing the statement below.

Although the United States spends more than $8,000 per person on health care, the quality of health care has been under scrutiny. Discuss a solution to the problem of rising health care costs and how to improve quality.

_____

_____

_____

_____

_____

_____

_____

_____

_____

_____

_____

_____

_____

_____

_____

_____

_____

_____

_____

_____

_____

_____

_____

Answer Key
PRACTICE TEST 1

VERBAL ABILITY

1. C	11. A	21. C	31. C
2. A	12. D	22. A	32. A
3. C	13. B	23. B	33. D
4. A	14. D	24. B	34. C
5. A	15. C	25. A	35. A
6. B	16. C	26. D	36. D
7. A	17. C	27. B	37. C
8. D	18. B	28. C	38. C
9. A	19. D	29. A	39. D
10. B	20. B	30. A	40. B

BIOLOGY

41. D	53. C	65. C	77. C
42. A	54. A	66. A	78. C
43. C	55. C	67. C	79. C
44. B	56. B	68. B	80. B
45. C	57. A	69. C	81. C
46. B	58. B	70. A	82. C
47. B	59. C	71. B	83. D
48. C	60. D	72. C	84. C
49. D	61. B	73. A	85. D
50. B	62. A	74. A	86. D
51. C	63. A	75. B	87. A
52. B	64. B	76. B	88. B

CHEMISTRY

89. A	101. B	113. C	125. B
90. C	102. B	114. B	126. D
91. A	103. A	115. D	127. B
92. A	104. D	116. B	128. B
93. C	105. A	117. B	129. A
94. A	106. A	118. A	130. B
95. A	107. B	119. C	131. B
96. C	108. B	120. B	132. C
97. C	109. B	121. C	133. A
98. B	110. B	122. B	134. C
99. C	111. D	123. D	135. D
100. B	112. C	124. B	136. B

Answer Key
PRACTICE TEST 1

QUANTITATIVE ABILITY

137. C	149. C	161. D	173. A
138. B	150. B	162. B	174. B
139. B	151. A	163. D	175. C
140. B	152. A	164. A	176. A
141. C	153. B	165. D	177. C
142. B	154. B	166. A	178. D
143. A	155. D	167. A	179. B
144. A	156. A	168. A	180. A
145. C	157. D	169. B	181. B
146. D	158. C	170. D	182. A
147. D	159. B	171. B	183. B
148. D	160. A	172. A	184. D

READING COMPREHENSION

185. B	197. C	209. A	221. B
186. D	198. D	210. D	222. D
187. B	199. A	211. A	223. A
188. C	200. B	212. A	224. B
189. C	201. D	213. C	225. A
190. D	202. C	214. B	226. C
191. D	203. A	215. D	227. C
192. D	204. C	216. A	228. D
193. C	205. C	217. C	229. D
194. B	206. B	218. A	230. B
195. B	207. A	219. C	231. C
196. D	208. C	220. D	232. D

EXPLANATORY ANSWERS

1. **(C)** The analogy here is based on synonyms, that is, words that have the same or nearly the same meaning. *Austere* and *dour* are both defined as stern; likewise *auspicious* and *hopeful* are both defined as suggesting good fortune. Answers A, B, and D are incorrect as *sovereign* is defined as ruler, *suspect* as doubtful, and *avarice* as greed.

2. **(A)** *Placate* and *pacify* have the same or nearly the same meaning, so you need to find the word that is synonymous with *confirm*. The answer is *ratify*. Answer B would be an antonym of *confirm*, while C and D do not fit the pattern of the analogy.

3. **(C)** The analogy is one of antonyms. You are looking for a word that means the opposite of *callow* (defined as immature), so the correct choice is C, *sophisticated* (defined as cultivated or experienced). Answers A, B, and D are synonyms of *callow*.

4. **(A)** This analogy involves causality. A *virus* causes a *cold*, just as a *deity* performs a *miracle*.

5. **(A)** This analogy involves the relationship of part to whole. The *margin* of a wound is the part analogous to the *rim* of a *volcano*.

6. **(B)** Here the analogy is based on the relationship of whole to part. A *book* is divided into parts, each of which is a *chapter*, and a *concerto* is divided into parts, each of which is a *movement*.

7. **(A)** Here the relationship is that of whole to part. The *small intestine* contains a part called the *duodenum*, and the *hand* contains *fingers*. Since an echidna is a spiny anteater, that is clearly not the correct choice. The other alternatives must be rejected as well since neither completes an analogy based on a whole-to-part relationship.

8. **(D)** In this example, the relationship is deceptively simple: purpose or use. We use a *needle* to *sew*, and we use a *hose* to *siphon*. Be careful not to choose the noun *lawn* erroneously; although we water the lawn with a hose, this word is not the correct choice in this case.

9. **(A)** This analogy involves purpose or use. A *barn* is used to house horses; an *aviary* is used to house birds.

10. **(B)** The correct answer is *egg* because this is an analogy of action to object. We *recycle* (action) *paper* (object), and *incubate* (action) an *egg* (object).

11. **(A)** Just as a *theory* is *refuted*, a *president* is impeached, so *impeach* is the correct choice. This analogy involves object to action.

12. **(D)** This analogy expresses the relationship of part to whole: the *ear* is part of the *corn* plant, and the *boll* is part of the *cotton* plant.

13. **(B)** *Debris* eventually becomes *compost* and can be used as fertilizer; *resin* eventually becomes *amber*. The analogy is one of sequence or time.

14. **(D)** In this analogy of characteristic or description, the *cheetah* is *sleek*, whereas the *seal* is *rotund*.

15. **(C)** A relationship of degree is implied here. The *flu* represents a disease with a much greater degree of severity than a *cold*. Likewise, a *depression* is a much greater economic problem than a recession.

16. **(C)** This is a grammatical analogy. You must find a verb that takes the preposition *out*, just as the verb *comment* takes the preposition *on*. The correct answer can only be *eke*.

17. **(C)** An analogy may express the relationship between a worker and tool. In this example, a *painter* uses a *palette*, and a *cook* uses a *spatula*.

18. **(B)** To understand this analogy of definition, it helps to know that an *ellipsis,* usually indicated by three successive dots . . . is an omission of words in a *sentence*. The correct answer is *pause*, a temporary cessation of utterance in a *speech*.

19. **(D)** Since a *Panama* is one of many kinds of *hat*, and a *Mako* is one of many kinds of *shark*, the relationship expressed is part to whole.

20. **(B)** Drums are part of a band; a goalie is part of a team. This is an analogy of part to whole.

21. **(C)** This is an analogy of synonyms. Despot and dictator both refer to a totalitarian ruler, and agitator and demagogue (answer C) both refer to a person who disturbs the peace. A cherub (answer A) is an angel. A narcissist (answer B) is someone who is completely self-centered. An epicure (answer D) is a person with a refined taste in food.

22. **(A)** This is an analogy of classification. Haiku and sonnet are both types of poetry, while concerto and madrigal (answer A) are both types of musical pieces. Answer B is an architectural school, and answers C and D are types of literary works.

23. **(B)** This is an analogy based on synonyms. Just as *canonize* and *exalt* are synonyms (defined as to raise or elevate), *mournful* and *lugubrious* have the same or nearly the same meaning (i.e., sorrowful or dismal). Answers A, C, and D are incorrect as *litigious* refers to being prone to lawsuits, *suspicious* refers to being questionable, and *contumacious* refers to being obstinate.

24. **(B)** This is an analogy of whole to part. A focuser is part of a telescope just as a condenser (answer B) is part of a microscope. A cathode (answer A) is part of a television, a microprocessor (answer C) is part of a computer, and an alternator (answer D) is part of an automobile engine.

25. **(A)** This grammatical analogy involves pairs of adverbs (*seemingly* and *ostensibly, thoroughly* and *completely*) with the same or nearly the same meaning. This example may also be considered an analogy of synonyms.

26. **(D)** The first blank is associated with evolution, relating to an introduction, development, or emergence of something that was not previously or originally available. After these modifications and deviations from the original state or condition occur (indicated by the first blank), the results can be deemed as dissimilar, irregular, or variant (indicated by the second blank). Based on the sentence's context, "mutation and variation" (Answer D) are the correct answer choices.

27. **(B)** The correct answer for the first blank will further describe a gentleman who is always "complaining and rude," indicating that it will be synonymous with "discourteous." Because the phrase "on the other hand" precedes the second blank (or the word we are looking for to replace the blank), we know that the blank will have a meaning that will be the opposite of the first blank. Furthermore, the correct word for the second blank will be synonymous with someone who is always "laughing and joking," also meaning "jovial" or "happy." Based on this, Answer B (cantankerous and mirthful) is the correct answer for this sentence.

28. **(C)** Because what Henry used to solve the problem and what he did NOT rely on seem to be in conflict, then we can conclude that the two correct words for the blanks will be opposing terms. Data collected through scientific study or experimentation are usually heralded as reliable and indisputable. This could be a clue as to why Henry used data to solve the problem and did NOT rely on something that was questionable, subjective, or that did not require the use of concrete reasoning. By reading each of the answer choices back into the sentence, Answer C (intuition and empirical) provides the answer choices that make the most sense.

29. **(A)** Because the story was described as having several twists and turns, answer A, *convoluted* (meaning twisted or complicated), is the best choice. *Dispassionate* (meaning free from emotion), *insipid* (meaning bland), and *placid* (meaning calm) would not be appropriate descriptors for a ghost story that had a "thrilling" ending.

30. **(A)** The use of *discourteous* suggests the senior partner exhibits negative qualities. *Imperious* is the only choice in the answer list with negative connotations due to its definition (domineering or overbearing). The young lawyer desires to leave her profession after working with the *imperious* senior partner, suggesting she is dissatisfied or *jaded*. Therefore, A is the correct answer.

31. **(C)** The first blank describes the remarks made during a sacred and dignified occasion that were offensive, and therefore probably inappropriate and disrespectful to many audience members. The second blank describes the type of damage these negative remarks potentially caused. Undoubtedly, the disdainful remarks changed the ceremony's solemn and formal tone, but we are not told in the sentence to what extent. It is possible that the damage was irreversible or unalterable, causing the ceremony to be ruined. Based on this and the answer choices provided, Answer C provides the best answer to complete this sentence.

32. **(A)** In this sentence, the word that fits in the blank describes a man who is free with his opinions as he is described as having "ample thoughts." Answer A (*profuse*) is the only answer listed that is synonymous with *ample*.

33. **(D)** The sentence indicates that Karen and her friends hold opposite views of the clothing store's ads. Because Karen's friends hold positive opinions, logically we can assume that Karen's opinion is negative. The only word in the answer list with a negative connotation is D, *meretricious*, which means gaudy. *Opulent* and *alluring* indicate something that is luxurious

and attractive, respectively. *Ephemeral* would not fit, as it means momentary or transient.

34. **(C)** The word for the first blank is further emphasized by the phrase "Without a doubt." Based on this, we can conclude that waiting until the solution has completely stabilized is of unquestionable importance and is required and mandatory. The word to be placed in the second blank in this sentence provides the connection between a completely stabilized solution and the risk of causing a violent chemical reaction. Until something regarding the solution is attained or achieved (indicated by the word to be placed in the second blank), a violent reaction may result. Based on this, we can conclude that the word in the second blank should be related to the solution being completely stable, balanced, or unchanged. Accordingly, "imperative" and "equilibrium" (found in Answer C) are the correct answers to complete this sentence.

35. **(A)** Because the word that goes into the first blank is preceded by the phrase "in contrast," we can conclude that the words to be placed in the two blanks describing the paintings in this sentence will have opposite meanings. Of the answer choices given, Answer A—"flamboyant" and "simplicity"—best matches this prediction. By reading each of the answer choices back into the sentence, these words make the most sense and best match the sentence's context.

36. **(D)** The word that goes into the blank in this sentence is in reference to our "best" (or most preferred and most beneficial) interest—in association with NOT acting too hastily. To act hastily means to act rapidly, swiftly, expeditiously, or immediately; therefore, to NOT act hastily means to wait or postpone. Thus, we can conclude that the action for the meeting "until next week" most likely means to "delay" or "reschedule"; Answer D (defer) is the best answer choice.

37. **(C)** The phrases "studying for several years" and "well-received research" indicate Dr. Smith has developed expertise on global economics. *Erudite* (defined as learned or scholarly) is a synonym for *expertise*, so answer C is correct. *Foppish* is defined as being vain, *inveterate* as deeply rooted, and *mawkish* as insipid or sentimental. None of these answer choices would be appropriate for the sentence.

38. **(C)** In this sentence we are told that the first description of multiple sclerosis was over 100 years ago, which denotes an ample and extended time frame. Because of the word "although," we can assume that something about the cause and cure still exists that should have been resolved or discovered, given the lengthy time period. Answer C (mystery and undiscovered) provides the only two answer choices that make sense for both blanks in this sentence.

39. **(D)** The context clues for the blank in this sentence are the phrases "early" and "begin to develop," which in this sentence describe a period in an individual's life span that is initial or introductory. Answer D (embryonic) most closely denotes a beginning or rudimentary formulation or development; therefore Answer D is the best answer choice.

40. **(B)** The word "sterile" in this sentence provides a clue. Sterile means to be clean, disinfected, or without germs. The sentence states that this is the type of rod that must be used to stir the experiment's solution in order to prevent something—indicated by the blank—from happening. Based on this we can predict that if a rod that is NOT sterile is used to stir the solution, the solution will become dirty, impure, or polluted. All of these words mean the same as "contaminate," which is Answer B.

41. **(D)** Fungi contain ergosterol in their plasma membranes. This sterol is unique to fungi and often a target of antifungal drugs.

42. **(A)** See figure below.

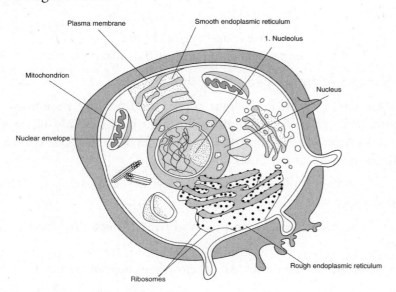

43. **(C)** No explanation needed.

44. **(B)** The cytoskeleton contains microtubules that are associated with cilia and flagella movement (along with motor proteins), whereas actin is associated with the forward movement of the leading edge of a cell.

45. **(C)** The rough endoplasmic reticulum contains ribosomes where new proteins are formed.

46. **(B)** Active transport is the process in which a cell transports a substance from a lower to a higher graduation. Simple diffusion is the net movement of dissolved particles down their concentration gradients, from a region of higher concentration to a region of lower concentration. Facilitated diffusion, also known as passive transport, is the net movement of dissolved particles down their concentration gradient.

47. **(B)** Mitochondria and chloroplasts are thought to have arisen from primitive prokaryotes. Mitochondria are the sites of cellular respiration by eukaryotic cells. Chloroplasts are the site of photosynthesis in plant cells.

48. **(C)** DNA replication is semi-conservative. The template strand pairs with the newly synthesized strand to produce two daughter molecules that contain one parental and one newly synthesized strand.

49. **(D)** Answer (D) does not describe the production of sex cells.

50. **(B)** A heterotroph (B) is an organism that obtains its carbon, as well as energy, from organic compounds. An autotroph (A) is a microorganism that uses only inorganic materials as its source of nutrients. The other choices, C and D, are irrelevant.

51. **(C)** The cross of Aa and Aa (choice C) will result in 25% red offspring.

	A	a
A	AA	Aa
a	Aa	aa

AA (homozygous blue),
Aa (heterozygous blue), and aa (homozygous red)

This cross will result in 75% blue and 25% red.

52. **(B)** Cones (A) provide daylight color vision and are responsible for visual acuity, while rods (B) respond to dim light for black-and-white vision. The iris (C) surrounds the pupil and regulates its diameter. The cornea (D) is the anterior portion of the outer layer of the eye.

53. **(C)** Normal red blood cells (erythrocytes) have an average life span of 120 days.

54. **(A)** White blood cells are formed and released into the blood to fight infection.

55. **(C)** Glucose is a monomer. All other options are polymers.

56. **(B)** Of the choices, the Golgi apparatus is the only one that modifies materials synthesized in the rough and smooth endoplasmic reticulum.

57. **(A)** Telophase. The order of the cell cycle is G_1 phase, S phase, G_2 phase, M phase (mitosis: prophase, metaphase, anaphase, telophase), and cytokinesis.

58. **(B)** No explanation needed.

59. **(C)** Clostridium are gram-positive, spore-forming bacilli.

60. **(D)** No explanation needed.

61. **(B)** Energy is released from ATP when a phosphate bond is broken.

62. **(A)** Respiration and heartbeat. Vision is controlled by the occipital lobe. Verbal communication is controlled by the frontal lobe of the brain.

63. **(A)** DNA ligase. DNA helicase (B) separates the two strands of DNA, while the DNA polymerases (C) and (D) work on building the new strand of DNA during DNA replication.

64. **(B)** No explanation needed.

65. **(C)** No explanation needed.

66. **(A)** No explanation needed.

67. **(C)** Mycoplasmas are microorganisms that lack cell walls and do not synthesize the precursor for peptidoglycan.

68. **(B)** Contraction of the heart is called systole (A), and relaxation of the heart is called diastole (B). Choices C and D are irrelevant.

69. **(C)** No explanation needed.

70. **(A)** Evolution refers to changes that occur in populations over time.

71. **(B)** The adrenal glands produce adrenaline and noradrenaline. The pineal gland produces melatonin and serotonin. The pancreas produces insulin and glucagon. Estrogen is produced by the ovaries in females, while testosterone is primarily produced by the testicles in males and ovaries in females.

72. **(C)** The ureter (A) passes waste from the kidneys to the bladder. The renal vein (B) carries blood away from the kidney. Lastly, the Loop of Henle (D) reabsorbs ions and molecules from the blood.

73. **(A)** The lysosome pH is acidic, around 5.0. The enzymes of the lysosome function well in this acidic environment. Mutant A has the pH closest to 5.0; therefore, it likely has the most function lysosome.

74. **(A)** Gas exchanges occur in the alveoli. The trachea and bronchi of the lungs carry the air to the alveoli.

75. **(B)** Cholesterol travels through the blood as HDLs and LDLs.

76. **(B)** No explanation needed.

77. **(C)** The other options are part of mitosis, a phase of the cell cycle that occurs very quickly compared to interphase.

78. **(C)** Carbon dioxide is released from blood to the air in the alveoli, the site where gas exchange occurs in the lungs.

79. **(C)** Vitamin C is the only water-soluble vitamin, the other options are fat soluble.

80. **(B)** The vestibular apparatus is the collection of receptors and associate structures in the ear that play a central role in maintaining balance in vertebrates.

81. **(C)** Blood cells are formed in bone marrow stem cells. Therefore, a bone marrow transplant (C) is the best for long term care. If you selected answer A, this treatment may work temporarily, but not long-term.

82. **(C)** A neutrophil is a white blood cell, or leukocyte. Megakaryocytes (D) form thrombocytes such as platelets (A). Red blood cells (B) are erythrocytes.

83. **(D)** The thyroid gland produces a hormone that controls the rate at which the body releases energy from food. When the blood levels of these hormones are at low levels, the hypothalamus releases a hormone called thyrotropin-releasing hormone (TRH) in the blood. In response to TRH, the pituitary gland releases thyroid-stimulating hormone (TSH). The thyroid gland responds to TSH by releasing two hormones that then increase the rate

of the release of energy from cells. Higher levels of thyroid hormones in the blood shut down the products of TRH and TSH by negative feedback.

84. **(C)** The immune response recognizes sequences in the viral proteins as foreign and makes antibodies specific for that sequence. In viruses, like HIV, frequent mutations change the protein sequences recognized by the immune system.

85. **(D)** No explanation needed.

86. **(D)** Viruses may contain double-stranded DNA, single-stranded DNA, single-stranded RNA, or double-stranded RNA. Examples include the herpes simplex virus, which contains double-stranded DNA, the influenza virus, which contains single-stranded RNA, the rotavirus, which contains double-stranded RNA, and bacteriophages which contain single-stranded DNA.

87. **(A)** No explanation needed.

88. **(B)** No explanation needed.

89. **(A)** The number of protons is the atomic number. Each element has a unique atomic number. Nucleons are the subatomic particles found in the nucleus, that is, the protons and neutrons.

90. **(C)** Molarity is defined as moles of solute divided by liters of solution.

$$M = \frac{\text{moles of solute}}{\text{liters of solution}} = \frac{\text{g/molecular weight}}{\text{liters of solution}}$$

Sugar, $C_6H_{12}O_6$, has a molecular weight of 180 g/mole. Substituting 18.0 g, 180 g/mole, and 0.500 liter into the above equation gives 0.200 M as the molarity of the solution.

$$M = \frac{18.0 \text{ g}/180 \text{ g}/\text{mole}}{0.500 \text{ liter}} = 0.200 \text{ M}$$

91. **(A)** The actual yield of the reaction, 32.0 g SO_2, is given. To calculate percent yield you must first calculate the theoretical yield which is the maximum possible yield of the reaction and then use the theoretical yield in the equation below to calculate percent yield.

$$\frac{\text{Actual yield}}{\text{Theoretical yield}} \times 100 = \% \text{ yield}$$

$$CS_2 + 3O_2 \rightarrow CO_2 + 2SO_2$$

$$\underline{\text{g } CS_2} \quad \rightarrow \quad \underline{\text{moles } CS_2} \quad \rightarrow \quad \underline{\text{moles } SO_2} \quad \rightarrow$$

$$38.0 \text{ gm} \qquad \frac{38.0 \text{ g}}{76 \text{ g/moles}} \qquad 0.50 \text{ mole } CS_2 \times \frac{2 \text{ moles } SO_2}{1 \text{ mole } CS_2}$$

$$0.50 \text{ mole} \qquad 1.00 \text{ mole } SO_2$$

g SO_2

$$1.00 \text{ mole } SO_2 \times \frac{64 \text{ g } SO_2}{1 \text{ mole } SO_2} = 64 \text{ g } SO_2 \qquad \% \text{ yield} = \frac{32 \text{ g}}{64 \text{ g}} \times 100 = 50\%$$

92. **(A)** DNA molecules are the permanent storage of nucleotide sequence information. RNA's are synthesized, used, and degraded.

93. **(C)** The synthesis of RNA is called transcription, the synthesis of protein is called translation, the synthesis of DNA is called replication, and translocation means the movement of something to a new place (it doesn't refer to a specific biochemical process although there is a step in translation in which the ribosome translocates).

94. **(A)** In a dilution problem, the number of moles of solute before dilution equals the number of moles of solute after dilution. Therefore:

Molarity × volume (before dilution) = Molarity × volume (after dilution)

$$2.0 \frac{\text{moles}}{\text{L}} (0.100 \text{ L}) = 4.0 \frac{\text{moles}}{\text{L}} (\text{volume})$$

$$0.05 \text{ L} = \text{volume required}$$

Dilute 50 mL of the 4.0 M solution with water to 100 mL to prepare the 2.0 M solution.

95. **(A)** The density of a gas, O_2 (mol. wt. = 32 g/mole), can be determined by a rearrangement of the ideal gas law.

$$PV = nRT \qquad PV = \frac{\#g}{\text{mol. wt.}} RT \qquad \frac{P(\text{mol. wt.})}{RT} = \frac{\#g}{V} = D$$

$$\frac{1.0 \text{ atm}(32 \text{ g/mole})}{0.082 \frac{\text{L-atm}}{\text{K-mole}}(273 + 15)\text{K}} = 1.35 \text{ g/L}$$

The densities of gases are reported as grams per liter because the same value as grams per milliliter would be a very small number. The volume of the gas is in liters because the value of R used is in liters.

96. **(C)** The partial pressure of a gas in a mixture of gases is equal to the mole fraction of the gas times the total pressure of the mixture. First, find the mole fraction of nitrogen and then find the partial pressure of nitrogen.

$$P_{\text{total}} \, x_{\text{nitrogen}} = P_{\text{nitrogen}}$$

$$x_{\text{nitrogen}} = \frac{\#\text{moles } N_2}{\# \text{ moles } N_2 + \# \text{ moles } O_2}$$

$$x_{\text{nitrogen}} = \frac{56/28}{56/28 + 64/32} = 0.50$$

1.6 atm (0.50) = 0.8 atm = P_{nitrogen} = partial pressure of nitrogen

97. **(C)** To solve this problem, let the units of the specific heat help you. The units are J/g°C, so if you multiply the specific heat by grams and °C temperature change, you should get joules. The unknown in this question is temperature change so set up the equation as follows:

$$10 \text{ J} = (5 \text{ g}) (0.385 \text{ J/g°C}) (x \text{ °C})$$

Solving for x gives 5.2°C and since joules of heat were absorbed, the temperature must have increased from 25°C to about 30°C.

98. **(B)** Answer (A) is false because it is the nucleotide sequence in mRNA that dictates the amino sequence of proteins. Answer (C) is false because codon and anticodon base pairing occurs during translation. Answer (D) is false because the amino acid incorporated is not a function of concentration, rather it is dictated by the nucleotide sequence of the mRNA.

99. **(C)** Remember that since the speed of light (c) is a constant, as the wavelength decreases, frequency increases (and vice versa). So the light with the highest frequency will be that with the lowest wavelength. A review of metric prefixes may aid in realizing that nm (nanometers) is the smallest of the units given as possible selections.

100. **(B)** A chloride ion has 8 valence electrons (a chlorine atom has 7 and when it becomes negatively charged by gaining an electron, it would have 8) and a sulfide ion also has 8 (a sulfur atom has 6 but the S^{2-} ion has 8).

101. **(B)** A basic oxide is a compound that, when it reacts with water, produces a base. Another name for a basic oxide is a basic anhydride. The oxide K_2O reacts with water to produce KOH according to the following equation:

$$K_2O + H_2O \rightarrow 2KOH$$

The other oxides, CO_2, SO_2, and P_2O_5 , are all acid oxides or acid anhydrides.

$$CO_2 + H_2O \rightarrow H_2CO_3$$
$$SO_2 + H_2O \rightarrow H_2SO_3$$
$$P_2O_5 + 3H_2O \rightarrow 2 \, H_3PO_4$$

102. **(B)** In order for hydrogen bonding to exist, the hydrogen must be bonded to nitrogen, oxygen, or fluorine: H — N, H — O, H — F. Hydrogen bonding is not possible between molecules of CH_4 because the hydrogen is bonded to carbon, C. Hydrogen bonding is possible, however, between molecules of H_2O, between molecules of CH_3OH, and between molecules of NH_3.

103. **(A)** Both are esters of glycerol and fatty acids, which are long-chain carboxylic acids.

104. **(D)** Conversion of gas to liquid is condensation and conversion of liquid to gas is evaporation. Evaporation requires heat input so it's endothermic but condensation releases heat so it is exothermic.

105. **(A)** Gases are usually most soluble in liquids at low temperature. As the temperature of a liquid increases, the gas molecules dissolved in it move faster

and escape more readily from the surface of the liquid. Low pressure on the surface of a liquid will not keep a gas dissolved in the liquid, but rather will allow it to escape from the liquid. High agitation or extreme stirring of the liquid will cause the gas molecules to move faster than they would otherwise move and consequently will decrease the solubility of a gas in a liquid.

106. **(A)** The sex hormones are produced from cholesterol.

107. **(B)** When two equilibrium reactions are added to give a third reaction, the equilibrium constant for the third reaction is calculated by multiplying the two equilibrium constants for each original reaction, (K^1) (K^2). Add equations, multiply equilibrium constants.

108. **(B)** The atomic number gives the number of protons and the atomic mass gives the sum of the protons and neutrons.

109. **(B)** With respect to proteins, the primary structure is the sequence of amino acids in the protein, the secondary structure is localized patterns that arise due to hydrogen bonding between peptide bonds in the protein, the tertiary structure is the overall folding pattern of the protein, and the quaternary structure is the association of multiple proteins (not all proteins exhibit quaternary structure). Beta sheets and alpha helices are the most common examples of a secondary structure.

110. **(B)** In determining the acidity of homologous compounds of members of the same family, as in HI, HBr, HCl, and HF, another concept besides electronegativity is invoked. HI is more acidic than HBr, which is more acidic than HCl, which is more acidic than HF. The larger the atom, I versus F, the more readily it can accommodate an extra electron and be stable. Therefore, I^- is more stable than F^- and consequently HI is more acidic than HF. Acidity increases as one progresses from top to bottom in a family, for example, HF < HCl < HBr < HI.

111. **(D)** A small amount of acid or base may be added to a buffer solution; however, the pH of the solution remains approximately the same as before the acid or base was added. A buffer consists of a weak acid and its conjugate base or of a weak base and its conjugate acid. Sulfuric acid, H_2SO_4, is a strong acid and consequently is not a buffer either alone or with one of its salts. Acetic acid, written as either HAc or CH_3COOH, is a weak acid and in combination with an acetate salt is a buffer solution.

112. **(C)** There are just a handful of common amino acids that are essentially 100% ionized at pH 7.4 (physiological pH) and they are lysine (has a primary amine in its side chain that is protonated and thus positively charged), aspartic acid, and glutamic acid (both have carboxylic acids in their side chains that are deprotonated and thus negatively charged).

113. **(C)** Beta decay is the expulsion of a nuclear electron resulting from the conversion of a neutron to a proton (meaning the atomic number will change but the atomic mass will not). With gamma emission alone, neither the atomic number nor the atomic mass changes (unless some other nuclear reaction also occurs). Alpha decay results in the change of both the atomic number and the

atomic mass (atomic mass is reduced by 4 and the atomic number reduced by 2). Nuclear fission is the splitting of the specie into two comparably sized nuclei.

114. **(B)** The First Law of Thermodynamics considers the conversion of energy from one form to another form without subsequent formation or loss of any of the energy. The Second Law of Thermodynamics states that entropy, the measure of disorder, increases in spontaneous reactions and remains the same in equilibrium systems. The Third Law of Thermodynamics says that the entropy for a perfect crystal is zero at absolute zero temperature. The statement that the Gibbs Free Energy is a measure of the spontaneity of a reaction is true. Refer to the explanation given to question 115.

115. **(D)** The Gibbs Free Energy measures energy changes which accompany a reaction. If the reaction releases usable energy, i.e., energy available to do work, the Gibbs Free Energy has a negative value and the reaction is spontaneous in the direction written. When the Gibbs Free Energy has a positive value, the reaction is not spontaneous in the direction written but is spontaneous in the opposite direction. When the Gibbs Free Energy equals zero, the reaction system is at equilibrium and no change occurs.

116. **(B)** Both solutes are called acids and have pKa's, so choice (C) is false. The stronger the acid, the larger the Ka and the lower the pKa (since pKa = –log Ka), so choices (A) and (D) are also false. Choice (B) is correct because acid B is the stronger acid (larger Ka) and a solution of it would contain more hydrogen ions lowering the pH (remember pH = –log [H$^+$] so as [H$^+$] increases, pH decreases).

117. **(B)** Substitution of a methyl group for a hydrogen on an arene is done using Friedel–Craft alkylation.

118. **(A)** LiAlH$_4$ is a hydride reducing agent. When added to an ester, a nucleophilic substitution first occurs converting the ester to an aldehyde, but then the aldehyde is attacked by a second hydride to convert it to the alcohol after protonation.

119. **(C)** Passive diffusion does not require ATP and nonpolar (lipophilic) species usually cross cell membranes via passive diffusion (because the interior of the membrane is also nonpolar).

120. **(B)** The formula C$_2$H$_6$ is the formula for the alkane ethane. The reaction of Br$_2$ with C$_2$H$_6$ has substituted one of the hydrogen atoms in ethane by a bromine atom. Whenever light or very high temperature is used in a reaction, the reaction usually occurs by a free radical mechanism. The reaction indicated is a free radical substitution reaction.

In a nucleophilic substitution reaction, one nucleophile replaces another in a reaction. In the following example, Br^{-1} + CH$_3$I → CH$_3$Br + I^{-1}, the nucleophilic bromide ion replaces I^{-1}. There is no change in the total number of hydrogen atoms in a nucleophilic substitution reaction while there is such a change in a free radical substitution reaction.

In an electrophilic elimination reaction, a base reacts with a molecule to cause the loss of HZ from the molecule, where Z can be a leaving group. In the following example

$$CH_3-\underset{\underset{Br}{|}}{\overset{\overset{CH_3}{|}}{C}}-CH_3 \;+\; NaOH \text{ (in alcohol)} \longrightarrow CH_3-\overset{\overset{CH_3}{|}}{C}=CH_2 + H_2O + NaBr$$

the hydroxide ion of sodium hydroxide, NaOH, removes the hydrogen bonded to one of the methyl carbon atoms to form water, H_2O. The sodium and bromide ions combine to form sodium bromide, NaBr. An alkene remains as the organic product. Refer to the answer given to question 121 for an explanation of an electrophilic addition reaction.

121. **(C)** The formula C_2H_4 is the formula for an alkene. The electrophile bromine, Br_2, adds atoms to C_2H_4 to produce the dibromide $C_2H_4Br_2$, 1,2-dibromoethane,

$$CH_2=CH_2 + Br_2 \longrightarrow \underset{\underset{Br}{|}}{\overset{\overset{Br}{|}}{CH_2}}-CH_2$$

122. **(B)** Enantiomers are a form of stereoisomers, i.e., compounds which have the same atom connections but different spacial (3D) arrangements. Enantiomers are two compounds having the same four different groups bonded to the stereocenter(s) in each compound, but because of the different positions in which these groups are placed relative to each other, i.e., because of different configurations, they are nonsuperimposable mirror images. Enantiomers are identical in almost all their physical and chemical properties, Fischer projections of the enantiomers of 1-chloro-1-iodoethane are shown below.

$$\underset{\underset{I}{|}}{\overset{\overset{CH_3}{|}}{H-C-Cl}} \qquad\qquad \underset{\underset{I}{|}}{\overset{\overset{CH_3}{|}}{Cl-C-H}}$$

Diastereomers are also a form of stereoisomers. They are stereoisomers which are not enantiomers. Diastereomers are two compounds, each having at least two different stereocenters or E/Z isomers of alkenes (see geomtetric isomerism on page 294). The diastereomers have the arrangement of the four different groups at one of the stereocenters identical in both molecules but the arrangement of another four different groups at the other stereocenter different in both compounds. In other words, diastereomers with two stereocenters have the same configuration at one of the stereocenters but opposite configurations at the other stereocenter. Diastereomers are nonsuperimposable and have different physical and chemical properties. Fischer projections of one pair of diastereomers of 2-bromo-3-chlorobutane are shown below.

$$
\begin{array}{ccc}
& CH_3 & \\
& | & \\
H - & C & - Cl \\
& | & \\
H - & C & - Br \\
& | & \\
& CH_3 &
\end{array}
\qquad\qquad
\begin{array}{ccc}
& CH_3 & \\
& | & \\
H - & C & - Cl \\
& | & \\
Br - & C & - H \\
& | & \\
& CH_3 &
\end{array}
$$

Geometric isomerism may occur in alkenes. It is not possible to freely rotate around a carbon-carbon double bond as it is around a carbon-carbon single bond. Therefore, when a carbon-carbon double bond is present in a compound, two different compounds, geometric isomers, may exist. In the example shown below:

$$
\begin{array}{cc}
CH_3 & CH_3 \\
\diagdown & \diagup \\
C & = C \\
\diagup & \diagdown \\
Cl & Cl
\end{array}
\qquad\qquad
\begin{array}{cc}
CH_3 & Cl \\
\diagdown & \diagup \\
C & = C \\
\diagup & \diagdown \\
Cl & CH_3
\end{array}
$$

the two chlorine atoms are on the same side of the double bond in one compound and on opposite sides of the double bond in the other compound. One could just as easily compare the position of the two methyl groups relative to the carbon-carbon double bond and arrive at the same conclusion. In order that geometric isomerism be present in alkenes, two identical groups cannot be bonded to the same carbon atom.

123. **(D)** Since a beta-hydroxy aldehyde product has been made in the presence of base, an aldol condensation has occurred. The product has 4 carbons so a 2-carbon aldehyde is the reactant.

124. **(B)** In infrared (IR) spectroscopy, the most significant bands are around 3300 cm^{-1} for O—H and N—H, around 2,100 cm^{-1} for triple bonds, and around 1,600–1,700 cm^{-1} for double bonds.

125. **(B)** Carbohydrates, like glucose, are oxidized through glycolysis and then the citric acid cycle produces ATP and reduced cofactors (NADH and FADH$_2$). More ATP is produced when the reduced cofactors are oxidized via oxidative phosphorylation. The monomers in protein synthesis are amino acids.

126. **(D)** Of the acid derivatives (includes acid halides, anhydrides, esters, and amides), the amides are the least reactive. In fact, the order of reactivity acid halides > anhydrides > esters > amides is helpful in remembering their reactions. Acid derivatives can be converted to anything less reactive than themselves but cannot be converted to derivatives more reactive. Thus, an amide cannot directly be converted to an ester.

127. **(B)** Proteins are polymers of alpha substituted amino acids which have the following generalized structure containing amide linkages.

$$
\underset{\substack{\text{several molecules of}\\\text{alpha amino acid}}}{R-\underset{\underset{NH_2}{|}}{CH}-\overset{\overset{O}{\|}}{C}-O-H}\ ---> \underset{\text{protein}}{-\overset{\overset{O}{\|}}{C}-\underset{\underset{H}{|}}{N}-\underset{\underset{H}{|}}{CH}-\overset{\overset{R}{|}}{\underset{\underset{O}{\|}}{C}}-\underset{\underset{R}{|}}{N}-\underset{\underset{H}{|}}{CH}-\overset{\overset{H}{|}}{\underset{\underset{H}{|}}{C}}-N-\underset{\underset{H}{|}}{CH}-}
$$

128. **(B)** It is not true that all bonds in benzene are equivalent in length. All of the C—C bonds are equivalent in length but the C—H bonds are a different length from the C—C bonds. Even though the C—C bonds in benzene may be represented by alternating single and double bonds, all of these C—C bonds are the same length because of delocalization of pi electrons, that is, resonance. All of the other statements about benzene are correct.

129. **(A)** The compound is named 3-methylpentanoic acid. The carbonyl carbon is numbered 1, so the carbon atom to which the methyl group is attached is carbon 3. The acid is named by removing the *-e* from pentane and adding *-oic acid*. The formulas for the other answers are shown below.

$$\underset{\substack{|\\CH_3}}{CH_3CH_2CH_2CHCOOH} \qquad \underset{\substack{|\\CH_3}}{CH_3CH_2CHCOOH} \qquad \underset{\substack{|\\CH_3}}{CH_3CHCH_2COOH}$$

2-methylpentanoic acid   2-methylbutanoic acid   3-methylbutanoic acid

130. **(B)** To name an alcohol, find the longest carbon chain containing the alcohol carbon, number the carbons of that chain such that the alcohol carbon has the lower number, and then identify any branches off the chain. That leads us to either (B) or (C) as the correct choice. Since there is a chiral center whose 3D arrangement has been specified in the structure, R or S can be designated. Assign priorities to the four groups attached to the chiral center based on atomic number. Here, the OH group would be number 1, the isopropyl group would be number 2, the methyl group would be number 3, and the hydrogen group would be number 4. Orient the molecule such that priority group number 4 is away from you and look at the other three groups. If they are arranged 1, 2, 3 clockwise, it's called R and if counterclockwise, it's S.

131. **(B)** $\% = \dfrac{\text{Part}}{\text{Whole}} \times 100$

$$\frac{8H}{(NH_4)_2\,SO_4} \times 100 = \frac{8}{132} \times 100 = 6.06\%$$

132. **(C)** An aldehyde is very easily oxidized and is converted to a carboxylic acid.

$$\underset{\text{RCH}}{\overset{\overset{\displaystyle O}{\|}}{}} \xrightarrow{[O]} \underset{\text{RCOH}}{\overset{\overset{\displaystyle O}{\|}}{}}$$

133. **(A)** 2.2 mL of pentanoic acid would be 2.046 g (2.2 mL × 0.93 g/mL), which is 0.020 moles of pentanoic acid (2.046 g × 1 mol/102 g). Thus 0.020 moles of sodium hydroxide would be needed (since stoichiometry is 1:1 in the equation), which is 0.80 g (0.020 moles × 40 g/mol).

134. **(C)** Molarity is defined as moles of solute divided by liters of solution.

$$M = \frac{\text{moles of solute}}{\text{liters of solution}} = \frac{\text{g/mol. wt.}}{\text{liters of solution}}$$

Sugar, $C_6H_{12}O_6$, has a molecular weight of 180 g/mole. Substitute 18 g, 180 g/mole, and 0.5 M into the above equation to obtain the volume of the solution.

$$M = \frac{18 \text{ g}/180 \text{ g}/\text{mole}}{x} = 0.5 \text{ M}$$

$$x = 0.2 \text{ L} = 200 \text{ mL}$$

135. **(D)** Nuclear fission is the breakdown of a larger nucleus, usually by bombarding it with neutrons, to produce smaller atoms and more neutrons. A great deal of energy is released in this process, which is the basis for the atomic bomb. Radioactive decay is the spontaneous emission of nuclear particles, e.g., alpha and beta particles, as well as gamma rays, by unstable nuclei. Carbon-14 dating is a method of determining the age of an object by comparing the amount of carbon-12 and the amount of radioactive carbon-14 present in the object. Nuclear fusion is the combination of small nucleii to produce a larger atom with the concomitant release of a large amount of energy. Nuclear fusion occurs on the sun. The hydrogen bomb is an example of nuclear fusion.

136. **(B)** Ozonolysis with reductive work up cleaves alkenes and alkynes. For alkenes, the double bond is cleaved and replaced with carbonyl groups on each carbon of the alkene. For alkynes, the triple bond is cleaved and replaced with carboxylic acid groups on each carbon of the alkyne. Acetic acid is CH_3CO_2H, so the reacting organic molecule must have been an alkyne and since two moles of acetic acid resulted, the alkyne must have had a methyl group on each alkyne carbon.

137. **(C)** Note that $\sqrt{32} + \sqrt{18} = \sqrt{16 \cdot 2} + \sqrt{9 \cdot 2} = 4\sqrt{2} + 3\sqrt{2} = 7\sqrt{2}$.

138. **(B)** Since the tank is already 4/5 full, the additional 7 gallons equals 1/5 of the tank's capacity. Thus, $7 = \frac{1}{5}x \Rightarrow x = 35$.

139. **(B)** To find the limit as x approaches ∞, notice that the expression $\dfrac{8x^6 + 5x^4 - x + 1000}{3x^6 + 21x^3 - 4}$ has the largest power of x in both the numerator and the denominator. Thus, as x approaches ∞, the expression $\dfrac{8x^6 + 5x^4 - x + 1000}{3x^6 + 21x^3 - 4}$ is dominated by these highest powered terms, i.e., $\dfrac{8x^6}{3x^6}$. The value of this resulting fraction approaches $\dfrac{8}{3}$ as x approaches ∞.

$$\lim_{x\to\infty}\left(\frac{8x^6 + 5x^4 - x + 1000}{3x^6 + 21x^3 - 4}\right) = \frac{8}{3}$$

140. **(B)** Given the function $f(x) = \dfrac{x+1}{10x}$, we solve for y in the equation

$$x = \frac{y+1}{10y}, \text{ that is,} \qquad x = \frac{y+1}{10y}$$
$$10xy = y + 1$$
$$10xy - y = 1$$
$$y(10x - 1) = 1 \Rightarrow y = \frac{1}{10x - 1}.$$

141. **(C)** $5^2 + 5^3 = 25 + 125 = 150$.

142. **(B)** There is a total of $11 + 10 + 4 = 25$ pieces of fruit, of which 21 are not lemons. The probability of **not** choosing a lemon is given by the formula:

$$\text{Probability} = \frac{\#\text{ of non-lemons}}{\#\text{ of fruit}} = \frac{21}{25} = 0.84 = 84\%$$

143. **(A)** The discriminant for this quadratic equation is given by $b^2 - 4ac = 5^2 - 4 \cdot 2 = 25 - 8 = 17 > 0$. Thus, there are two real roots.

144. **(A)** We complete the square on the given equation as follows.

$x^2 + y^2 - 12x + 14y + 9 = 0$
$x^2 - 12x + 36 + y^2 + 14y + 49 = -9 + 36 + 49$
$(x - 6)^2 + (y + 7)^2 = 76$
$(x - 6)^2 + (y + 7)^2 = \left(\sqrt{76}\right)^2$

Now use the fact that a circle with equation $(x - h)^2 + (y - k)^2 = r^2$ has center point (h, k) and radius equal to r. In the given equation, we have $(x - 6)^2 + (y + 7)^2 = \left(\sqrt{76}\right)^2$. Thus, the radius equals $\sqrt{76}$.

145. **(C)** The curve intersects the x-axis when $f(x) = 0$.

$$2x^3 - 6x = 0$$

$$2x(x^2 - 3) = 0 \Rightarrow x = 0, \ x = \pm\sqrt{3}$$

So the region is bounded on the left by $x = -\sqrt{3}$ and on the right by $x = 0$.

The exact area of the shaded region is given by the definite integral

$$\int_{-\sqrt{3}}^{0} \left(2x^3 - 6x\right) dx$$

Using the Fundamental Theorem of Calculus yields

$$\int_{-\sqrt{3}}^{0} \left(2x^3 - 6x\right) dx = \frac{2}{4}x^4 - \frac{6}{2}x^2 \Big]_{-\sqrt{3}}^{0} = \frac{1}{2}x^4 - 3x^2 \Big]_{-\sqrt{3}}^{0}$$

$$= \left(\frac{1}{2}(0)^4 - 3(0)^2\right) - \left(\frac{1}{2}\left(\sqrt{3}\right)^4 - 3\left(\sqrt{3}\right)^2\right)$$

$$= 0 - \left(\frac{9}{2} - 9\right) = 4.5$$

146. **(D)** There are 6 numbers divisible by 3 or 4, that is, 3, 4, 6, 8, 9, and 12.

We use the formula: Probability $= \dfrac{6}{12} = 0.5 = 50\%$.

147. **(D)** We use the Fundamental Theorem of Calculus for integrals.

$$\int_{1}^{2} \left(5x^4\right) dx = \frac{5x^5}{5}\Big|_{1}^{2} = x^5\Big|_{1}^{2} = 2^5 - 1^5 = 32 - 1 = 31.$$

148. **(D)** We simplify the expression as follows.

If $x < 6$, then $x - 6 < 0$. Thus, $|x - 6| = -(x - 6)$. Therefore,

$$\frac{x^2 - 7x + 6}{|x - 6|} = \frac{(x - 6)(x - 1)}{-(x - 6)} = -(x - 1) = -x + 1.$$

149. **(C)** We simplify the expression as follows.

$$\frac{x^2 - 11x + 24}{x - 8} = \frac{(x - 8)(x - 3)}{x - 8} = x - 3$$

150. **(B)** We use the quadratic formula.

$$x = \frac{-b \pm \sqrt{b^2 - 4ac}}{2a} = \frac{-1 \pm \sqrt{1^2 - 4 \cdot 6 \cdot 1}}{2 \cdot 6} = \frac{-1 \pm \sqrt{-23}}{12}$$

Since $\sqrt{-23}$ is not a real number, the equation has no real solutions.

151. **(A)** Each point on the graph of $y = 5f(x + 2) - 3$ is obtained by transforming the points on the graph of $y = f(x)$ as follows. Subtract 2 from each x coordinate; multiply each y coordinate by 5 and then subtract 3.

152. **(A)** Note that $\log_7(49) = x$ is equivalent to the equation $7^x = 49$. This equation has solution $x = 2$.

153. **(B)** Note that

$$\lim_{x \to 4}\left(\frac{x^2 - 10x + 24}{4 - x} \right) = \lim_{x \to 4}\left(\frac{(x - 4)(x - 6)}{4 - x} \right) =$$

$$\lim_{x \to 4}\left(\frac{(x - 4)(x - 6)}{-(x - 4)} \right) = \lim_{x \to 4}(-(x - 6)) = -(4 - 6) = 2$$

154. **(B)** Add $8 + 35 + 8 + 9 + 5 + 10 + 7 + 3 + 12 = 97$. Then, divide 97 by 9, which is the total amount of numbers in the set; therefore, $97 \div 9 = 10.77$.

155. **(D)** The total rental cost is given by the daily cost plus the mileage cost. Daily cost = (\$30 per day)(7 days) = \$210. Mileage cost = (\$0.14 per mile)(x miles) = \$0.14x.

156. **(A)** The probability of heads on a coin toss is $\frac{1}{2}$. Since there are four tosses,

each with a probability of $\frac{1}{2}$ for heads, we have:

$$\frac{1}{2} \cdot \frac{1}{2} \cdot \frac{1}{2} \cdot \frac{1}{2} = \frac{1}{16}$$

157. **(D)** The desired instantaneous rate of change is given by the derivative of the function evaluated at $t = 3$.

$$f'(t) = 4(2t \cdot e^{t^2 - 9}) = 8t \cdot e^{t^2 - 9}$$

When $t = 3$, $f'(3) = 8(3) \cdot e^{3^2 - 9} = 24 \cdot e^0 = 24$.

158. **(C)** To compute $(f + g)(x)$, add the function formulas for f and g, then combine like terms.

$$(f + g)(x) = x^2 + 2x - 1 + 2x + 1 = x^2 + 4x$$

159. **(B)** We solve the equation as follows.

$$4(x + 3)(x - 2) = 4x^2 + x$$
$$4(x^2 + x - 6) = 4x^2 + x$$
$$4x^2 + 4x - 24 = 4x^2 + x$$
$$4x - 24 = x$$
$$3x = 24 \Rightarrow x = 8$$

160. **(A)** Each time a die is rolled, there are two possible outcomes: an even number or an odd number. Therefore, the probability that the die will land on an odd number is 50%.

161. **(D)** Note that $\dfrac{5}{9} - \dfrac{3}{10} = \dfrac{5 \cdot 10 - 3 \cdot 9}{9 \cdot 10} = \dfrac{50 - 27}{90} = \dfrac{23}{90}$.

162. **(B)** The mode of a list of numbers is the number that occurs most frequently. The number 6, which occurs four times, is the mode of the given data set.

163. **(D)** There are 2 ways that the sum of the numbers shown can equal 5, that is, 1 + 4 and 2 + 3. Note that there are 6 possible outcomes for each die in the pair. Therefore, to calculate the possible combinations for the pair, we multiple $6 \cdot 6 = 36$. So, the probability that the sum of the numbers shown equals 5 is $\dfrac{2}{36} = \dfrac{1}{18}$. Thus, the probability that the sum of the numbers shown is NOT equal to 5 is $1 - \dfrac{1}{18} = \dfrac{17}{18}$.

164. **(A)** We can use the *Power Rule* for integrals to integrate term-by-term.

$$\int (x + 2)\, dx = \int x\, dx + \int 2\, dx$$
$$= \int x\, dx + 2 \int x^0\, dx$$
$$= \frac{1}{2} x^2 + 2x + C$$

165. **(D)** The highest point on the graph has a y coordinate equal to 300.

166. **(A)** The highest point on the graph occurs when the x coordinate equals 3.

167. **(A)** The quadratic equation $10x^2 + \pi x + q = 0$ has a double root when the discriminant equals zero. So we solve $b^2 - 4ac = \pi^2 - 4 \cdot 10 \cdot q = 0$.

$$\pi^2 - 40q = 0$$
$$\pi^2 = 40q \Rightarrow q = \frac{\pi^2}{40}$$

168. **(A)** The given function will be undefined for any x-value that causes the denominator to equal zero. Setting the denominator equal to zero yields

$$x^2 + 9x + 18 = 0$$
$$(x + 6)(x + 3) = 0$$
$$x = -6, \ x = -3$$

Thus, the domain for f must exclude $x = -6$ and $x = -3$.

169. **(B)** Note that $9^3 \cdot 9^{-1} = 9^{3-1} = 9^2 = 81$.

170. **(D)** The total number of ways to choose 3 girls and 1 boy is given by the formula $\underbrace{{}_5C_3}_{\substack{\text{choose} \\ \text{3 girls}}} \cdot \underbrace{{}_3C_1}_{\substack{\text{choose} \\ \text{1 boy}}} = \dfrac{5!}{3!2!} \cdot \dfrac{3!}{1!2!} = 10 \cdot 3 = 30$. The total number of ways to

choose 4 people is given by the formula ${}_8C_4 = \dfrac{8!}{4!4!} = \dfrac{1680}{24} = 70$.

Thus, probability $= \dfrac{30}{70} = \dfrac{3}{7}$.

171. **(B)** A quadratic function $f(x) = ax^2 + bx + c$ will have its vertex at the

point $\left(-\dfrac{b}{2a}, f\left(-\dfrac{b}{2a} \right) \right)$.

$$f(x) = 9x^2 + 18x - 7 \Rightarrow = -\dfrac{b}{2a} = -\dfrac{18}{2(9)} = -\dfrac{18}{18} = -1$$
$$f(-1) = 9(-1)^2 + 18(-1) - 7 = 9 - 18 - 7 = -16$$

Thus, the vertex is $(-1, -16)$.

172. **(A)** We compute the derivative $f'(x) = 12x^2 + 7$, and then evaluate $f'(-1) = 12(-1)^2 + 7 = 12 + 7 = 19$.

173. **(A)** We solve the equation as follows.

$$\ln(2w + 9x) = 4$$
$$e^{\ln(2w + 9x)} = e^4$$

$$2w + 9x = e^4 \Rightarrow 9x = e^4 - 2w \Rightarrow x = \dfrac{e^4 - 2w}{9}$$

174. **(B)** We have the ratio $\dfrac{3 \text{ apples}}{7 \text{ oranges}} \Rightarrow \dfrac{3 \cdot 3 \text{ apples}}{7 \cdot 3 \text{ oranges}} = \dfrac{9 \text{ apples}}{21 \text{ oranges}}$.

175. **(C)** Note that $\dfrac{2 + \sqrt{3}}{2 - \sqrt{3}} \cdot \dfrac{1 + \sqrt{3}}{2 + \sqrt{3}} = \dfrac{4 + 4\sqrt{3} + 3}{4 - 3} = \dfrac{7 + 4\sqrt{3}}{1} = 7 + 4\sqrt{3}$.

176. **(A)** Consider the Venn diagram.

The total number of employees = 260 + 235 + 65 + 55 = 615.

177. **(C)** Note that $\lim\limits_{x \to 5.1}\left(\dfrac{f(x) - f(5.1)}{x - 5.1}\right) = f'(5.1) =$ the slope of the tangent

line to the graph when $x = 5.1$. Since the graph has a horizontal tangent line at this point, the slope = 0 there.

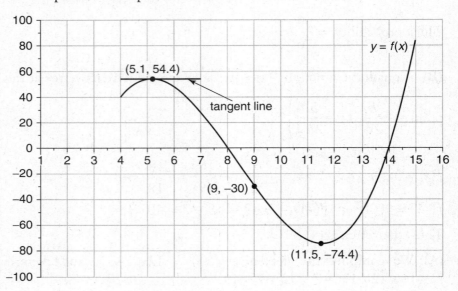

178. **(D)** A logarithmic function is undefined unless the input value is strictly greater than zero. Thus, we solve $2x - 7 > 0$ and obtain $x > 3.5$.

179. **(B)** $P(x) = 35x^2 + 420x - 50$ is a quadratic function whose graph is a parabola that opens up since the coefficient of the x^2 term is positive. This means that the function has a minimum value at the vertex of the parabola.

The minimum value occurs at the vertex, that is, when

$$x = -\frac{b}{2a} = -\frac{420}{2(35)} = -6.$$

Thus, the minimum value of the given function is

$$P(-6) = 35(-6)^2 + 420(-6) - 50 = -1,310.$$

180. **(A)** We simplify the expression as follows:

$$\frac{\sqrt{x-h}-\sqrt{x}}{h}\cdot\left(\frac{\sqrt{x-h}+\sqrt{x}}{\sqrt{x-h}+\sqrt{x}}\right)=\frac{x-h-x}{h\left(\sqrt{x-h}+\sqrt{x}\right)}=\frac{-h}{h\left(\sqrt{x-h}+\sqrt{x}\right)}$$

$$=-\frac{1}{\sqrt{x-h}+\sqrt{x}}$$

181. **(B)** The *Quotient Rule* for logarithms states that

$$\log(M)-\log(N)=\log\left(\frac{M}{N}\right)$$

$$\log(75)-\log(3)=\log\left(\frac{75}{3}\right)$$

$$=\log(25)$$

182. **(A)** The truck must travel 48 miles in 45 minutes = 0.75 hour. We have the formula

$$\text{speed}=\frac{\text{distance}}{\text{time}}=\frac{48\text{ miles}}{0.75\text{ hr}}=64\text{ mph}$$

183. **(B)** A circle with equation $(x-h)^2+(y-k)^2=r^2$ has radius equal to r. In this problem $r^2=36\Rightarrow r=6$.

184. **(D)** We solve the equation as follows.

$$\frac{x}{x+3}+\frac{x}{x+2}=2$$

$$\frac{x(x+2)+x(x+3)}{(x+3)(x+2)}=2$$

$$x(x+2)+x(x+3)=2(x+3)(x+2)$$

$$x^2+2x+x^2+3x=2x^2+10x+12$$

$$5x=10x+12$$

$$-5x=12\Rightarrow x=-\frac{12}{5}$$

The numbers in the margins of the reprinted passages indicate the statements in which the answer to the questions can be found.

Passage 1

185 Bronchial asthma is a common disease of children and adults. Although the clinical manifestations of asthma have been known since antiquity, it is a disease that still defies precise definition. The word *asthma* is of Greek origin and means "panting."

193 More than 2000 years ago, Hippocrates used the word *asthma* to describe episodic shortness of breath; however, the first detailed description of the asthmatic patient was made by Aretaeus in the second century. Since that time *asthma* has been used

186 to describe any disorder with episodic shortness of breath or dyspnea; thus, the terms *cardiac asthma* and *bronchial asthma* have been used to delineate the etiologies of the

192 dyspnea. These terms are now obsolete and asthma refers to a disorder of the respiratory system characterized by episodes of difficulty in breathing. An Expert Panel of the National Institutes of Health National Asthma Education Program (NAEP) has defined asthma as a lung disease characterized by (1) airway obstruction that is reversible (but not completely so in some patients) either spontaneously or with

187 treatment; (2) airway inflammation; and (3) increased airway responsiveness to a variety of stimuli. This descriptive definition for asthma is attributed to our lack of knowledge of the precise pathogenic defect that results in the clinical syndrome we recognize as asthma. The current definition does allow for the important heterogene-

189 ity of the clinical presentation of asthma. New technologies have added substantially to our understanding of the interrelationships of immunology, biochemistry, and physiology to the clinical presentation of asthma, and further research may yet uncover a specific genetic defect associated with asthma. Until such time, asthma will continue to defy exact definition.

191 An estimated 10 million persons in the United States have asthma (about 5% of the population). The reported prevalence increased 29% from 1980 to 1987 to 40.1 per 1000 population. African-Americans have a 19% higher incidence of asthma than whites and are twice as likely to be hospitalized. The estimated cost of asthma in the United States in 1990 was $6.2 billion. The largest single direct medical expenditure was for inpatient hospital services (emergency care), reaching almost $1.5 billion, followed by prescription medications ($1.1 billion). The costs of medication increased 54% between 1985 and 1990. In total, 43% of the economic impact was associated with emergency room use, hospitalization, and death. Asthma accounted for 1% of all ambulatory care visits according to the National

190 Ambulatory Medical Care Survey and results in more than 450,000 hospitalizations per year.

185. **(B)** As stated in the passage, bronchial asthma is a common disease of children and adults that defies precise definition.

186. **(D)** The passage states *cardiac asthma* and *bronchial asthma* are now two obsolete terms that delineated the etiologies of dyspnea.

187. **(B)** The passage states that the NAEP defines asthma as a lung disease characterized by: (1) airway obstruction that is reversible, but not completely in some patients, either spontaneously or with treatment; (2) airway inflammation; and (3) increased airway responsiveness to a variety of stimuli.

188. **(C)** The passage states that the total cost of asthma in the United States in 1990 was $6.2 billion. Cost of prescription medications accounted for $1.1 billion of the total amount. Subtracting $1.1 billion from $6.2 billion equals $5.1 billion.

189. **(C)** Wheezing and episodes of shortness of breath (B) and the interrelationship of immunology, biochemistry, and physiology (D) are already understood, and answer A is irrelevant. Researchers hope to uncover a specific genetic defect in asthma.

190. **(D)** No explanation necessary.

191. **(D)** The passage states that the estimated number of persons in the United States who have asthma is 10 million.

192. **(D)** Answers A, B, and C are incorrect choices, since "panting" (A) and dyspnea of cardiac (B) or bronchial etiology (C) are obsolete definitions. Answer D represents the current definition of asthma.

193. **(C)** The passage states that more than 2,000 years ago Hippocrates used the word *asthma* to describe episodic shortness of breath.

194. **(B)** The passage provides some facts about the prevalence of asthma in the United States.

Passage 2

Hypercalcemia, increased serum calcium concentrations, occurs in approximately 15% of individuals with cancer. Occurrences of this condition have been reported in 195 most types of malignancies. The most effective management of treating this life- 198 threatening disease is successful treatment of the malignancy. Unfortunately, successful treatment of the cancer may not be possible. In these cases, treatment goals should include correcting intravascular depletion, enhancing renal excretion of cal- 199 cium, and inhibiting bone resorption. First line treatment of acute hypercalcemia includes the administration of normal saline and furosemide. Since many patients suffering from acute hypercalcemia are dehydrated, the administration of normal 200 saline is warranted. In addition to treating dehydration, normal saline helps to increase renal excretion of calcium. The optimal administration of normal saline is dependent on the severity of hypercalcemia, the degree of dehydration, and the clinical status of the patient. An infusion rate of 400 mL per hour of normal saline is typical. Furosemide, a diuretic, is useful in the treatment of hypercalcemia due to its ability to enhance urinary excretion and, more importantly, calcium excretion. Additionally, furosemide protects patients from becoming volume overloaded due to

197 the administration of the normal saline. <u>It is very important that patients be adequately hydrated prior to the administration of furosemide in order to get maximum benefits.</u> Intravenous doses of 100 mg of furosemide every 2 hours may be used. Although normal saline and furosemide are the most commonly used agents to treat acute cancer hypercalcemia, only a modest decrease in calcium levels are achieved from this regimen. <u>The use of normal saline and furosemide may be sufficient for the</u>

201 <u>management of mild to moderate hypercalcemia, but it is commonly insufficient for treating severe hypercalcemia.</u>

195. **(B)** Hypercalcemia has been reported in most types of malignancies. Answers A, C, and D are incorrect because they refer only to specific kinds of malignancies.

196. **(D)** The passage is not concerned with the pathogenesis of cancer-related hypercalcemia (A); it does not cover all the uses of normal saline and furosemide (B); nor does it deal with the general characteristics or severity of cancer-related hypercalcemia (C). The focus is first line agents (normal saline and furosemide) used to manage acute cancer-related hypercalcemia.

197. **(C)** To obtain maximum benefits from the administration of furosemide, it is important to hydrate the patient before administering the diuretic. Answers A, B, and D are not mentioned in the passage.

198. **(D)** The passage states that cancer-related hypercalcemia is most effectively managed by successful treatment of the malignancy. Both normal saline (A) and furosemide (B) are agents used in first line treatment of cancer-related hypercalcemia when successful treatment of the cancer may not be possible. Dialysis (C) is not mentioned in the passage.

199. **(A)** The passage states that treatment goals should include enhancing renal excretion of calcium (B), inhibiting bone resorption (C), and correcting intravascular depletion (D). However, administrating calcium carbonate (A) is not mentioned in the passage.

200. **(B)** The passage states that since many patients suffering from acute hypercalcemia are dehydrated, the administration of normal saline is warranted.

201. **(D)** The last sentence of the passage clearly states that a normal saline-furosemide regimen alone is insufficient for treating severe hypercalcemia. However, it is usually effective in mild cancer-related hypercalcemia (A), mild hypercalcemia (B), and moderate hypercalcemia (C).

Passage 3

Gastroesophageal reflux disease (GERD) is a common medical disorder seen by health care practitioners of all specialties. It is generally chronic in nature, and long-term therapy may be required. <u>While the mortality associated with GERD is very</u>

202 <u>low (1 death per 100,000 patients), the quality of life experienced by the patient can be greatly diminished.</u>

GERD refers to any symptomatic clinical condition or histologic alteration that results from episodes of gastroesophageal reflux. Gastroesophageal reflux refers to the retrograde movement of gastric contents from the stomach into the esophagus. Many people experience some degree of reflux, especially after eating, which may be considered a benign physiologic process. <u>When the esophagus is repeatedly exposed</u> 204 <u>to refluxed material for prolonged periods of time, inflammation of the esophagus (i.e., reflux esophagitis) can occur.</u> It is important to realize that gastroesophageal reflux must precede the development of GERD or reflux esophagitis. <u>In severe cases,</u> <u>reflux may lead to a multitude of serious complications including esophageal stric-</u> 203 <u>tures, esophageal ulcers, motility disorders, perforation, hemorrhage, aspiration,</u> <u>and Barrett's esophagus.</u> While mild disease is often managed with life-style changes and antacids, more intensive therapeutic intervention with histamine (H_2) antagonists, sucralfate, prokinetic agents, or proton pump inhibitors is generally required for patients with more severe disease. <u>In general, response to pharmacologic inter-</u> 206 <u>vention is dependent on the efficacy of the agent, dosage regimen employed,</u> <u>duration of therapy, and severity of the disease.</u> <u>Following discontinuation of ther-</u> 205 <u>apy, relapse is common and long-term maintenance therapy may be required.</u> Historically, surgical intervention has been reserved for patients in whom conventional treatment modalities fail. However, the recent development of laparoscopic antireflux surgical procedures has led to a reevaluation of the role of surgery in the long-term maintenance of GERD. <u>Some clinicians have suggested that laparoscopic</u> 208 <u>antireflux surgery may be a cost-effective alternative to long-term maintenance ther-</u> <u>apy in young patients.</u> <u>However, long-term comparative trials evaluating the cost</u> 207 <u>effectiveness of the various treatment modalities are warranted.</u>

The pathogenesis of gastroesophageal reflux is related to the complex balance between defense mechanisms and aggressive factors. Understanding both the normal protective mechanisms and the aggressive factors that may contribute to or promote gastroesophageal reflux helps one to design rational therapeutic treatment regimens. <u>Gastric acid, pepsin, bile acids, and pancreatic enzymes are considered</u> <u>aggressive factors and may promote esophageal damage upon reflux into the esoph-</u> 209 <u>agus. Thus, the composition (potency) and volume of the refluxate are aggressive</u> <u>factors that may lead to esophageal injury.</u> Conversely, normal protective mechanisms include anatomic factors, lower esophageal sphincter pressure, esophageal clearing, mucosal resistance, and gastric emptying. Rational therapeutic regimens in the treatment of gastroesophageal reflux are designed to maximize normal defense mechanisms and/or attenuate the aggressive factors.

202. **(C)** According to the passage, the mortality rate of GERD is 1 death per 100,000 patients.

203. **(A)** One possible complication of reflux is perforation. Mucosal resistance (B), gastric emptying (C), and lower esophageal sphincter pressure (D) are all cited in the passage as normal protective mechanisms.

204. **(C)** The passage states when the esophagus is repeatedly exposed to refluxed material for prolonged periods of time, inflammation of the esophagus (i.e., reflux esophagitis) can occur.

205. **(C)** The passage states that following discontinuation of therapy, relapse is common and long-term maintenance therapy may be required.

206. **(B)** Efficacy of the agent plays a part in GERD patients' response to pharmacologic intervention.

207. **(A)** The passage states that long-term comparative trials evaluating the cost effectiveness of various treatment modalities for GERD are warranted.

208. **(C)** The passage states that laparoscopic antireflux surgery has been suggested as a possible cost-effective alternative therapy.

209. **(A)** Gastric acid and pancreatic enzymes are aggressive factors and may promote esophageal damage upon reflux into the esophagus. The factors in answer C are protective, and the factors in answer B are a combination of aggressive (bile acids) and protective (esophageal clearing). Answer D is unrelated to the passage.

Passage 4

Many people in the United States are diagnosed with diabetes mellitus. Type 2 diabetes is the most common type of diabetes and it is associated with a significant amount of morbidities and mortalities. Type 2 diabetes is classified as an endocrine disorder characterized by defects in insulin secretion as well as in insulin action. In type 2 diabetes patients, a defect also exists in insulin receptor binding. These defects lead to increased serum glucose concentrations or hyperglycemia.

Sulfonylureas are one of the most popular classes of agents used to treat type 2 diabetes. One of the agents to treat type 2 diabetes is acarbose, an oral alpha-glucosidase inhibitor. Acarbose interferes with the hydrolysis of dietary disaccharides and complex carbohydrates, thereby delaying absorption of glucose and other monosaccharides. Acarbose is available for oral administration only. To be most effective, it should be taken at the beginning of a meal. The recommended starting dose is 25 mg three times daily and doses as high as 200 mg three times a day have been safely used. The most common adverse experiences associated with the use of acarbose are abdominal cramps, flatulence, diarrhea, and abdominal distension. Most of the adverse effects are due to the unabsorbed carbohydrates undergoing fermentation in the colon. Acarbose has also been associated with decreased intestinal absorption of iron, thereby possibly leading to anemia. The occurrence of hypoglycemia when using acarbose in combination with other agents used to lower serum glucose is great. Glucose should be administered to treat hypoglycemia in patients taking acarbose because sucrose may not be adequately hydrolyzed and absorbed. The effectiveness of this agent to lower serum glucose concentrations in patients with type 2 diabetes has been clearly demonstrated in clinical trials. Acarbose provides another option for treating type 2 diabetes.

210. **(D)** Whereas "endocrine in nature" (A), "hyperglycemia" (B), and "may be due to a defect in insulin receptor binding" (C) are stated in, or may be inferred from, the passage, "results in iron deficiencies" is not listed as a characteristic of type 2 diabetes. Rather, it is mentioned as a possible adverse effect of acarbose.

211. **(A)** The passage states that a sulfonylurea agent is one of the most popular classes of agents used to treat type 2 diabetes. Glucose (B), sucrose (C), and fructose (D) all represent types of sugar.

212. **(A)** The passage states that to be most effective, acarbose should be taken at the beginning of a meal.

213. **(C)** Hyperglycemia (A) is a characteristic of type 2 diabetes; anemia (B) is a possible adverse effect of acarbose, but not one of the most common side effects; rash (D) is not mentioned in the passage. Gastrointestinal discomfort is stated to be the most common side effect of acarbose.

214. **(B)** The passage states that glucose is the best choice for patients taking acarbose. A sulfonylurea agent (A) is the most popular class of agents used to treat type 2 diabetes. Sucrose (C) is mentioned in the passage as a sugar that the patient may not be able to adequately hydrolyze and absorb, and fructose (D) is not mentioned at all.

215. **(D)** Although low serum glucose concentration (A), gastrointestinal discomfort (B), and decreased iron absorption (C) are all described in the passage as possible adverse effects associated with the use of acarbose, obstruction of the urinary tract is not mentioned.

216. **(A)** The passage states that sulfonylureas are one of the most popular classes of agents used to treat type 2 diabetes and that using acarbose in combination with other agents may lead to hypoglycemia. Glucose (B), iron (C), and increased caloric intake (D) are not described as having this effect.

217. **(C)** Since the passage does not cover the topic of diabetes in the United States, answer A cannot be the correct choice. Nor does the passage deal with all the various agents used to treat type 2 diabetes, so answer B is ruled out. Answer D is too specific; the passage does deal with some adverse effects of acarbose, but it covers much more than that. The best title for the passage is The Use of Acarbose in the Treatment of Type 2 Diabetes.

Passage 5

Osteoporosis, the most common skeletal disorder associated with aging, is a significant cause of mortality and morbidity among the elderly. The two most common types of osteoporosis are type I (postmenopausal) osteoporosis and type II (senile) osteoporosis. Type I osteoporosis is due to a drastic decline in bone mass during the first five years of menopause and a slower rate of bone loss in subsequent years. Type II osteoporosis is characterized by a gradual, age-related loss of bone in females and males over the age of 65 years. By far, osteoporosis is most prevalent in the post-   218
menopausal population. In addition to menopausal-associated hormonal changes,   219
other risk factors for osteoporosis in women include low calcium intake, medical
factors such as oophorectomy, and life-style factors such as inactivity and cigarette
smoking. In osteoporosis, osteoclasts excavate areas in bone that the bone forming   223
cells, the osteoblasts, are unable to fully reconstitute. Often this defective bone loses   224

compressive strength, thereby leading to an increased risk of fracture. <u>Osteoporosis</u>
221 <u>evolves as a silent disease with no obvious early warning signs.</u> Many patients suffering from osteoporosis are not aware of their condition until a fracture occurs. This disease is responsible for at least 1.5 million fractures in Americans each year,
222 with annual costs to the United States health care system of approximately <u>$10 billion. Other consequences of osteoporosis include pain and spinal deformities such</u>
220 <u>as dorsal kyphosis and dowager's or widow's hump.</u> In addition, a decrease in appetite, fatigue, and weakness may be present. As the population continues to age, the cost of treating osteoporosis and its associated complications are predicted to
222 <u>double over the next 30 years.</u>

218. **(A)** Since the passage states that osteoporosis is associated with aging, infants (C) and teenagers (D) are clearly incorrect. Young males (B) is also incorrect; males with osteoporosis are described as over the age of 65. Postmenopausal women are the population in whom osteoporosis most commonly occurs.

219. **(C)** Age (A), low calcium intake (B), and cigarette smoking (D) are all mentioned or implied as risk factors; however, weight-bearing exercises is not. In fact, answer C is the opposite of one of the stated risk ractors, inactivity.

220. **(D)** The passage mentions dowager's hump as a consequence of osteoporosis. Height gain (A) is clearly not the best choice, since a decline in bone mass is more likely to lead to height loss. Oophorectomy (C) is mentioned in the passage as a risk factor for osteoporosis; hypertension (B) is irrelevant.

221. **(B)** The passage states that osteoporosis evolves as a silent disease with no obvious early warning signs.

222. **(D)** The passage states that the current cost of treating osteoporosis is approximately $10 billion. The last sentence in the passage states that the cost of treating osteoporosis and its associated complications is predicted to double over the next 30 years; thus $20 billion is the correct answer.

223. **(A)** The passage states that osteoclasts excavate areas in bone. Osteoblasts (B) are also discussed in the passage, but they are the cells that form bone. The other two choices, osteomasts (C) and osteotrasts (D) are not mentioned in the passage and are therefore irrelevant.

224. **(B)** Osteoblasts are responsible for forming bone. As stated in the passage, osteoclasts remove bone. Again, osteomasts (C) and osteotrasts (D) are irrelevant.

Passage 6

Although phenytoin may be used to treat cardiac arrhythmias, migraines, and 225
trigeminal neuralgia, the primary use of phenytoin is to treat seizure disorders. 226
Phenytoin, one of the most important agents used to manage seizures, works similarly of other hydantoin-derivative anticonvulsants. It decreases seizure activity by
stabilizing neuronal membranes and by increasing efflux or decreasing influx of 227
sodium ions across cell membranes in the motor cortex during generation of nerve
impulses. Phenytoin is commercially available as oral suspension, tablets, and capsules. It is also available as an injection. The dosage of phenytoin varies according to
the frequency of seizures, the type of seizures, and the patient's tolerance for pheny- 228
toin. Therefore, it is extremely important to monitor the patient for seizure activity
as well as to monitor phenytoin serum concentrations. Phenytoin has a narrow ther- 229
apeutic window and monitoring of serum concentrations is necessary. Therapeutic
serum concentrations of phenytoin are usually 10–20 mcg per mL (millimeter) and
depend on the assay method used. Serum concentrations above 20 mcg per mL often
result in toxicity. Adverse reactions associated with dose-related toxicities include 231
blurred vision, lethargy, rash, fever, slurred speech, nystagmus, and confusion. In
some patients, seizure control is not achieved when plasma concentrations are within
the therapeutic concentration range and therefore clinical response of the patient is
more meaningful than plasma concentrations. Generally, therapeutic steady state 232
serum concentrations are achieved within 30 days of therapy with an oral dosage of
300 mg daily in adults. Following an intravenous administration of 1000–1500 mg,
at a rate not exceeding 50 mg per minute, therapeutic concentrations can be attained
within 2 hours. Rapid administration of intravenous phenytoin may result in adverse 230
effects such as decreased blood pressure and other cardiac complications. The use of
phenytoin has been associated with osteomalacia, thrombocytopenia, and gastrointestinal upset.

225. **(A)** Trigeminal neuralgia is treated with phenytoin. Arthritis (B) is not mentioned in the passage; osteomalacia (C) is mentioned as a possible adverse
effect; and nystagmus (D) is mentioned as an adverse reaction associated with
toxicity.

226. **(C)** The first sentence clearly states that phenytoin is most commonly used
to treat seizure disorders. Cardiac arrythmias (A) and migraines (B) are mentioned as other possible uses; arthritis (D) is not mentioned in the
passage.

227. **(C)** Neither answer A nor answer B appears in the passage, and answer D
states the opposite of the correct answer.

228. **(D)** Although phenytoin serum concentration (A), number of seizures (B),
and adverse events (C) are listed as factors that affect the dosage of phenytoin, puncture sites available are not mentioned in the passage.

229. **(D)** Answer A incorrectly implies that phenytoin produces seizures; answer
B incorrectly states that there is no known difference between the serum con-
centrations known to produce desirable and undesirable effects; and answer
C refers to migraines rather than to seizures.

230. **(B)** A higher rate of administration may lower blood pressure. Answer A is irrelevant; answer C is inaccurate; and answer D refers to a condition (rash) that may be associated with phenytoin toxicity but not with the rapid administration of intravenous phenytoin.

231. **(C)** Blurred vision (A), lethargy (B), and mental confusion (D) are mentioned in the passage as adverse reactions associated with drug-related toxicities. There is no reference to dysuria.

232. **(D)** The passage states only that the therapeutic steady state serum concentration may be achieved within 30 days with an oral dosage of 300 mg daily of phenytoin. Therefore, 5 days (A), 24 hours (B), and 6 days (C) are all inaccurate.

Practice Test 2

This second sample PCAT is not a copy of an actual PCAT, but it has also been designed to closely represent the types of questions that may be included in an actual exam. Proceed with this practice exam as if you were taking the actual PCAT, adhering to the time allowed for each section in the table below.

Section	Time Allowed*
1. Verbal Ability	25 minutes
2. Chemistry	35 minutes
3. Biology	35 minutes
4. Reading Comprehension	50 minutes
5. Quantitative Ability	45 minutes
6. Writing (Essay)	30 minutes

*Please note: The order of the subjects (test sections) may vary from test to test.

Answer Sheet
PRACTICE TEST 2

Verbal Ability (1–40)

1 (A) (B) (C) (D)	11 (A) (B) (C) (D)	21 (A) (B) (C) (D)	31 (A) (B) (C) (D)
2 (A) (B) (C) (D)	12 (A) (B) (C) (D)	22 (A) (B) (C) (D)	32 (A) (B) (C) (D)
3 (A) (B) (C) (D)	13 (A) (B) (C) (D)	23 (A) (B) (C) (D)	33 (A) (B) (C) (D)
4 (A) (B) (C) (D)	14 (A) (B) (C) (D)	24 (A) (B) (C) (D)	34 (A) (B) (C) (D)
5 (A) (B) (C) (D)	15 (A) (B) (C) (D)	25 (A) (B) (C) (D)	35 (A) (B) (C) (D)
6 (A) (B) (C) (D)	16 (A) (B) (C) (D)	26 (A) (B) (C) (D)	36 (A) (B) (C) (D)
7 (A) (B) (C) (D)	17 (A) (B) (C) (D)	27 (A) (B) (C) (D)	37 (A) (B) (C) (D)
8 (A) (B) (C) (D)	18 (A) (B) (C) (D)	28 (A) (B) (C) (D)	38 (A) (B) (C) (D)
9 (A) (B) (C) (D)	19 (A) (B) (C) (D)	29 (A) (B) (C) (D)	39 (A) (B) (C) (D)
10 (A) (B) (C) (D)	20 (A) (B) (C) (D)	30 (A) (B) (C) (D)	40 (A) (B) (C) (D)

Chemistry (41–88)

41 (A) (B) (C) (D)	53 (A) (B) (C) (D)	65 (A) (B) (C) (D)	77 (A) (B) (C) (D)
42 (A) (B) (C) (D)	54 (A) (B) (C) (D)	66 (A) (B) (C) (D)	78 (A) (B) (C) (D)
43 (A) (B) (C) (D)	55 (A) (B) (C) (D)	67 (A) (B) (C) (D)	79 (A) (B) (C) (D)
44 (A) (B) (C) (D)	56 (A) (B) (C) (D)	68 (A) (B) (C) (D)	80 (A) (B) (C) (D)
45 (A) (B) (C) (D)	57 (A) (B) (C) (D)	69 (A) (B) (C) (D)	81 (A) (B) (C) (D)
46 (A) (B) (C) (D)	58 (A) (B) (C) (D)	70 (A) (B) (C) (D)	82 (A) (B) (C) (D)
47 (A) (B) (C) (D)	59 (A) (B) (C) (D)	71 (A) (B) (C) (D)	83 (A) (B) (C) (D)
48 (A) (B) (C) (D)	60 (A) (B) (C) (D)	72 (A) (B) (C) (D)	84 (A) (B) (C) (D)
49 (A) (B) (C) (D)	61 (A) (B) (C) (D)	73 (A) (B) (C) (D)	85 (A) (B) (C) (D)
50 (A) (B) (C) (D)	62 (A) (B) (C) (D)	74 (A) (B) (C) (D)	86 (A) (B) (C) (D)
51 (A) (B) (C) (D)	63 (A) (B) (C) (D)	75 (A) (B) (C) (D)	87 (A) (B) (C) (D)
52 (A) (B) (C) (D)	64 (A) (B) (C) (D)	76 (A) (B) (C) (D)	88 (A) (B) (C) (D)

Answer Sheet
PRACTICE TEST 2

Biology (89–136)

89 Ⓐ Ⓑ Ⓒ Ⓓ	101 Ⓐ Ⓑ Ⓒ Ⓓ	113 Ⓐ Ⓑ Ⓒ Ⓓ	125 Ⓐ Ⓑ Ⓒ Ⓓ
90 Ⓐ Ⓑ Ⓒ Ⓓ	102 Ⓐ Ⓑ Ⓒ Ⓓ	114 Ⓐ Ⓑ Ⓒ Ⓓ	126 Ⓐ Ⓑ Ⓒ Ⓓ
91 Ⓐ Ⓑ Ⓒ Ⓓ	103 Ⓐ Ⓑ Ⓒ Ⓓ	115 Ⓐ Ⓑ Ⓒ Ⓓ	127 Ⓐ Ⓑ Ⓒ Ⓓ
92 Ⓐ Ⓑ Ⓒ Ⓓ	104 Ⓐ Ⓑ Ⓒ Ⓓ	116 Ⓐ Ⓑ Ⓒ Ⓓ	128 Ⓐ Ⓑ Ⓒ Ⓓ
93 Ⓐ Ⓑ Ⓒ Ⓓ	105 Ⓐ Ⓑ Ⓒ Ⓓ	117 Ⓐ Ⓑ Ⓒ Ⓓ	129 Ⓐ Ⓑ Ⓒ Ⓓ
94 Ⓐ Ⓑ Ⓒ Ⓓ	106 Ⓐ Ⓑ Ⓒ Ⓓ	118 Ⓐ Ⓑ Ⓒ Ⓓ	130 Ⓐ Ⓑ Ⓒ Ⓓ
95 Ⓐ Ⓑ Ⓒ Ⓓ	107 Ⓐ Ⓑ Ⓒ Ⓓ	119 Ⓐ Ⓑ Ⓒ Ⓓ	131 Ⓐ Ⓑ Ⓒ Ⓓ
96 Ⓐ Ⓑ Ⓒ Ⓓ	108 Ⓐ Ⓑ Ⓒ Ⓓ	120 Ⓐ Ⓑ Ⓒ Ⓓ	132 Ⓐ Ⓑ Ⓒ Ⓓ
97 Ⓐ Ⓑ Ⓒ Ⓓ	109 Ⓐ Ⓑ Ⓒ Ⓓ	121 Ⓐ Ⓑ Ⓒ Ⓓ	133 Ⓐ Ⓑ Ⓒ Ⓓ
98 Ⓐ Ⓑ Ⓒ Ⓓ	110 Ⓐ Ⓑ Ⓒ Ⓓ	122 Ⓐ Ⓑ Ⓒ Ⓓ	134 Ⓐ Ⓑ Ⓒ Ⓓ
99 Ⓐ Ⓑ Ⓒ Ⓓ	111 Ⓐ Ⓑ Ⓒ Ⓓ	123 Ⓐ Ⓑ Ⓒ Ⓓ	135 Ⓐ Ⓑ Ⓒ Ⓓ
100 Ⓐ Ⓑ Ⓒ Ⓓ	112 Ⓐ Ⓑ Ⓒ Ⓓ	124 Ⓐ Ⓑ Ⓒ Ⓓ	136 Ⓐ Ⓑ Ⓒ Ⓓ

Reading Comprehension (137–184)

137 Ⓐ Ⓑ Ⓒ Ⓓ	149 Ⓐ Ⓑ Ⓒ Ⓓ	161 Ⓐ Ⓑ Ⓒ Ⓓ	173 Ⓐ Ⓑ Ⓒ Ⓓ
138 Ⓐ Ⓑ Ⓒ Ⓓ	150 Ⓐ Ⓑ Ⓒ Ⓓ	162 Ⓐ Ⓑ Ⓒ Ⓓ	174 Ⓐ Ⓑ Ⓒ Ⓓ
139 Ⓐ Ⓑ Ⓒ Ⓓ	151 Ⓐ Ⓑ Ⓒ Ⓓ	163 Ⓐ Ⓑ Ⓒ Ⓓ	175 Ⓐ Ⓑ Ⓒ Ⓓ
140 Ⓐ Ⓑ Ⓒ Ⓓ	152 Ⓐ Ⓑ Ⓒ Ⓓ	164 Ⓐ Ⓑ Ⓒ Ⓓ	176 Ⓐ Ⓑ Ⓒ Ⓓ
141 Ⓐ Ⓑ Ⓒ Ⓓ	153 Ⓐ Ⓑ Ⓒ Ⓓ	165 Ⓐ Ⓑ Ⓒ Ⓓ	177 Ⓐ Ⓑ Ⓒ Ⓓ
142 Ⓐ Ⓑ Ⓒ Ⓓ	154 Ⓐ Ⓑ Ⓒ Ⓓ	166 Ⓐ Ⓑ Ⓒ Ⓓ	178 Ⓐ Ⓑ Ⓒ Ⓓ
143 Ⓐ Ⓑ Ⓒ Ⓓ	155 Ⓐ Ⓑ Ⓒ Ⓓ	167 Ⓐ Ⓑ Ⓒ Ⓓ	179 Ⓐ Ⓑ Ⓒ Ⓓ
144 Ⓐ Ⓑ Ⓒ Ⓓ	156 Ⓐ Ⓑ Ⓒ Ⓓ	168 Ⓐ Ⓑ Ⓒ Ⓓ	180 Ⓐ Ⓑ Ⓒ Ⓓ
145 Ⓐ Ⓑ Ⓒ Ⓓ	157 Ⓐ Ⓑ Ⓒ Ⓓ	169 Ⓐ Ⓑ Ⓒ Ⓓ	181 Ⓐ Ⓑ Ⓒ Ⓓ
146 Ⓐ Ⓑ Ⓒ Ⓓ	158 Ⓐ Ⓑ Ⓒ Ⓓ	170 Ⓐ Ⓑ Ⓒ Ⓓ	182 Ⓐ Ⓑ Ⓒ Ⓓ
147 Ⓐ Ⓑ Ⓒ Ⓓ	159 Ⓐ Ⓑ Ⓒ Ⓓ	171 Ⓐ Ⓑ Ⓒ Ⓓ	183 Ⓐ Ⓑ Ⓒ Ⓓ
148 Ⓐ Ⓑ Ⓒ Ⓓ	160 Ⓐ Ⓑ Ⓒ Ⓓ	172 Ⓐ Ⓑ Ⓒ Ⓓ	184 Ⓐ Ⓑ Ⓒ Ⓓ

Answer Sheet

PRACTICE TEST 2

Quantitative Ability (185–232)

185 Ⓐ Ⓑ Ⓒ Ⓓ	197 Ⓐ Ⓑ Ⓒ Ⓓ	209 Ⓐ Ⓑ Ⓒ Ⓓ	221 Ⓐ Ⓑ Ⓒ Ⓓ
186 Ⓐ Ⓑ Ⓒ Ⓓ	198 Ⓐ Ⓑ Ⓒ Ⓓ	210 Ⓐ Ⓑ Ⓒ Ⓓ	222 Ⓐ Ⓑ Ⓒ Ⓓ
187 Ⓐ Ⓑ Ⓒ Ⓓ	199 Ⓐ Ⓑ Ⓒ Ⓓ	211 Ⓐ Ⓑ Ⓒ Ⓓ	223 Ⓐ Ⓑ Ⓒ Ⓓ
188 Ⓐ Ⓑ Ⓒ Ⓓ	200 Ⓐ Ⓑ Ⓒ Ⓓ	212 Ⓐ Ⓑ Ⓒ Ⓓ	224 Ⓐ Ⓑ Ⓒ Ⓓ
189 Ⓐ Ⓑ Ⓒ Ⓓ	201 Ⓐ Ⓑ Ⓒ Ⓓ	213 Ⓐ Ⓑ Ⓒ Ⓓ	225 Ⓐ Ⓑ Ⓒ Ⓓ
190 Ⓐ Ⓑ Ⓒ Ⓓ	202 Ⓐ Ⓑ Ⓒ Ⓓ	214 Ⓐ Ⓑ Ⓒ Ⓓ	226 Ⓐ Ⓑ Ⓒ Ⓓ
191 Ⓐ Ⓑ Ⓒ Ⓓ	203 Ⓐ Ⓑ Ⓒ Ⓓ	215 Ⓐ Ⓑ Ⓒ Ⓓ	227 Ⓐ Ⓑ Ⓒ Ⓓ
192 Ⓐ Ⓑ Ⓒ Ⓓ	204 Ⓐ Ⓑ Ⓒ Ⓓ	216 Ⓐ Ⓑ Ⓒ Ⓓ	228 Ⓐ Ⓑ Ⓒ Ⓓ
193 Ⓐ Ⓑ Ⓒ Ⓓ	205 Ⓐ Ⓑ Ⓒ Ⓓ	217 Ⓐ Ⓑ Ⓒ Ⓓ	229 Ⓐ Ⓑ Ⓒ Ⓓ
194 Ⓐ Ⓑ Ⓒ Ⓓ	206 Ⓐ Ⓑ Ⓒ Ⓓ	218 Ⓐ Ⓑ Ⓒ Ⓓ	230 Ⓐ Ⓑ Ⓒ Ⓓ
195 Ⓐ Ⓑ Ⓒ Ⓓ	207 Ⓐ Ⓑ Ⓒ Ⓓ	219 Ⓐ Ⓑ Ⓒ Ⓓ	231 Ⓐ Ⓑ Ⓒ Ⓓ
196 Ⓐ Ⓑ Ⓒ Ⓓ	208 Ⓐ Ⓑ Ⓒ Ⓓ	220 Ⓐ Ⓑ Ⓒ Ⓓ	232 Ⓐ Ⓑ Ⓒ Ⓓ

Writing

For the essay portion of the test, please compose your response on a separate sheet of paper.

VERBAL ABILITY

40 QUESTIONS (#1–#40)

TIME: 25 MINUTES

Directions: Select the word that **best** completes the analogy.

1. MECHANIC : WRENCH :: GARDENER :
   - (A) Lawn
   - (B) Grass seed
   - (C) Annuals
   - (D) Trowel

2. CHARLATAN : FAKE :: PATRIOT :
   - (A) Honest
   - (B) Loyal
   - (C) Honorable
   - (D) Charming

3. ORACLE : FORESIGHT :: SAGE :
   - (A) Wisdom
   - (B) Talent
   - (C) Wealth
   - (D) Clarity

4. ZIPPER : FASTEN :: ESCALATOR :
   - (A) Embed
   - (B) Lift
   - (C) Shuffle
   - (D) Camp

5. SHALLOW : DEPTH :: APATHETIC :
   - (A) Monopoly
   - (B) Apology
   - (C) Trying
   - (D) Caring

6. BUILDING : BLUEPRINT :: REPORT :
   - (A) Outline
   - (B) Canvas
   - (C) Table
   - (D) Artist

7. ANTISEPTIC : GERMS :: WATER :
   - (A) Sterilized
   - (B) Disinfectant
   - (C) Thirst
   - (D) Cook

8. SLUGGISH : ENERGY :: SATIATED :
   - (A) Dissatisfied
   - (B) Slothful
   - (C) Wary
   - (D) Hunger

9. NEOPHYTE : EXPERIENCED :: INVALID :
   - (A) Sickly
   - (B) Healthy
   - (C) Compliant
   - (D) Wealthy

10. BUS : PASSENGERS :: FREIGHTER :
    - (A) Requirement
    - (B) Tires
    - (C) Plane
    - (D) Cargo

11. ARCANE : ESOTERIC :: IRASCIBLE :
    - (A) Occult
    - (B) Fractious
    - (C) Joyful
    - (D) Unknowable

12. EMBARGO : TRADE :: HELMET :
    - (A) Injury
    - (B) Respite
    - (C) Football
    - (D) Hearing

13. REDOLENT : AROMATIC :: SEQUESTER :
    - (A) Cloister
    - (B) Sedition
    - (C) Curative
    - (D) Satirical

14. METER : LENGTH :: POUND :

(A) Inch
(B) Yard
(C) Heavy
(D) Weight

15. ANACONDA : SNAKE :: BASKETBALL :

(A) Serve
(B) Sport
(C) Shorts
(D) Ball

16. BRUISE : SKIN :: STAIN :

(A) Muscle
(B) Bone
(C) Fabric
(D) Veneer

17. SPHYGMOMANOMETER : BLOOD
PRESSURE :: THERMOMETER :

(A) Temperature
(B) Fahrenheit
(C) Ampere
(D) Air

18. OEDIPUS COMPLEX : FREUD ::
UNCERTAINTY PRINCIPLE :

(A) Hindenberg
(B) Heisenberg
(C) Jung
(D) Newton

19. HINDENBERG : BLIMPS :: LUSITANIA :

(A) Tragedies
(B) Oceans
(C) Icebergs
(D) Ocean liners

20. VIROLOGY : VIRUSES ::
KINESIOLOGY :

(A) Human movement
(B) Nature of existence
(C) Nature of knowledge
(D) Animal behavior

21. ANTHROPOMORPHIC : HUMAN ::
THERIOMORPHIC :

(A) Inhuman
(B) Evolution
(C) Egypt
(D) Animal

22. QUELL : SUCCEED :: SUCCINCT :

(A) Prolix
(B) Proscribe
(C) Profligate
(D) Prodigal

23. NUCLEAR MEMBRANE : CELL ::
HYPOTENUSE :

(A) Algebra
(B) Hippocrates
(C) Triangle
(D) Pythagoras

24. BASS : TREBLE :: ACME :

(A) Pitch
(B) Rhythm
(C) Peak
(D) Nadir

25. IMPERCEPTIBLE : TANGIBLE :: MILD :

(A) Tiny
(B) Severe
(C) Bland
(D) Magnified

Directions: Select the word or set of words that makes the most sense when inserted into the sentence and that best fits the meaning of the sentence as a whole.

26. The senator was _____ and unyielding, as she refused to give up her filibuster of a proposal she _____ disagreed with.

    (A) sallow; ruefully
    (B) penitent; plaintively
    (C) refractory; vehemently
    (D) pacifistic; irreverently

27. The well-read scholar is considered a _____ due to the breadth and depth of his knowledge of several, wide-ranging academic topics.

    (A) puritan
    (B) polymath
    (C) sycophant
    (D) supplicant

28. By planning ahead, you may be able to _____ some of the _____ events that may spoil your camping trip.

    (A) circumvent; unforeseen
    (B) circumscribe; suggested
    (C) oppose; progressive
    (D) misconstrue; catastrophic

29. The _____ during their trip to the beach were pleasant, unlike the hurricane-force winds they experienced when visiting the same spot last year.

    (A) monsoons
    (B) gales
    (C) squalls
    (D) zephyrs

30. One example of _____ is Greek mythology because it was _____ on the belief that many gods exist.

    (A) polytheism; established
    (B) triennial; extended
    (C) monotheism; legalized
    (D) truancy; admitted

31. Not all tree fungi are detrimental to trees; there are some instances where both the fungi and the tree live together in a _____ existence where both organisms _____.

    (A) psychotic; succumb
    (B) triangular; synchronize
    (C) symbiotic; benefit
    (D) superimposed; cooperate

32. The couple were unsure of where they wanted to go on their honeymoon and _____ over the three choices presented by their travel agent.

    (A) vaunted
    (B) reneged
    (C) vacillated
    (D) reposed

33. The puzzled and impatient listener _____ a question before the speaker could _____ the presentation.

    (A) interjected; conclude
    (B) projected; preclude
    (C) postponed; transmit
    (D) interceded; supervise

34. You don't have to _____ the message exactly as it was spoken; you may _____ it in your own words.

    (A) delegate; convene
    (B) communicate; paraphrase
    (C) suggest; eradicate
    (D) provide; devalue

35. When the facilitator asked her to make a few _____ remarks about the conference's festivities, she was _____.

   (A) sporadic; illuminated
   (B) indecisive; thorough
   (C) impromptu; unprepared
   (D) devised; equipped

36. The fortress in which the group of villagers took refuge was considered _____, and their fears of the violent raiders diminished considerably.

   (A) inimical
   (B) implacable
   (C) ignominious
   (D) impregnable

37. She had a contemptuous and _____ attitude toward the volunteers, and it seemed as though she thought of them as _____ and inferior.

   (A) submissive; superficial
   (B) condescending; substandard
   (C) perceptive; incriminating
   (D) contentious; cosmopolitan

38. Do not include _____ and irrelevant information; please keep your reports as _____ as possible.

   (A) rhetorical; sufficient
   (B) incessant; ideological
   (C) extraneous; succinct
   (D) affable; sardonic

39. One of the _____ aspects of his dynamic presentation was his ability to _____ the listless children so that they wanted to fully participate.

   (A) sanctimonious; compel
   (B) luminous; chastise
   (C) absolute; acquire
   (D) salient; captivate

40. This initial class is _____; it is imperative that you complete it so that you will be able to _____ to the next class.

   (A) malignant; transfer
   (B) inevitable; propagate
   (C) mandatory; advance
   (D) undetermined; transcend

STOP

End of Verbal Ability section. If you have any time left, you may go over your work in this section only.

CHEMISTRY

48 QUESTIONS (#41–#88)

TIME: 35 MINUTES

Directions: Choose the **best** answer to each of the following questions.

41. The class of biomolecules that is primarily characterized by its hydrophobicity is

    (A) proteins.
    (B) nucleic acids.
    (C) carbohydrates.
    (D) lipids.

42. Human immunodeficiency virus (HIV) infection is managed by several classes of drugs. One of those classes is the nucleoside reverse transcriptase inhibitors (NRTIs). These agents are nucleosides and, after conversion to the corresponding triphosphate nucleotides, they inhibit reverse transcriptase, the enzyme needed by HIV to transcribe its RNA genome into DNA. The NRTIs are useful in this situation because they disrupt the production of proviral DNA. Because they are structurally similar to the nucleotides used in the synthesis of cellular nucleic acids, they may also affect DNA/RNA synthesis in uninfected cells causing undesired side effects. Fortunately, the affinity for NRTIs of the normal cellular enzymes involved in DNA/RNA synthesis is much lower than the affinity of the viral reverse transcriptase for them. Even so, patients receiving NRTIs often experience side effects related to their impact on the synthesis of normal cellular DNA.

    Which statement describes nucleotides?

    (A) They are polymerized to form proteins.
    (B) They contain purines and/or pyrimidines.
    (C) They contain glucose.
    (D) Their polymerization is called translation.

43. How many protons are indicated in the following symbol for the lithium ion, $_3^7\text{Li}^{+1}$?

    (A) 3
    (B) 7
    (C) 10
    (D) 4

44. When a solute is dissolved in a solvent, which of the following is true concerning the solution?

    (A) The boiling point will increase.
    (B) The freezing point will increase.
    (C) The osmotic pressure will decrease.
    (D) The solution will conduct electricity if the solute is a nonelectrolyte.

45. In the synthesis of protein from the nucleotide sequence in the mRNA, what is the term used to describe the group of three nucleotides that corresponds to an amino acid?

    (A) rRNA
    (B) codon
    (C) tRNA
    (D) anticodon

46. Many drugs contain chiral centers. When a chiral center is synthesized in the laboratory, both forms of the chiral center (R and S) are produced. Usually one form is biologically active, while the other is biologically inert since cellular molecules can discriminate between the two forms. For example, the molecule responsible for the smell of rye bread and spearmint oil, carvone, exists in two forms—the R form in spearmint oil and the S form in caraway, a component in rye bread. The nose quickly distinguishes these two forms because the receptors in the nose are able to discriminate between them. The same is true with drug molecules. Zyrtec (cetirizine), a drug used to treat allergies, contains a chiral center, and the preparation sold over-the-counter in drugstores is a mixture of both the R and S forms. The drug product levocetirizine (Xyzal) contains only the active form of cetirizine and is available only with a prescription.

What is the name of the following compound?

(A) (1S, 3S)-3-methyl-1-chlorocyclohexane
(B) (1S, 3R)-3-methyl-1-chlorocyclohexane
(C) (1R, 3S)-3-methyl-1-chlorocyclohexane
(D) (1R, 3R)-3-methyl-1-chlorocyclohexane

47. What is the product of the following reaction?

(A)

(B) CO$_2$H

(C) CO$_2$H

(D)

48. How many moles of carbon dioxide, CO_2, are present in 22 grams CO_2? (O = 16 amu, C = 12 amu)

(A) 0.80
(B) 0.50
(C) 2.00
(D) 1.30

49. What is the percentage yield of the following reaction if 1.0 gram of hydrogen, H_2, reacts with excess chlorine, Cl_2, to produce 18.3 grams of hydrogen chloride, HCl? (Cl = 35.5 amu, H = 1 amu)

$$H_2 + Cl_2 \rightarrow 2\ HCl$$

(A) 100%
(B) 75%
(C) 50%
(D) 25%

50. How many moles of copper, Cu, are present in 1.2×10^6 atoms of Cu? (Avogadro's Number $= 6 \times 10^{+23}$, Cu = 63.5 amu)

    (A) $5.0 \times 10^{+17}$
    (B) $2.0 \times 10^{+4}$
    (C) 5.3×10^{-5}
    (D) 2.0×10^{-18}

51. Carboxylic acid derivatives are a class of organic functional, groups that include the acid halides, the anhydrides, the esters, the amides, the acylphosphates, and the thioesters. All of the members of this class have a carbonyl containing a partial positive carbon. This carbon is susceptible to nucleophilic attack. The reactivity of the carbonyl carbon is dependent on the level of partial positive charge as well as steric factors. Because halides are more electronegative than carbon and not able to efficiently stabilize the partial positive carbon through resonance, the carbonyl carbon of acid halides has the greatest partial positive charge of the functional groups in this class. For this reason, reactions involving the acid halides occur quickly making them a desirable reagent in organic synthesis. Many organic transformations can be accomplished using acid halides, but because atmospheric water is nucleophilic, they will quickly be hydrolyzed to the corresponding carboxylic acid when exposed to air.

    What functional group results from the following reaction?

    $(CH_3)_2NH + CH_3CH_2COCl \rightarrow$

    (A) Amine
    (B) Enamine
    (C) Amide
    (D) Imine

52. Which of the following reactions is a neutralization reaction?

    (A) $Mg + 2HCl \rightarrow MgCl_2 + H_2$
    (B) $2HCl + CaCO_3 \rightarrow CaCl_2 + H_2O + CO_2$
    (C) $BaCl_2 + Na_2SO_4 \rightarrow BaSO_4 + 2NaCl$
    (D) $2KClO_3 \rightarrow 2KCl + 3O_2$

53. What is the oxidation number of phosphorus, P, in PO_4^{-3}?

    (A) -8
    (B) -3
    (C) $+8$
    (D) $+5$

54. Protein function is destroyed by denaturation that

    (A) causes the cleavage of peptide bonds.
    (B) results in the loss of secondary structure.
    (C) does not affect hydrogen bonding.
    (D) digests the protein.

55. How many grams of sodium hydroxide, NaOH, are required to produce 800 milliliters of a 2.0 molar, 2.0 M, solution? (Na = 23 amu, O = 16 amu, H = 1 amu)

    (A) 8.0
    (B) 64
    (C) $1.6 \times 10^{+3}$
    (D) $6.4 \times 10^{+4}$

56. An autoclave has an initial pressure of 1.0 atmosphere and initial temperature of 27°C. The autoclave is heated until the final pressure inside the autoclave equals 5.0 atmospheres. What is the final temperature in degrees Celsius of the oven?

    (A) 1500
    (B) 1227
    (C) 135
    (D) 1000

57. To which biomolecular class does the following molecule belong?

(A) Nucleic acids
(B) Proteins
(C) Lipids
(D) Carbohydrates

Use the periodic table below in order to answer questions 58–65.

58. What is the electron configuration of the magnesium atom, Mg?

(A) $1s^2 2s^2 2p^6 3s^2$
(B) $1s^2 2s^2 2p^6$
(C) $1s^2 2s^2 2p^6 3s^2 3p^4$
(D) $1s^2 2s^2$

59. Which reagent would accomplish the following conversion?

(A) H_2SO_4
(B) $K^+ \ ^-OC(CH_3)_3$
(C) NH_3
(D) $LiAlH_4$

60. What is the product of the following reaction?

(A)

(B)

(C)

(D)

61. Which statement describes the compound, copper (II) sulfide?

    (A) It is a covalent compound.
    (B) The oxidation number of copper is +1.
    (C) The formula is Cu_2S.
    (D) It is expected to be insoluble in water.

62. Which structure for a substance with the formula $C_5H_{10}O_2$ is consistent with the following ^1H NMR data?

    δ 1.2 ppm, doublet, 6H
    δ 2.0 ppm, singlet, 3H
    δ 5.0 ppm, septet, 1H

    (A)

    (B)

    (C)

    (D)

63. Resonance is the term used to describe the delocalization of pi or unshared electrons within molecules. When drawing the Lewis structure for compounds exhibiting resonance, a collection of Lewis structures is required, with each having the same sigma bonding framework but differing in the location of pi and unshared electrons. The actual molecule, called the resonance hybrid, is a hybrid of all of the individual resonance structures. It is not necessarily an average of the structures since depending on the stability of each structure, the contribution of each to the hybrid may vary. Resonance stabilizes molecules by distributing charge or radical character among several atoms. Drawing a collection of resonance structures involves beginning with a Lewis structure and "pushing" pi and unshared electrons using a curved arrow format.

    Which is a resonance structure of the following ion?

    (A)

    (B)

    (C)

    (D)

64. Which of the following bonds is most polar?

 (A) N — F
 (B) C — F
 (C) S — Cl
 (D) N — O

65. Which of the following compounds displays hydrogen bonding?

 (A) H_2
 (B) H_2S
 (C) NH_3
 (D) CH_4

66. What is the molality of a solution that is 12 M (formula weight of solute is 33) and has a density of 1.2 g/ml?

 (A) 15 m
 (B) 12 m
 (C) 10 m
 (D) Cannot be determined

67. Lipids are involved in all of the following biological processes or structures EXCEPT

 (A) cell membrane construction.
 (B) hormones.
 (C) protein synthesis.
 (D) storage of carbon chains.

68. How would 100 mL of a 1.5 M NaBr solution be prepared? (Na = 23 amu, Br = 80 amu)

 (A) Dissolve 103 g of NaBr in 100 mL of water
 (B) Dissolve 15.5 g of NaBr in 100 mL of water
 (C) Dissolve 1.5 g of NaBr in enough water to make a final volume of 100 mL
 (D) Dissolve 15.5 g of NaBr in enough water to make a final volume of 100 mL

69. Phosholipids are found in cell membranes and are characterized by

 (A) a triester of glucose.
 (B) the presence of a nonpolar phosphate group.
 (C) their arrangement in a bilayer that has a nonpolar interior.
 (D) extensive arrangements in alpha helices.

70. In an aqueous environment, proteins assume an overall conformation driven by

 (A) their nucleotide sequence.
 (B) the positioning of hydrophilic side chains toward the interior of the conformation.
 (C) a variety of forces including hydrogen bonding.
 (D) the formation of a double helix.

71. Which is expected to have the lowest boiling point?

 (A)

 (B)

 (C)

 (D)

72. Which of the following is the process by which acetyl groups are oxidized?

 (A) The citric acid cycle
 (B) Glycolysis
 (C) Beta-oxidation
 (D) Oxidative phosphorylation

73. Molecular geometry has an impact on molecular polarity. For example, since CO_2 is a linear molecule, the polarity of each of the carbon-oxygen bonds is balanced, making the molecule overall nonpolar. Water, on the other hand, is not linear and is polar. Its molecular geometry is described as bent with a predicted bond angle near 109 degrees, the tetrahedral bond angle. This is true because when the Lewis structure of water is examined, there are 4 sets of electrons around the oxygen atom and, according to the Valence Shell Electron Pair Repulsion Theory, those 4 sets will spread out as far apart as possible, giving a tetrahedral geometry for the sets. When the molecular geometry is identified, however, only the positions of the atoms are considered, giving a bent molecular geometry.

    What is the geometry of ammonia, NH_3?

    (A) Trigonal planar
    (B) Trigonal pyramidal
    (C) Tetrahedral
    (D) Trigonal bipyramidal

74. Which reagent(s) will accomplish the following conversion?

    (A) 1. $Hg(OAc)_2$, H_2O
        2. $NaBH_4$

    (B) 1. BH_3
        2. H_2O_2, OH^-

    (C) MCPBA

    (D) 1. OsO_4
        2. $NaHSO_3$

75. What is the hybridization state of the carbon, C, atom in $H_2C = CH_2$?

    (A) sp
    (B) sp^2
    (C) sp^3
    (D) sp^3d^2

76. What is the pH of a solution in which the hydrogen ion concentration equals 1×10^{-5} M (moles/liter)?

    (A) 5
    (B) 9
    (C) 6
    (D) 7

77. Which of the following statements about the behavior of gases is NOT true?

    (A) Gases generally behave the same way regardless of their identity.
    (B) If the volume of a gas is increased, the pressure will decrease if the temperature remains constant.
    (C) If the temperature of a gas is decreased, the molecular motion of the gas particles will increase.
    (D) The average kinetic energy of gas particles is directly proportional to the Kelvin temperature.

78. A solution of the following salt, sodium acetate, CH_3COONa, in water will be

    (A) acidic
    (B) basic
    (C) nearly neutral
    (D) independent of pH

79. Which of the following solutions is a buffer solution?

    (A) Hydrochloric acid and sodium chloride, $HCl + NaCl$
    (B) Acetic acid and sodium acetate, $CH_3COOH + CH_3COONa$
    (C) Nitric acid and sodium nitrate, $HNO_3 + NaNO_3$
    (D) Sulfuric acid and sodium sulfate, $H_2SO_4 + Na_2SO_4$

80. Which statement describes the carbon-carbon bonds in ethene?

    (A) The pi bond is the overlap of hybrid orbitals.
    (B) The sigma bond is weaker than the pi bond.
    (C) The pi bond electron density resides above and below the sigma bond.
    (D) The sigma bond involves the overlap of p orbitals.

81. According to the kinetic molecular theory, in which of the following states of matter do atoms or molecules have the greatest freedom of motion?

    (A) Solid
    (B) Gas
    (C) Liquid
    (D) All states have the same freedom of motion.

82. Which compound could be used to react with ethyl magnesium bromide followed by protonation to form 3-pentanol?

    (A)

    (B)

    (C)

    (D)

    CHO

83. Which of the following is methyl 2-methylbutanoate?

    (A)

    (B)

    (C)

    (D)

84. The process by which protein is synthesized in the cell involves all of the following EXCEPT

    (A) mRNA
    (B) Ribosomes
    (C) tRNA
    (D) RNA polymerase

85. In the thermodynamic equation
$$\Delta G = \Delta H - T \Delta S$$
ΔG represents the change in free energy in a reaction, ΔH the change in enthalpy, and ΔS the change in entropy. The reaction is spontaneous when ΔG is

    (A) +
    (B) −
    (C) 0
    (D) The sign of ΔG has no significance.

86. Which of the following reactions shows an increase in entropy?

    (A) $2KClO_3$ (s) → $2KCl$ (s) + $3O_2$ (g)
    (B) H_2O (g) → H_2O (l)
    (C) $2H_2$ (g) + O_2 (g) → $2H_2O$ (l)
    (D) PCl_3 (l) + Cl_2 (g) → PCl_5 (s)

87. A change in which of the following factors causes a change in the equilibrium constant of the reversible reaction shown?

    $$A + B \leftrightarrow C + D \qquad K = \frac{[C][D]}{[A][B]}$$

    (A) Temperature
    (B) Volume
    (C) Concentration
    (D) Catalyst

88. Which of the following is a nuclear reaction?

    (A) Beta decay
    (B) Delta decay
    (C) Neutralization
    (D) Nuclear resonance

Practice Test 2

STOP

End of Chemistry section. If you have any time left, you may go over your work in this section only.

BIOLOGY

48 QUESTIONS (#89–#136)

TIME: 35 MINUTES

Directions: Choose the **best** answer to each of the following questions.

89. The chromosome number is reduced from diploid to haploid in cell division by

    (A) meiosis.
    (B) mitosis.
    (C) hapnosis.
    (D) triosis.

90. In animal x, black hair (B) is dominant over white hair (b). If a homozygous black-hair is crossed with a white-hair, the hair color of white is expected in what percent of the offspring?

    (A) 0%
    (B) 25%
    (C) 75%
    (D) 100%

91. What structure in a cell controls the exchange of materials between the inside of the cell and the extracellular environment?

    (A) Nucleus
    (B) Endoplasmic reticulum
    (C) Cell wall
    (D) Plasma membrane

92. A tumor that has spread through the bloodstream and formed a second tumor in a new location is what type of tumor?

    (A) Malignant
    (B) Metastatic
    (C) Benign
    (D) Sarcomic

93. The three types of cellular RNA polymerases in eukaryote cells transcribe different types of genes. What does RNA polymerase II produce?

    (A) Transfer RNA
    (B) Messenger RNA
    (C) Ribosomal RNA
    (D) Satellite RNA

94. Tetanus is associated with which type of pathogen?

    (A) Virus
    (B) Bacteria
    (C) Fungus
    (D) Protozoa

95. Which of the following represent the proper sequence for the stages of mitosis?

    (A) Prophase, Metaphase, Anaphase, Telophase
    (B) Prophase, Anaphase, Telophase, Metaphase
    (C) Anaphase, Telophase, Prophase, Metaphase
    (D) Anaphase, Prophase, Telophase, Metaphase

96. Exergonic reactions are defined as

    (A) anabolic.
    (B) building substrates into new products.
    (C) requiring energy.
    (D) releasing energy.

97. An endocrine gland

    (A) has a duct.
    (B) does not depend on the blood for transport of its secretions.
    (C) secretes hormones through a duct.
    (D) secretes hormones directly into the blood rather than through a duct.

98. A small population of new mothers experience postpartum depression after the birth of a child. Symptoms can include prolonged sadness, loss of appetite, and, most notably, difficulty bonding with or caring for the baby. Most symptoms subside after approximately six months.

    A new mother has reported the aforementioned symptoms and is also having trouble producing milk from her mammary glands during breastfeeding. Which of the following may be an underlying physiological explanation for all of these symptoms?

    (A) Higher than normal levels of estrogen
    (B) Lower than normal levels of oxytocin
    (C) Higher than normal levels of progesterone
    (D) Lower than normal levels of estrogen

99. During development, different embryonic cells express different sets of genes resulting in

    (A) gene mutation.
    (B) developmental abnormalities.
    (C) genetic recombination.
    (D) the formation of different cell types.

100. Calcitonin

    (A) is produced by the pancreas.
    (B) levels increase when blood calcium levels decrease.
    (C) causes blood calcium levels to decrease.
    (D) is produced by the gallbladder.

101. Parathyroid hormone secretion increases in response to

    (A) a decrease in blood calcium.
    (B) increased production of parathyroid-stimulating hormone from the anterior pituitary.
    (C) increased secretion of parathyroid-releasing hormone from the hypothalamus.
    (D) an increase in blood calcium.

102. The adrenal medulla secretes epinephrine

    (A) when blood glucose levels are high.
    (B) during deep sleep.
    (C) during times of stress.
    (D) during times of inactivity.

103. Which type of blood is the universal recipient?

    (A) O
    (B) B
    (C) A
    (D) AB

104. The valve between the right atrium and right ventricle is

    (A) Bicuspid (mitral) valve
    (B) Tricuspid valve
    (C) Atrioventricular valve
    (D) Chamber valve

105. Given the blood vessels below:

    1. aorta
    2. inferior vena cava
    3. pulmonary trunk
    4. pulmonary vein

    Choose the arrangement that lists the vessels in the order a red blood cell would encounter them in going from the systemic veins back to the systemic arteries.

    (A) 1, 3, 4, 2
    (B) 2, 3, 4, 1
    (C) 2, 4, 3, 1
    (D) 3, 2, 1, 4

106. Oxygen is mostly transported in the blood

    (A) in white blood cells.
    (B) bound to albumin.
    (C) bound to gamma globulins.
    (D) bound to the heme portion of hemoglobin.

107. What cytoskeletal element supports the nuclear envelop in animal cells?

(A) Actin
(B) Microtubules
(C) Intermediate filament
(D) Cell cortex

108. Which of the following statements is true concerning vitamins?

(A) They function as coenzymes.
(B) Most can be synthesized by the body.
(C) They are normally broken down before they can be used by the body.
(D) A, D, E, and K are water-soluble vitamins.

109. Trichotillomania and hoarding are forms of obsessive compulsive disorder (OCD) best described as

(A) immunological disorders.
(B) mental disorders.
(C) intestinal disorders.
(D) reproductive disorders.

110. In the reaction versus substrate concentration graph below, the curve plateaus because

(A) a noncompetitive inhibitor is present.
(B) a competitive inhibitor is present.
(C) the active site is saturated with substrate.
(D) all the substrate has been converted to product.

111. In a heterozygous monohybrid cross, the dominant trait would be expressed _____ of the time.

(A) 0 percent
(B) 25 percent
(C) 75 percent
(D) 100 percent

112. Which of the following is the specialized absorptive structure in the intestine?

(A) Alveoli
(B) Villi
(C) Bowman's capsule
(D) Nephron

113. Crossing over is more likely to occur between genes that are

(A) close together on the chromosome.
(B) on different chromosomes.
(C) located on the X chromosome.
(D) far apart on a chromosome.

114. Human skin develops from

(A) ectoderm.
(B) mesoderm.
(C) endoderm.
(D) trophoderm.

115. A personal trainer at a university is very interested in helping obese college students lose weight. He has developed a new exercise routine that he hypothesizes will maximize weight loss. He recruits fifty overweight students and places them on his special exercise regimen. He recruits another fifty obese students to serve as the control group. Both groups are told to maintain their normal diets.

A nutrition professor in the Health Science department hears about the study and asks the personal trainer if she can collect urine samples from the participants at the start of the study and again at the end of the study. The professor tests the urine for the presence of vitamins. The data from the study is below.

	Average weight before (lbs)	Average weight after (lbs)	Urine analysis before	Urine analysis after
Experimental group	303	276	Vitamin C	Vitamin C, A, and D
Control group	315	316	Vitamin C	Vitamin C

Which of the following best describes the results?

(A) Students in the experimental group lost body fat and likely changed their diet to include more vitamin rich foods.

(B) Students in the experimental group lost body fat and fat-soluble vitamins were released.

(C) Students in the control group gained body fat and likely changed their diet to include less vitamin rich foods.

(D) Students in the experimental group gained body fat and fat-soluble vitamins were released.

116. In minks, the gene for brown fur (B) is dominant to the gene for silver fur (b). Which set of genotypes represents a cross that could produce offspring with silver fur from parents that both have brown fur?

(A) Bb × Bb
(B) BB × Bb
(C) BB × bb
(D) Bb × bb

117. HIV (human immunodeficiency virus) infects mostly

(A) CT-cells
(B) D-killer cells
(C) T-helper cells
(D) R-cells

118. Carbohydrate digestion begins in the _____ with the action of the enzyme _____.

(A) mouth; amylase
(B) stomach; pepsin
(C) small intestine; cholecystokinin
(D) large intestine; water

119. What are the basic nutrients the body must have?

(A) Calcium, carbohydrates, protein, fats, vitamins, minerals, water
(B) Carbohydrates, protein, fats, vitamins, minerals, water
(C) Salt, carbohydrates, protein, fats, vitamins, minerals, water
(D) Magnesium, carbohydrates, proteins, fats, vitamins, minerals, water

120. _____ is a condition where a person's concerns about dieting, food restriction, fear of becoming overweight, and dissatisfaction with body image interfere with normal daily life.

(A) Binge-eating disorder
(B) Bulimia nervosa
(C) Affective-eating disorder
(D) Disordered eating patterns

121. A major function of white blood cells is to fight

    (A) pain.
    (B) infections.
    (C) glucose intolerance.
    (D) hormone imbalances.

Figure 1.

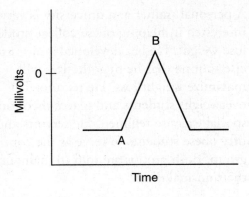

Figure 2.

122. All cells in the body require oxygen and sugar to undergo cellular respiration to produce ATP. Some cells require more ATP than others; therefore, they respire more than others.

    Above is a graph (Figure 1) of oxygen consumption vs. Tissue A and Tissue B. Based on the graph, which of the following statements best describes the cells of Tissue A?

    (A) Tissue A has either a greater number of mitochondria, larger mitochondria, or more enzymatic activity.
    (B) Tissue A has a lesser number of mitochondria, smaller mitochondria, or less enzymatic activity.
    (C) Tissue A has a lesser number of mitochondria, medium-sized mitochondria, or less enzymatic activity.
    (D) Tissue A has to have a smaller nucleus.

123. In Figure 2, the ascending portion of the action potential observed in the cell in the graph is caused by

    (A) fluoride efflux out of the cell.
    (B) potassium influx into the cell.
    (C) sodium efflux out of the cell.
    (D) sodium influx into the cell.

124. The pancreas produces which two hormones?

    (A) Melatonin and serotonin
    (B) Adrenalin and noradrenaline
    (C) Insulin and glucagon
    (D) Estrogen and testosterone

125. Hormones are distributed throughout the body by means of the

    (A) gallbladder.
    (B) blood.
    (C) pancreas.
    (D) stomach.

Figure 3.

126. During inhalation, oxygen is brought into the lungs. That oxygen diffuses into the blood and binds to hemoglobin (Hb) on red blood cells. The red blood cells then travel through the body to oxygen-depleted cells where oxygen unbinds from Hb and enters the cells.

You are interested in the "unloading" of oxygen at cells in the body. You decide to conduct a study with three animals: an elephant, a cat, and a mouse. You take a measure of each animal's saturation of Hb with oxygen (%) as it relates to the partial pressure of oxygen (mm Hg). The data is shown in Figure 3 above. In Figure 3, for an animal's hemoglobin to unload more readily it must

(A) have a high metabolic rate and high oxygen requirements.
(B) have a low metabolic rate and low oxygen requirements.
(C) have an intermediate oxygen requirement.
(D) not require oxygen.

127. You are studying penicillin production and secretion in the fungus *Penicillium chryso-genum*. You discover a strain of the fungus that does not secrete penicillin. You sequence genes associated with penicillin production, and there are no mutations present. You determine that the fungus is able to produce penicillin but is unable to secrete it. A mutation in which of the following proteins would lead to the observed phenotype?

(A) Vesicle tethering SNARE
(B) DNA condensin
(C) Actin
(D) RNA polymerase

128. Neurotransmitters trigger a new action potential in a postsynaptic neuron via

(A) voltage-gated channels.
(B) ligand-gated channels.
(C) stress-gated channels.
(D) stretch-gated channels.

129. The sugars associated with glycolipids and glycoproteins are important in

(A) cell division.
(B) protein production.
(C) cell recognition.
(D) cell movement.

130. Red blood cells possess a large amount of _____ to transport oxygen.

(A) albumin proteins
(B) cholesterol
(C) nuclei
(D) globin proteins

Practice Test 2

131. The interaction of _____ and
     _____ cause the shortening of
     sacromeres during muscle contractions.

     (A) kinesin; microtubules
     (B) kinesin; actin
     (C) myosin; microtubules
     (D) myosin; actin

132. Which form of diabetes may not require
     insulin injections for disease management?

     (A) Type 1
     (B) Type 2
     (C) Type 3
     (D) Type 4

133. This process occurs when double strands of
     a DNA segment separate and RNA
     nucleotides pair with DNA nucleotides.

     (A) Transcription
     (B) Translation
     (C) Transduction
     (D) Transmetric

134. Apoptosis describes a process of

     (A) cell specialization.
     (B) cell death.
     (C) cell differentiation.
     (D) cell proliferation.

Figure 4.

135. In Figure 4, the number 1 points to the

     (A) lag phase.
     (B) decline phase.
     (C) stationary phase.
     (D) logarithmic phase.

136. One bacterial cell is placed in a nutrient
     broth test tube at 12 noon. Its generation
     time is 30 minutes, and its growth occurs by
     binary fission. By 2:00 P.M., the size of the
     population of bacteria in the test tube is

     (A) 4.
     (B) 8.
     (C) 16.
     (D) 32.

STOP

*End of Biology section. If you have any time left,
you may go over your work in this section only.*

READING COMPREHENSION

48 QUESTIONS (#137–#184)

TIME: 50 MINUTES

> **Directions:** Read each of the following passages, and choose the **best** answer to each of the questions that follows each passage.

Passage 1

A dreaded disease is striking California's coast live oaks with the ferocity of an oak-tree Ebola virus, causing the trees to sprout sores, hemorrhage sap, and become infested with beetles and various fungi. The trees die within a few weeks of their first symptoms.

A pathologist at the University of California, Davis, announced that his team had found the cause of the disease dubbed "Sudden Oak Death." The tree-slayer is a new member of the genus Phytophthora, whose name means "plant destroyer." Its kin include pathogens responsible for the Irish potato famine and die-offs in Australian eucalyptus forests and European oak groves. "We don't know if the new species was just recently introduced, or if it has always been here and something else has changed that has allowed it to go crazy," one pathologist says.

The first trees to succumb to the plague 5 years ago were tan oaks, which often grow in the understory of redwood forests. Last year the disease began hitting large numbers of coast live oaks, the signature species in scenic coastal woodlands. Alarmingly, the pathogen has begun to blight another species, the black oak.

Knowing the culprit doesn't make the outlook much brighter. "Fungicides can save individual oaks," says one pathologist, "but we can't go to Mount Tamalpais and spray 10,000 trees." And prevention is largely limited to warning people not to carry oak firewood to uninfected areas. The Sierra Nevada hosts black oaks, and pathologists fear the deadly spores could strike groves in beloved Yosemite Valley.

From "Culprit Named in Sudden Oak Death," Science, Vol 289, August 2000. Page 859. Reprinted with permission from AAAS.

137. "Sudden Oak Death" causes trees to

(A) grow multiple trunks and become infested with mold.
(B) sprout sores, hemorrhage sap, and become infested with beetles and various fungi.
(C) lose all leaves, branches and wilt.
(D) hemorrhage at the tips, spout new branches, and become infested with termites.

138. This plague began

(A) 5 years ago.
(B) 10 years ago.
(C) 15 years ago.
(D) 2 years ago.

139. The cause of this disease is

(A) phytohemagglutinin.
(B) phytosterol.
(C) phytophthora.
(D) phytoalexin.

140. The first trees to succumb were

(A) tan oaks.
(B) coast live oaks.
(C) black oaks.
(D) European oaks.

141. The greatest fear of this plague is that it will strike

(A) redwood forests.
(B) Yosemite Valley.
(C) Australian eucalyptus forests.
(D) coastal woodlands.

142. The tree species that have been affected by the tree virus are

(A) the tan oak, coast live oak, and the black oak.
(B) the redwood oak, the tan oak, and the firewood oak.
(C) the Mount St. Helen's live oak.
(D) the Irish and Australian coastal oak.

143. According to the passage, treatment of the pathogen affecting California's oaks

    (A) can be done easily now that the cause has been identified
    (B) is possible using fungicides, but is difficult to disperse on a large scale.
    (C) is impossible as no known cure has been developed.
    (D) can only be accomplished during the winter months when the spread of the pathogen slows due to lower temperatures.

144. Coast live oaks are a characteristic oak species in

    (A) redwood forests.
    (B) Yosemite Valley.
    (C) Sierra Nevada.
    (D) scenic coastal woodlands.

Passage 2

Non-adherence to medication therapy results in numerous adverse effects such as increased hospitalizations and even death. Additionally, it costs the U.S. healthcare system billions of dollars each year. It is important to assess patients' adherence to medications.

Improper medication adherence encompasses an assortment of behaviors. These include not having a prescription filled, forgetting or intentionally not taking a medication, consuming an incorrect amount of a medication, taking a medication at the wrong time, ceasing therapy too soon, or continuing therapy after advised to discontinue. All forms of improper medication taking behavior may jeopardize health outcomes.

Measuring medication-taking behavior is often difficult. The ideal method of measurement should be simultaneously unobtrusive (to avoid patient sensitization and maximize cooperation), objective (to produce discrete and reproducible data for each subject), and practical (to maximize portability and minimize cost). Refill records, pill counts, electronic medication dispensers/caps, patient surveys (interviews), blood-drug level monitoring, and urine

assay for drug metabolites can be used as clues to identify improper medication use.

Before altering therapy based on the assumption that a patient is taking a medication as prescribed, practitioners should ascertain patient's medication taking behavior. This becomes especially important when modifying dosages of medications. Due to the advantages and disadvantages of each measurement, it is important for practitioners to use a combination of methods to assess a patient's medication usage behavior and relate these findings to the patient's clinical presentation.

145. The ideal method of medication adherence measurement should be

    (A) simultaneously functional, easy, and reliable.
    (B) simultaneously fun, personalized, and fancy-free.
    (C) simultaneously practical, objective, and unobtrusive.
    (D) simultaneously advantageous, creative, and unpretentious.

146. According to the passage, current techniques for assessing a patient's medication usage include

    (A) blood-drug level monitoring, pill counts, refill records, and half-life tables.
    (B) refill records, patient interviews, electronic medication dispensers, and nucleic acid levels.
    (C) pill counts, electronic medication dispensers, patient interviews, x-ray, and refill records.
    (D) blood-level drug monitoring, refill records, electronic medication dispensers, and urine assays for drug metabolites.

147. Improper medication adherence

   (A) encompasses taking a medication too soon, not taking enough of the drug, and forgetting to take the medication.
   (B) results in few adverse effects.
   (C) results in little cost to the U.S. health care system.
   (D) is easily measured.

148. Before altering therapy based on the assumption that the medication is being taken as prescribed, practitioners should

   (A) assess the patient's behavior concerning taking their medication.
   (B) check the patient's blood glucose levels and ask about their dietary intake.
   (C) discern the patient's refill rate and whether they were on schedule.
   (D) decide if the patient is in the maintenance phase of adherence.

149. The most appropriate title for the passage would be

   (A) Factors Impacting U.S. Health Care Costs
   (B) Interventions to Ameliorate Medication Nonadherence
   (C) Prevention of Medication Nonadherence
   (D) Defining and Measuring Medication Nonadherence

150. It is important to assess patients' adherence to medication because

   (A) if they are not adherent then their medication will not work.
   (B) it can result in adverse effects such as increased hospitalizations and perhaps death.
   (C) it costs the U.S. government trillions in lawsuits each year.
   (D) maintenance of adherence contributes to an increase in suicides.

Passage 3

As many as 50 million Americans have high blood pressure, defined as a systolic blood pressure ≥140 mm Hg and a diastolic blood pressure ≥90 mm Hg. Although blood pressure generally increases with age, the onset of hypertension most often occurs in the third, fourth, or fifth decade of life. The prevalence of hypertension in the elderly population (age ≥65 years) is approximately 63% in whites and 76% in blacks. In younger generations (35 to 45 years of age), the prevalence is markedly different with 44% among black men, 37% among black women, 26% among white men, and 17% among white women.

A specific cause of sustained hypertension cannot be found in the vast majority of individuals with high blood pressure. Genetic factors have been suggested to play a role in essential hypertension due to the fact that high blood pressure may be hereditary. Evidence that a single gene may account for specific subtypes of hypertension has also been suggested. Genetic traits include high angiotensin levels, increased aldosterone and other adrenal steroids, and high sodium-lithium countertransport. More direct approaches for preventing or treating hypertension could be achieved by identifying individuals with these traits. Factors such as sodium excretion and transport rates, blood pressure response to plasma volume expansion, electrolyte homeostasis, and glomerular filtration rate help explain the predisposition for a person to develop hypertension.

Anti-hypertensive drug therapy should be individualized according to various patient characteristics and fundamental pathophysiologic circumstances. Dietary intake has been shown to be similar in all races but blacks ingest less potassium and calcium than whites. Supplemental potassium and calcium has shown to cause a modest reduction in blood pressure in some studies. Therefore, it would seem reasonable to ascertain the affects of increasing the amount of potassium and calcium in the diet as part of the non-pharmacologic regulation of hypertension. The initial treatment for hypertension is lifestyle changes unless target-organ damage is present. These changes include sodium restriction, weight reduction, increased physical activity, and ethanol reduction or abstinence. In terms of target-organ damage, diuretics and beta-blockers are first-line therapy. Control of blood pressure and prevention of cardio-vascular morbidity and mortality are the goals of antihypertensive therapy. By maintaining arterial blood pressure below 140 mm Hg systolic and 90 mm Hg diastolic and by controlling other risk factors such as smoking, hyperlipidemia, and diabetes, morbidity and mortality may be averted.

151. The onset of hypertension most often occurs in which decades?

    (A) Third and fifth
    (B) Third, fourth, and fifth
    (C) Fourth, fifth, and sixth
    (D) Fifth, sixth, and seventh

152. Based on the information presented in the first paragraph, one may conclude

    (A) hypertension is a rarely diagnosed disease state.
    (B) hypertension is more prevalent among white individuals compared with their black counterparts in both the elderly and younger populations.
    (C) hypertension is more prevalent among black individuals compared with their white counterparts in both the elderly and younger populations.
    (D) hypertension rarely occurs prior to the sixth decade of life.

153. According to the passage, initial treatment for hypertension is lifestyle changes which include

    (A) smoking cessation, weight reduction, decreased physical activity, and ethanol restriction.
    (B) sodium restriction, weight reduction, increased physical activity, and ethanol reduction or abstinence.
    (C) ethanol reduction or abstinence, sodium restriction, reduced mental activity or stress, and gaining weight.
    (D) weight reduction, increase sodium intake, ethanol reduction, and increase stress.

154. Two of the factors that help provide an explanation of hypertensive development are centered around

    (A) diuretic usage and abstinence.
    (B) electrolyte homeostasis and sodium excretion.
    (C) increased calcium intake and proper medication adherence.
    (D) decreased medication therapy costs and decreased steroid usage.

155. Genetic factors have been suggested to play a role in essential hypertension based on the fact that

    (A) parents can get it from their children.
    (B) if ancestors have high angiotensin levels they have a higher rate of morbidity.
    (C) geneticists know which gene causes hypertension.
    (D) high blood pressure may be hereditary.

156. Anti-hypertensive therapy should be individualized according to

    (A) patient characteristics and fundamental pathophysiologic circumstances.
    (B) number of offspring and dietary habits stemming from care of those offspring.
    (C) features found in their family tree.
    (D) the climate of the state where the patient lives.

157. Morbidity and mortality associated with hypertension may be averted if an individual can maintain an arterial blood pressure of

    (A) 155 mm Hg systolic and 77 mm Hg diastolic.
    (B) 136 mm Hg systolic and 99 mm Hg diastolic.
    (C) 160 mm Hg systolic and 98 mm Hg diastolic.
    (D) 135 mm Hg systolic and 85 mm Hg diastolic.

158. How many Americans currently suffer from high blood pressure?

    (A) As many as 60 billion
    (B) As many as 50 billion
    (C) As many as 50 million
    (D) As many as 40 million

Passage 4

We humans sense old age through feeling those creaky joints or observing those graying hairs but, according to Apfeld and Kenyon reporting in a recent issue of Nature, the nematode worm senses its age by smelling and tasting the environment. These investigators show that worms with defective olfactory organs (that would normally detect odor molecules in the environment) live longer than their comrades with a keener sense of smell. By comparing these worms with other mutant nematodes that live an unusually long time, the researchers found clues to how a reduced ability to "smell the roses" might lengthen life-span.

The worm's olfactory sense organs—amphids on the head and plasmids on the tail—are composed of a cluster of nerve cells, the ends of which are modified into cilia. The cilia are encircled by a sheath and a socket cell that form a pore in the worm's skin through which the tips of the cilia protrude. Odor molecules and soluble compounds bind to G protein-coupled receptors (similar to the olfactory and taste receptors of mammals) located at the tip of each cilium. Worms with a poor sense of smell—because their olfactory organs have defective or absent cilia, blocked pores, or damaged sheaths—live much longer, yet are otherwise normal (for example, their feeding and reproductive behaviors are unchanged). Mutations in TAX-4—a channel regulated by cyclic GMP that sits under the G protein-coupled receptor and transduces the sensory signals into electrical impulses—also imbue the worm with a longer life.

But mutations in the worm's olfactory machinery are not the only defects that extend its life-span. In an earlier study, Kenyon's group found that defects in the reproductive system could prolong life by decreasing the activity of DAF-2 (a receptor for an insulin-like molecule) and increasing the activity of DAF-16 (a transcription factor). By looking at worms defective in both sensory perception and reproduction, Apfeld and Kenyon worked out a putative pathway through which smell might influence a worm's longevity.

An environmental signal, perhaps produced by bacteria (the worm's favorite food), binds to G protein-coupled olfactory receptors on sensory cilia activating TAX-4, which then incites electrical activity in the sensory neurons. This activity triggers secretory vesicles in the neurons to release insulin-like molecules, which bind to DAF-2 and activate the insulin-like signaling pathway. This then switches on genes that will ensure the worm dies at the usual age of 2 weeks. A reduced ability to sense olfactory cues would result in a decrease in DAF-2 activation and an increase in life-span.

This chain of events is not proven, but insulin-like molecules that might bind to DAF-2 have been identified in the nematode. Such a pathway would also make physiological sense. After all, if food is scarce it may behoove the worm to live longer to ensure that it has the chance to produce its full quota of off-spring. A scarcity of food also promotes longevity in rodents and primates. But so far it seems that in these more complicated creatures a poor sense of smell is not a harbinger of a ripe old age.

———————

From "Nota Bene: Sensing Old Age" by Orda Smith, Science, Vol 287, January 2000. Page 54. Reprinted with permission from AAAS.

159. A worm usually lives to the "old age" of

(A) 3 weeks.
(B) 5 weeks.
(C) 1 week.
(D) 2 weeks.

160. TAX-4 is

(A) a channel regulated by cyclic GMP which sits beneath the G protein-coupled receptor and transduces the sensory signals into electrical impulses.
(B) a cyclic regulated AMP which lies above the G protein-coupled receptor and transduces the neurological signals into electrical impulses.
(C) a liability which the nematode has to deal with four times the amount of cyclic GMP next to the G protein-coupled receptor.
(D) a receptor for an insulin-like molecule which activate the insulin-like pathway.

161. A nematode worm detects its age by

(A) a biological stopwatch which notes sunrise and sunset.
(B) burrowing through the soil at speeds up to 0.01 mph.
(C) whether it has had the chance to produce its full quota of offspring.
(D) smelling and tasting the environment.

162. The worm's olfactory sense organs are composed of

(A) a cluster of nervous tissue surrounded by a sheath which protects it.
(B) socket cells that are embedded in the head and tail of the worm.
(C) a cluster of nerve cells of which the ends are modified into cilia.
(D) their individual mouths and noses which are covered with cilia.

163. What other traits in the worm extend its lifespan?

(A) Defects in the circulatory system.
(B) Mutations in the excretory system.
(C) Alterations in the lymphatic system.
(D) Aberrations in the reproductive system.

164. DAF-2 is

(A) a receptor for an insulin-like molecule.
(B) a transcription factor.
(C) a transduction factor.
(D) a binding site for a glucose molecule.

165. A logical pathway by which smell might influence a worm's longevity was achieved by studying

(A) worms flawed in both circulatory and sensory perception.
(B) worms defective in both reproduction and sensory perception.
(C) worms deficient in only the reproductive system.
(D) worms impaired in the nervous and circulatory system.

166. Secretory vesicles in the neurons are stimulated by what to release insulin-like molecules?

(A) TAX-4 excites electrical activity.
(B) DAF-2 activates the insulin-like pathway.
(C) DAF-16 regulates the electrical activity.
(D) TAX-2 initiates the secretory vesicles.

167. A scarcity of food is known to promote longevity in

    (A) nematodes.
    (B) nematodes and rodents.
    (C) nonprimates and nematodes.
    (D) rodents and primates.

168. The reduced ability to sense olfactory cues results in

    (A) a decrease in life-span and an increase in DAF-2 activation.
    (B) a decrease in DAF-2 activation and an increase in lifespan.
    (C) a decrease in TAX-4 which incites electrical activity.
    (D) a decrease in DAF-16 which creates more gene activity.

Passage 5

Presidents of the United States are not like you and me. A personality assessment presented at the American Psychological Association conference in Washington, D.C., shows that, compared to the public they serve, presidents are more likely to be extroverted, assertive, and disagreeable. They're also less modest and straightforward.

"Says who? Historians who have written book-length biographies of Oval Office occupants. Psychologist Steve Rubenzer of the Mental Health and Mental Retardation Authority of Harris County in Houston, Texas, and colleagues asked the biographers to fill out three standard personality inventories on their subjects, basing answers on the presidents' behavior during the 5 years preceding their reigns. The researchers compared the presidents' scores to population norms and compared the profiles of successful commanders-in-chief with those history hasn't smiled upon.

"Great" presidents, such as Jefferson and Lincoln, they find, "are attentive to their emotions, willing to question traditional values ... imaginative, and more interested in art and beauty than less successful Chief Executives." They're also more assertive, stubborn, and "tender-minded," which is a measure of concern for the less fortunate. Rubenzer hasn't ana-

lyzed the current presidential contenders yet—he prefers to have at least three "unbiased" historians fill out the forms for each president or presidential wanna-be.

From "Presidential Personalities," Science, Vol 289, August 2000. Page 859. Reprinted with permission from AAAS.

169. This personality assessment was presented at a conference of which group?

    (A) The American Pharmacists Association
    (B) The Annual Physicians Association
    (C) The American Psychological Association
    (D) The Association of Practicing Psychiatrists

170. This data was collected from

    (A) historians.
    (B) presidents.
    (C) psychologists.
    (D) historiographers.

171. Steve Rubenzer and his team of researchers

    (A) are historians who write biographies.
    (B) are from Houston, Texas.
    (C) are from Washington, D.C.
    (D) work in the Oval Office.

172. The standard personality inventories that were completed by the biographers were based on

    (A) the comparisons of current presidential contenders.
    (B) the presidents' behaviors during the five years after their term of office.
    (C) biased population norms.
    (D) the presidents' behaviors during the five years before their term of office.

173. According to the passage, "great" presidents include those such as

    (A) Kennedy and Roosevelt.
    (B) Jefferson and Lincoln.
    (C) Bush and Wilson.
    (D) Adams and Carter.

174. In this article, use of the word *tender-minded* meant

    (A) less stubborn.
    (B) more concerned for the less-fortunate.
    (C) more apathetic toward the environment.
    (D) less concerned for the more-fortunate.

175. According to Rubenzer, how many historians should fill out the forms for each presidential contender or presidential wanna-be?

    (A) Three
    (B) Two
    (C) As many as possible, as long as they are biased.
    (D) One

176. Presidents are more likely to be

    (A) disagreeable, extroverted, and assertive.
    (B) agreeable, apathetic, and introverted.
    (C) unwilling to question traditional values.
    (D) less interested in art and beauty.

Passage 6

Drug interactions, a common type of drug-related problem, are categorized as pharmacokinetic, pharmacodynamic, or a combination of both. Pharmacokinetic drug interactions include changes in absorption, distribution, excretion, and metabolism; whereas, pharmacodynamic drug interactions may lead to antagonist or synergistic effects. Not all drug interactions are undesirable; in fact, many drug interactions are used to produce desirable effects. Patients who take drugs with narrow therapeutic indices and drugs that interfere with the pharmacokinetic properties of other drugs are at increased risk of experiencing a drug interaction. Also, patients who take multiple medications per day or take multiple doses of medications per day are at increased risk. Because renal transplant patients take immunosuppressive agents that have narrow therapeutic indices and are subjected to multiple medications per day, they are vulnerable to experiencing adverse drug events. To prevent adverse drug interactions, an alternative therapy should be considered when possible or the dose or schedule of the drugs should be adjusted to reduce the occurrence of an adverse experience. Additionally, adequate monitoring to prevent and detect adverse effects is an essential part of patient care.

A common pharmacokinetic interaction involves drugs that interfere with the absorption of other medications. Drugs that bind and decrease the gastrointestinal absorption of another drug, such as cholestyramine decreasing the absorption of tacrolimus, typically can be prevented by administering the agents two to three hours apart from each other. Prokinetic agents interfere with the rate of absorption. Since many transplant patients take prokinetic agents, such as metochlopromide, this may increase the bioavailability of other medications. This is of significant importance since immunosuppressive agents have narrow therapeutic indices and toxicity may result from this interaction. If the prokinetic agent cannot be avoided, careful monitoring (e.g., serum drug levels, clinical presentation of patient) and adjustments should be made to prevent immunosuppressant toxicity.

177. The passage indicates that prokinetic agents

    (A) interfere with the rate of metabolism.
    (B) affect all interactions in the gastrointestinal tract.
    (C) interfere with the rate of absorption.
    (D) should be monitored and adjusted.

178. Drug interactions are characterized as

    (A) pharmacokinetic only.
    (B) pharmacokinetic, pharmacodynamic, or a combination of both.
    (C) pharmacodynamic only.
    (D) pharmacosynthetic only.

179. Toxicity can result from a prokinetic agent being administered with an immunosuppressive agent because

    (A) cholestyramine has a narrow therapeutic index.
    (B) patients have to take immunosuppressive agents multiple times per day.
    (C) the prokinetic agent may increase the bioavailability of the immunosuppressive agent.
    (D) all drug interactions are undesirable.

180. Pharmacokinetic drug interactions include

    (A) changes in allocation, circulation, and dispersion.
    (B) changes in absorption, distribution, excretion, and metabolism.
    (C) reactions which affect composition of other medications.
    (D) cumulative and additive effects.

181. Patients that are at increased risk of experiencing a drug interaction include

    (A) patients who take multiple medications per day or multiple doses of medications per day.
    (B) patients who take drugs with wide therapeutic indices.
    (C) patients who take drugs that do not interfere with the pharmacokinetic properties of other drugs.
    (D) patients who are taking medications for a brief time period.

182. In this passage, an example of a drug that binds and decreases the gastrointestinal absorption of another drug is

    (A) tacrolimus.
    (B) metochlopromide.
    (C) sirolimus.
    (D) cholestyramine.

183. To prevent adverse drug reactions

    (A) consult neighbors regularly.
    (B) consider an alternate therapy or alter the dose or schedule of the drugs.
    (C) time medication regimens with meals.
    (D) increase water intake.

184. If the prokinetic agent cannot be avoided, to prevent immunosuppressant toxicity

    (A) carefully arrange the patient's medication consumption schedule.
    (B) monitor compliance to see if the prokinetic factor is really necessary.
    (C) monitor serum levels and the clinical presentation of the patient and make appropriate adjustments.
    (D) do not educate the patient on the types of adverse drug reactions which may occur.

STOP

End of Reading Comprehension section. If you have any time left, you may go over your work in this section only.

Practice Test 2

QUANTITATIVE ABILITY

48 QUESTIONS (#185–#232)

TIME: 45 MINUTES

Directions: Choose the **best** answer to each of the following questions.

185. Evaluate the integral $\int_{2}^{3}(10x^4)\,dx$.

    (A) 550
    (B) 760
    (C) 650
    (D) 422

186. What is the median value for the sequence {8, 24, 3, 9, 11, 16, 42, 5, 6}?

    (A) 22
    (B) 18
    (C) 9
    (D) 21

187. Eighty-six degrees Fahrenheit =

    (A) 30 degrees Celsius
    (B) 15 degrees Celsius
    (C) 20 degrees Celsius
    (D) 30 degrees Celsius

188. Given that $\ln(a) = 12$ and $\ln(b) = 3$,

    $\ln\left(\dfrac{a}{b}\right) =$

    (A) 9
    (B) 4
    (C) $\ln(9)$
    (D) $\ln(4)$

189. One tablespoonful contains 15 mL of volume. If a patient takes one tablespoonful three times a day, how many days supply will be provided by a 12 ounce bottle? (One ounce = 30 mL)

    (A) 6
    (B) 8
    (C) 12
    (D) 16

190. What is the mean value for the sequence {4, 5, 11, 18, 20, 22, 34, 35, 38}?

    (A) 20.77
    (B) 25.77
    (C) 30.77
    (D) 35.77

191. Given the function $f(x) = \dfrac{x^3}{4+x}$,

    compute $\dfrac{dy}{dx}$.

    (A) $\dfrac{12x - 2x^3}{(4+x)^2}$

    (B) $\dfrac{12x^2 + 2x^3}{(4+x)^2}$

    (C) $\dfrac{2x^3 - 12x^2}{(4+x)^2}$

    (D) $\dfrac{-2x^3 - 12x^2}{(4+x)^2}$

192. If a square plot of land 210 feet on one side contains one acre, approximately how many square feet are in the one acre of land?

    (A) 44,100
    (B) 28,400
    (C) 2,860
    (D) 840

193. Given the function, $f(x) = \dfrac{x}{x^2 + 3}$

    compute $\dfrac{dy}{dx}$.

    (A) $\dfrac{3x^2 + 3}{(x^2 + 3)^2}$

    (B) $\dfrac{3 - x^2}{(x^2 + 3)^2}$

    (C) $\dfrac{3 + x^2}{(x^2 + 3)^2}$

    (D) $\dfrac{1}{2x}$

194. $10^2 + 9^2 =$

    (A) 90^4
    (B) 19^4
    (C) 1.81×10^2
    (D) 1^4

195. Determine the length of the line segment with endpoints (6, 8) and (−2, 5).

    (A) $\sqrt{55}$

    (B) $\sqrt{185}$

    (C) $\sqrt{73}$

    (D) $\sqrt{153}$

196. John has $6.60 in quarters and dimes. He has twice as many quarters as dimes. How many quarters does he have?

    (A) 11
    (B) 20
    (C) 18
    (D) 22

197. Simplify the expression $\dfrac{1}{x} + \dfrac{1}{y}$.

    (A) $\dfrac{2}{xy}$

    (B) $\dfrac{y + x}{xy}$

    (C) $\dfrac{2}{x + y}$

    (D) $\dfrac{x}{y}$

198. Given the function $f(x) = 3x - 1$, determine the formula for $f^{-1}(x)$.

    (A) $f^{-1}(x) = \dfrac{1}{3x - 1}$

    (B) $f^{-1}(x) = \dfrac{x + 1}{3}$

    (C) $f^{-1}(x) = \dfrac{x - 1}{3}$

    (D) $f^{-1}(x) = \dfrac{1}{3x + 1}$

For problems 199–201, consider the given graph of the function $y = f(x)$.

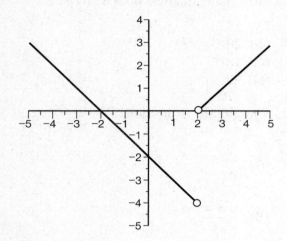

199. $\displaystyle\lim_{x \to 2^+} f(x) =$

(A) 0 and –4
(B) Does not exist
(C) 0 or –4
(D) 0

200. $\displaystyle\lim_{x \to 2^-} f(x) =$

(A) –4
(B) Does not exist
(C) 0 or –4
(D) 0 and –4

201. $\displaystyle\lim_{x \to 2} f(x) =$

(A) –4
(B) Does not exist
(C) 0
(D) 0 and –4

202. $\log(mn) =$

(A) $\log(m) - \log(n)$
(B) $\log(m) + \log(n)$

(C) $\log\left(\dfrac{m}{n}\right)$

(D) $\dfrac{\log(m)}{\log(n)}$

203. A truck travels at a steady speed of 100 kilometers per hour from 12 noon until 6 P.M. How many miles will be driven?

(A) 968
(B) 600
(C) 372
(D) 106

204. Thirty-two percent of 800 equals

(A) 256
(B) 266
(C) 246
(D) 236

205. $\displaystyle\int_{e}^{e^2}\left(\dfrac{6}{x}\right) dx =$

(A) 6

(B) $\dfrac{6}{e^2} - \dfrac{6}{e}$

(C) 18

(D) $\dfrac{6}{e^2} + \dfrac{6}{e}$

206. Determine the derivative for the function $f(x) = e^{2x} \cdot \sin(x)$.

    (A) $2e^{2x} \cdot \sin(x) - e^{2x} \cdot \cos(x)$
    (B) $2e^{2x} \cdot \sin(x) + e^{2x} \cdot \cos(x)$
    (C) $e^{2x} \cdot \sin(x) + e^{2x} \cdot \cos(x)$
    (D) $e^{2x} \cdot \sin(x) - e^{2x} \cdot \cos(x)$

207. $\lim\limits_{x \to \infty} \left(\dfrac{8x^6 + 4x^2 - 10x + 5}{7x^6 + 12x^3} \right) =$

    (A) ∞
    (B) Undefined
    (C) 1
    (D) $\dfrac{8}{7}$

208. A man is tossing a coin. The first three tosses have been heads. What are the chances that heads will occur on the fourth toss?

    (A) 50%
    (B) 25%
    (C) 12.5%
    (D) 6.25%

209. The height h of a projectile is given by $h(x) = -0.006x^2 + 12x$, where x is the horizontal distance the projectile travels. The projectile hits the ground after it has traveled a horizontal distance of

    (A) 100 feet
    (B) 1,000 feet
    (C) 200 feet
    (D) 2,000 feet

210. A store reduces the selling price of an item by 30%. The new price is $210. What was the original price?

    (A) $320
    (B) $240
    (C) $300
    (D) $280

211. Event A has a probability of $\dfrac{5}{9}$. What is the probability that event A does NOT occur?

    (A) $\dfrac{4}{9}$

    (B) $-\dfrac{5}{9}$

    (C) $\dfrac{9}{5}$

    (D) Not enough information

212. Calculate the value of x in the expression $4x = \dfrac{1}{2}$.

    (A) $\dfrac{1}{42}$

    (B) $\dfrac{1}{24}$

    (C) $\dfrac{1}{16}$

    (D) $\dfrac{1}{8}$

For questions 213 and 214, consider the data shown in the table below.

Drug Prescribed	# of patients
Drug A	730
Drug B	185
Drug C	90
Drug D	466
Other	29

213. What percentage of patients received prescriptions for Drug A or Drug B?

    (A) 40%
    (B) 65%
    (C) 60%
    (D) 75%

214. What percentage of patients did NOT receive a prescription for Drug D?

    (A) 69%
    (B) 31%
    (C) 47%
    (D) 53%

215. Digoxin injection is supplied in ampules of 500 micrograms per 2 mL. What quantity must a nurse administer to provide a dose of 0.25 milligrams?

    (A) 0.2 mL
    (B) 0.5 mL
    (C) 1.0 mL
    (D) 2.0 ml

216. Determine the slope of the line passing through the points (10, 3) and (4, –6).

    (A) $\dfrac{3}{2}$

    (B) $-\dfrac{3}{2}$

    (C) $\dfrac{2}{3}$

    (D) $-\dfrac{2}{3}$

For question 217, consider the given graph of the function $y = f(x)$.

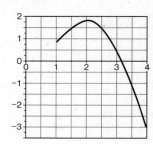

217. Identify the graph of the function $y = f(x - 3)$.

    (A)

    (B)

    (C)

    (D)

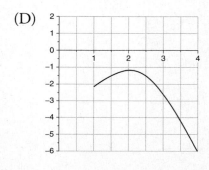

218. A patient's creatine clearance rate (CrCl) can be calculated by using the following formula:

$$CrCl = \frac{140 - \text{age in years}}{72 \cdot SCr} \cdot \text{(ideal body weight in kilograms)}$$

What is the CrCl for a 58-year-old patient who has a SCr of 2.6 and an ideal body weight of 76 kg?

(A) 23
(B) 33
(C) 30
(D) 37

219. If the range of the function f is given by $(10,\infty)$, determine the domain for f^{-1}.

(A) $(10,\infty)$
(B) $(-\infty,10)$
(C) $\left(\frac{1}{10},\infty\right)$
(D) $\left(-\infty,\frac{1}{10}\right)$

For questions 220–223, consider the given graph of the function $y = f(x)$.

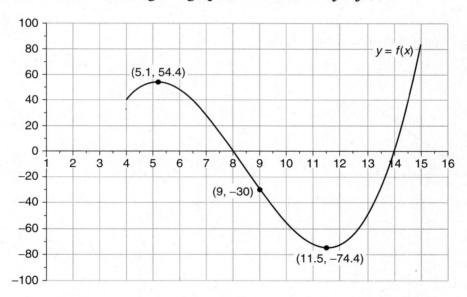

220. Choose the interval for which $f'(x) > 0$.

(A) $x > 11.5$
(B) $4 < x < 8$
(C) $x > -74.4$
(D) $0 < x < 40$

221. Identify the x-value(s) for which $f''(x) < 0$.

(A) $9 > x > \infty$
(B) $-\infty < x < 9$
(C) $9 < x < \infty$
(D) $-\infty > x > 9$

222. Identify the relative maxima (if any) for f.

(A) $(5.1, 54.4)$
(B) $(9, -30)$
(C) None
(D) $(11.5, -74.4)$

223. $\lim\limits_{x \to 8}\left(\dfrac{f(x) - f(8)}{x - 8}\right) =$

(A) 0
(B) A positive number
(C) A negative number
(D) Not enough information

224. Determine the average rate of change of the function $f(x) = x^3$ on the interval $2 \le x \le 4$.

    (A) 28
    (B) 56
    (C) 36
    (D) 38

225. What is the value of $\sqrt{45} + \sqrt{80}$?

    (A) $4\sqrt{125}$

    (B) $5\sqrt{35}$

    (C) $4\sqrt{9}$

    (D) $7\sqrt{5}$

226. What is the slope of the line shown in the graph below?

    (A) 1
    (B) 2
    (C) 4
    (D) 10

227. What is the median of the following values:
    10, 12, 9, 10, 11, 9, 9, 10, 8, 12?

    (A) 2
    (B) 9.5
    (C) 10
    (D) 12

228. How many three-letter codes can be formed from the set $\{A, B, C, D, E,\}$? Repeated letters are allowed.

    (A) 60
    (B) 120
    (C) 80
    (D) 125

229. Determine the x-coordinate of the points, if any, where the graph of $f(x) = \dfrac{x}{x+2}$ has a horizontal tangent line.

    (A) When $x = -2$
    (B) When $x = 0$
    (C) When $x = 2$
    (D) Never

230. Identify the graph that demonstrates an exponential relationship between the variables x and y.

    (A)

    (B)

    (C)

    (D)

231. Event *A* has a probability of 0.35. Event *B* has a probability of 0.22. The probability that events *A* and *B* both occur is 0.09. What is the probability that either event *A* or event *B* occurs?

   (A) 0.57
   (B) 0.52
   (C) 0.48
   (D) 0.66

232. Find the exact value of the shaded area bounded above by the graph of $f(x) = \dfrac{3}{x}$ and below by the *x*-axis from $x = 1$ to $x = \sqrt{e}$.

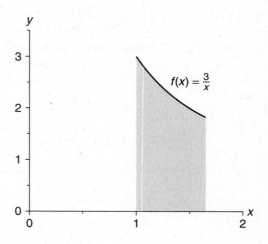

   (A) $\ln(1.5)$
   (B) $\dfrac{2}{3}$
   (C) 1.5
   (D) $\ln\left(\dfrac{2}{3}\right)$

STOP

End of Quantitative Ability section. If you have any time left, you may go over your work in this section only.

ESSAY

TIME: 30 MINUTES

Directions: Write a well-constructed essay addressing the statement below.

In recent years, the U.S. Congress has had difficulty reaching a consensus regarding legislation to address the issue of illegal immigration and the more than 11 million illegal immigrants residing in the United States. Discuss a solution to the problem of illegal immigration in the United States.

_____

_____

_____

_____

_____

_____

_____

_____

_____

_____

_____

_____

_____

_____

_____

_____

_____

_____

_____

Answer Key
PRACTICE TEST 2

VERBAL ABILITY

1. **D**	11. **B**	21. **D**	31. **C**
2. **B**	12. **A**	22. **A**	32. **C**
3. **A**	13. **A**	23. **C**	33. **A**
4. **B**	14. **D**	24. **D**	34. **B**
5. **D**	15. **B**	25. **B**	35. **C**
6. **A**	16. **C**	26. **C**	36. **D**
7. **C**	17. **A**	27. **B**	37. **B**
8. **D**	18. **B**	28. **A**	38. **C**
9. **B**	19. **D**	29. **D**	39. **D**
10. **D**	20. **A**	30. **A**	40. **C**

CHEMISTRY

41. **D**	53. **D**	65. **C**	77. **C**
42. **B**	54. **B**	66. **A**	78. **B**
43. **A**	55. **B**	67. **C**	79. **B**
44. **A**	56. **B**	68. **D**	80. **C**
45. **B**	57. **D**	69. **C**	81. **B**
46. **A**	58. **A**	70. **C**	82. **D**
47. **C**	59. **B**	71. **C**	83. **A**
48. **B**	60. **C**	72. **A**	84. **D**
49. **C**	61. **D**	73. **B**	85. **B**
50. **D**	62. **D**	74. **B**	86. **A**
51. **C**	63. **A**	75. **B**	87. **A**
52. **B**	64. **B**	76. **A**	88. **A**

BIOLOGY

89. **A**	101. **A**	113. **D**	125. **B**
90. **A**	102. **C**	114. **A**	126. **A**
91. **D**	103. **D**	115. **B**	127. **A**
92. **B**	104. **B**	116. **A**	128. **B**
93. **B**	105. **B**	117. **C**	129. **C**
94. **B**	106. **D**	118. **A**	130. **D**
95. **A**	107. **C**	119. **B**	131. **D**
96. **D**	108. **A**	120. **D**	132. **B**
97. **D**	109. **B**	121. **B**	133. **A**
98. **B**	110. **C**	122. **A**	134. **B**
99. **D**	111. **C**	123. **D**	135. **D**
100. **C**	112. **B**	124. **C**	136. **C**

Answer Key
PRACTICE TEST 2

READING COMPREHENSION

137. **B**	149. **D**	161. **D**	173. **B**
138. **A**	150. **B**	162. **C**	174. **B**
139. **C**	151. **B**	163. **D**	175. **A**
140. **A**	152. **C**	164. **A**	176. **A**
141. **B**	153. **B**	165. **B**	177. **C**
142. **A**	154. **B**	166. **A**	178. **B**
143. **B**	155. **D**	167. **D**	179. **C**
144. **D**	156. **A**	168. **B**	180. **B**
145. **C**	157. **D**	169. **C**	181. **A**
146. **D**	158. **C**	170. **A**	182. **D**
147. **A**	159. **D**	171. **B**	183. **B**
148. **A**	160. **A**	172. **D**	184. **C**

QUANTITATIVE ABILITY

185. **D**	197. **B**	209. **D**	221. **B**
186. **C**	198. **B**	210. **C**	222. **A**
187. **A**	199. **D**	211. **A**	223. **C**
188. **A**	200. **A**	212. **D**	224. **A**
189. **B**	201. **B**	213. **C**	225. **D**
190. **A**	202. **B**	214. **A**	226. **A**
191. **B**	203. **C**	215. **C**	227. **C**
192. **A**	204. **A**	216. **A**	228. **D**
193. **B**	205. **A**	217. **B**	229. **D**
194. **C**	206. **B**	218. **B**	230. **D**
195. **C**	207. **D**	219. **A**	231. **C**
196. **D**	208. **A**	220. **A**	232. **C**

EXPLANATORY ANSWERS

1. **(D)** In this worker-to-tool analogy, the gardener uses a trowel just as the mechanic uses a wrench. (If you chose A, you may have mistaken this for an analogy of association, but you need to select the name of a specific tool instead.)

2. **(B)** This is an analogy of characteristics or description. A *charlatan* is considered a *fake* or a fraud, just as a *patriot* is considered *loyal* to his or her country.

3. **(A)** This is an analogy of characteristics or description. An oracle by definition has foresight and a sage has wisdom.

4. **(B)** This is an analogy of "used to" or "serves to" relationship. A zipper is used to fasten and an escalator is used to lift.

5. **(D)** This is an analogy of a "lack of" or "without" relationship where one word means lack of or without the other. Shallow is lack of depth and apathetic is lack of caring.

6. **(A)** This is an analogy of characteristic or description in which the blueprint is the plan of the building and the outline is the plan of a report.

7. **(C)** This is an analogy of characteristic or description. An antiseptic helps to eliminate germs, water helps to eliminate thirst.

8. **(D)** This is an analogy of a "lack of" or "without" relationship. Sluggish means lack of energy and satiated means lack of hunger.

9. **(B)** This is an analogy of a "lack of" or "without" relationship. A neophyte is without experience and an invalid is not healthy.

10. **(D)** This is an analogy of characteristic or description. A bus carries passengers and a freighter carries cargo.

11. **(B)** This is an analogy of synonyms. *Arcane* and *esoteric* are both defined as mysterious. Likewise, *irascible* and *fractious* are both defined as grouchy.

12. **(A)** This is an analogy of characteristic or description. An embargo prevents trade and a helmet prevents injury.

13. **(A)** This is an analogy of synonyms. *Redolent* and *aromatic* are both defined as having a pleasing fragrance, as *sequester* and *cloister* are both defined as being in seclusion. Regarding the incorrect answer choices, *sedition* refers to behavior that prompts rebellion, *curative* refers to a remedy that cures an illness, and *satirical* refers to expressing ridicule through satire.

14. **(D)** This is an analogy of "used to" or "serves to" relationship. A meter is used to measure length and a pound is used to measure weight.

15. **(B)** This is a part-to-whole analogy. An anaconda is a type of snake and basketball is a type of sport. To help clarify this kind of analogy, think of the group of all snakes and the group of all sports as "wholes," of which the anaconda and basketball are merely parts.

16. **(C)** This is an analogy of characteristics or description. A bruise is a mark on the skin and a stain is a mark on fabric.

17. **(A)** This is an analogy of purpose or use. A sphygmomanometer is used to measure blood pressure, and a thermometer is used to measure temperature.

18. **(B)** This is an analogy of association. The Oedipus complex is associated with Freud, and the uncertainty principle is associated with the physicist Heisenberg.

19. **(D)** In this part-to-whole analogy, the Hindenberg is an example of a blimp, and the Lusitania is an example of an ocean liner. (The fact that both met tragic fates is not relevant here.)

20. **(A)** This is an analogy of classification. Virology is the study of viruses, and kinesiology is the study of human movement (A). Ontology is the study of the nature of existence (answer B), epidemiology is the study of the nature of knowledge (answer C), and ethology is the study of animal behavior (answer D).

21. **(D)** The word anthropomorphic means having a human shape or human characteristics; theriomorphic means having an animal shape or animal characteristics. This analogy is based on the definitions of words.

22. **(A)** This is an analogy of antonyms. Quell is defined as defeat, while succeed is defined as achieving a favorable outcome, and succinct is defined as brief, while prolix (answer A) is defined as being wordy. Answers B, C, and D are not applicable to the analogy as proscribe (answer B) means condemn, profligate (answer C) means corrupt, and prodigal (answer D) means wasteful.

23. **(C)** In this analogy of part to whole, the nuclear membrane is part of a cell, and the hypotenuse is part of a triangle.

24. **(D)** Since bass and treble represent opposite ends of a portion of the spectrum of sound, this can be considered either an analogy of antonyms or an analogy of degree. Acme and nadir also represent opposites.

25. **(B)** This analogy may be considered one of antonyms or of degree, since the pairs of terms (imperceptible and tangible, mild and severe) represent opposite extremes.

26. **(C)** The use of unyielding suggests the senator was behaving in a stubborn manner. "Refractory" is defined as stubborn. Likewise, her refusal to end her filibuster suggests she has strong or forceful beliefs regarding the proposal. "Vehemently" is a synonym for forceful. Answer A would not be appropriate as "sallow" refers to a pale or unhealthy appearance and "ruefully" is a synonym of regretful. The first word in answer B, "penitent," also suggests regret or remorse, while the second word suggests being depressed or downcast. Answer D is incorrect as "pacifistic" means peaceful (which the senator certainly was not) and "irreverent" means facetious or impertinent.

27. **(B)** The sentence suggests the scholar possesses a great deal of knowledge on several subjects. As such, the best fit for the blank would be "polymath," a person of great and varied learning. "Puritan" (a person who practices a strict

moral code), "sycophant" (a person who is a flatterer), and "supplicant" (a person who asks for something humbly) are incorrect.

28. **(A)** "Planning ahead" is the key phrase that connects the correct word for the first blank and the type of events that may occur and spoil a camping trip (the correct word for the second blank). Generally speaking, a camping trip can be characterized as an informal, improvised event. Planning ahead is typically done to try to avoid or bypass some of the unpredictable events that may happen. Thus, based on the answer choices provided, Answer A is the correct choice for this sentence completion.

29. **(D)** The sentence suggests the visitors to the beach experienced the opposite of very strong ("hurricane-like") winds. Thus, "zephyrs," which refer to gentle breezes, would be the best choice. The other answers all refer to strong or violent winds or storms.

30. **(A)** An example of the correct word for the first blank in this sentence completion is Greek mythology, which is somehow related to the concept or theory of the existence of multiple gods or holy beings (religion). Since the prefix "poly" means "many" or "much," we can conclude that the word for the first blank will describe something that is founded or based (synonymous with the correct word for the second blank) on the idea of numerous gods. Based on the answer choices listed and by reading each of the choices into both blanks in the sentence, Answer A is the best match and makes the most sense, given the sentence's context.

31. **(C)** The correct word for the first blank in this sentence will further describe the type of existence where the tree and fungi live together or cohabitate; however, we must also look closely at the two parts that make up this sentence. The first part of this sentence tells us that not all fungi are detrimental to trees, that is, harmful, hurtful, or damaging. The second part provides an alternative or counter-example to what has been stated in the first part. Thus, the correct word for the second blank will contradict what was said previously, meaning "advantageous" or "helpful." Answer C is the correct response for both blanks in this sentence completion. "Symbiotic" is made up of the words "sym" (meaning "together") and "bio" (meaning "life" or "living"), and "benefit" is synonymous with "good contributions" and "valuable."

32. **(C)** The use of "unsure" in the sentence suggests the couple were indecisive about their honeymoon destination. "Vacillated" is defined as showing indecision. The other answer choices make no sense in the sentence as "vaunted" means boasted about, "reneged" means to go back on, and "reposed" means relaxation.

33. **(A)** In this sentence the listener has made some action associated with a question directed toward the presentation's speaker. Since the listener is described as both puzzled and impatient, we can assume that the listener could not wait to ask his or her question, and therefore interrupted the speaker in order to do so. Typically, questions are solicited and answered by

a speaker when their presentation has finished or been completed. Thus, Answer A (interjected and conclude) is the correct answer.

34. **(B)** In this sentence, the correct word will relate to an action regarding the message where it does not have to be "exactly as it was spoken." Since the express purpose of taking a message is so that it can be given, meaning "relayed" or "disclosed to a designated recipient," we can assume that the correct word for the first blank will also have the same meaning. Continuing on in the sentence, there are additional instructions that may be done for this message (the second blank's correct word): "in your own words." If a verbal communication is not worded "exactly as spoken," then it is typically said to be "rephrased" or "reworded." Based on this, to "disclose" the message means to "communicate" it, and if the message was not exactly as spoken, then it was "paraphrased," and Answer B is the correct answer for this sentence.

35. **(C)** By reading each of the answer choices into this sentence, Answer C makes the most sense, given the sentence's context. "Impromptu" remarks are ones that are improvised or unrehearsed. The unexpected and spontaneous nature of the facilitator's request most likely caught this woman off guard and unready, which best matches the word "unprepared" given in this answer choice. Answer C is the best response to complete both blanks in this sentence.

36. **(D)** The villagers believed themselves safe from the raiders while they remained inside the fortress. They therefore believed the raiders could not find a way into the fortress. The best fit for the blank is that the fortress was "impregnable," or able to resist attack. The other answer choices make no sense in the sentence as "inimical" means hostile, "implacable" means inflexible, and "ignominious" means dishonorable.

37. **(B)** The correct word for the first blank will describe a negative attitude characterized by contempt, disdain, and superiority. This is further compounded by the thought of the volunteers as "inferior," meaning "underneath" or "lowly" (indicated by the correct response for the second blank). Looking closer at the word parts in the answers listed can provide additional clues that lead to the correct responses. The word prefix "con" means "against" or "opposing." To "condescend" means to be "against lowering oneself," and in this sentence's context, it means to have a high or elevated attitude. The prefix "sub" means "below" or "lesser." The word "substandard" means "of a lesser quality" or to be "below acceptable levels." Based on this, the best matches for both of the sentence blanks are found in Answer B—condescending and substandard.

38. **(C)** In this sentence, information that should not be included in the report will be synonymous with "irrelevant" (meaning "nonessential" or "without bearing or importance"). Generally speaking, you would NOT include information that is unimportant or not pertinent if you want to make the report as short and concise as possible, instead of long and verbose. Accordingly,

Answer C—extraneous and succinct—provides the best answer choices for both blanks in this sentence.

39. **(D)** The correct word that will complete the first blank in this sentence will describe one of the obvious, distinct, or prominent aspects of a charismatic and vivacious presentation. Furthermore, there is something so appealing about the man's presentation ability that he was able to engage or stimulate the interest of apathetic and lethargic children (indicated by the word that will complete the second blank). This presenter brought about a significant change in the children's demeanor to the point where they wanted to fully participate. Based on these conclusions, Answer D (salient and captivate) provides the best match for both blanks in this sentence.

40. **(C)** In this sentence, the completion of the initial class is characterized as "imperative"—vital, crucial, or non-negotiable. Oftentimes, an initial or pre-liminary class can provide such fundamental and essential information that it is deemed to be required. Furthermore, classes such as these must be completed in order to move on, progress, or proceed to any subsequent classes. Based on this, Answer C (mandatory and advance) provides the best match for both blanks in this sentence.

41. **(D)** Of the major classes of biomolecules, the lipids are characterized by their hydrophobicity (or lipophilicity) due to their structural nonpolarity. The other biomolecular classes (proteins, carbohydrates, and nucleic acids) have more polar features (like carbon-oxygen bonds, carbon-nitrogen bonds, oxygen-hyrogen bonds, and nitrogen-hydrogen bonds) and are therefore more hydrophilic (lipophobic).

42. **(B)** Nucleotides are composed of a purine or pyrimidine (a heterocyclic arene: the purines are guanine and adenine; the pyrimidines are uracil, thymine, and cytosine), a ribose/deoxyribose and at least one phosphate group. They are polymerized to make the nucleic acids (DNA and RNA). Their polymerization is called replication (for DNA) and transcription (for RNA).

43. **(A)** In the symbol for the lithium ion, $_3^7\text{Li}^{+1}$, the bottom number, 3, is the number of protons. One could obtain the number of neutrons, 4, by subtracting the number of protons, 3, from the number of protons plus neutrons, 7.

44. **(A)** When a solute is dissolved in a solvent some of the physical properties of the solvent are affected—the boiling point, the freezing point, and the osmotic pressure. The impact on these properties is a function of the number of solute particles dissolved and not the specific identity of the particles themselves and are called colligative properties. Dissolved solutes raise the boiling point, lower the freezing point, and raise the osmotic pressure. The conduction of electricity by a solution is dependent on the presence of ions in solutions. If a given solute dissolves in the solvent resulting in the presence of ions, then the solution will conduct electricity and the solute is said to be an electrolyte.

45. **(B)** In translation or protein synthesis, the nucleotide sequence (or base sequence) in a messenger RNA (mRNA) determines the order of amino acids in the resulting protein. Each of the three nucleotides or bases is called a codon and each codon "codes" for the incorporation of a specific amino acid in the growing protein. The term *anticodon* refers to the corresponding nucleotide sequence in the tRNA that carries the particular amino acid to the ribosome where protein synthesis occurs.

46. **(A)** This molecule has two chiral centers. The one with the chlorine has chlorine as priority 1, the side of the ring closest to the methyl as priority 2, the other side of the ring as priority 3, and the hydrogen as priority 4. Positioning the hydrogen away from you gives 1, 2, 3 as counterclockwise and thus S at that chiral center. The other chiral center has priority 1 as the side of the ring closest to the chlorine, priority 2 as the other side of the ring, priority 3 as the methyl group, and priority 4 as the hydrogen. Again, positioning the hydrogen away from you (which it already is in the structure given), the other three are arranged as 1, 2, 3 in a counterclockwise manner and thus also S.

47. **(C)** When $KMnO_4$ is reacted with any alkyl benzene having at least one benzylic hydrogen (the benzylic position is the carbon adjacent to the ring), benzoic acid results.

48. **(B)** Moles may be defined as grams/molar mass.

$$\text{Moles} = \frac{\text{Grams}}{\text{Molar Mass}}$$

The molar mass of carbon dioxide, CO_2, is

$$1\ C = 1(12) = 12$$

$$2\ O = 2(16) = 32$$

$$12 + 32 = 44\ \frac{\text{grams}}{\text{mole}}$$

Dividing 22 grams by $44\ \frac{\text{grams}}{\text{mole}}$ gives 0.50 mole.

49. **(C)** Percentage yield is defined as $100 \times \dfrac{\text{actual yield}}{\text{theoretical yield}}$.

Theoretical yield is the number of grams calculated as being possible to produce in a reaction. Actual yield is the number of grams actually isolated in a reaction.

$$H_2 + Cl_2 \rightarrow 2\ HCl$$

From the balanced equation above it can be seen that 1 mole of hydrogen reacts with 1 mole of chlorine to produce 2 moles of hydrogen chloride. In the problem, grams of hydrogen are given and they react with excess chlorine. Therefore, hydrogen is the limiting reagent and is used to calculate the theoretical yield. Theoretical yield may be calculated as follows:

$$\text{grams } H_2 \rightarrow \text{moles } H_2 \rightarrow \text{moles } Cl_2 \rightarrow \text{grams HCl}$$

Refer to explanation to question 48 for definition of moles.

Grams H_2

1.0

Moles H_2

$$\frac{1.0 \text{ gram}}{2 \text{ grams per mole}} = 0.5 \text{ moles } H_2$$

Moles HCl

$$0.5 \text{ moles } H_2 \times \frac{2 \text{ moles HCl}}{1 \text{ mole } H_2} = 1.0 \text{ mole HCl}$$

Grams HCl

$$1.0 \text{ mole HCl} \times \frac{36.5 \text{ grams HCl}}{1 \text{ mole HCl}} = 36.5 \text{ grams HCl} \left(\text{theoretical yield}\right)$$

$$\text{Percentage yield} = \frac{\text{Actual Yield}}{\text{Theoretical Yield}} \times 100 = \frac{18.3 \text{ grams HCl}}{36.5 \text{ grams HCl}} \times 100$$

$$= 50\%$$

50. **(D)** There are 6×10^{23} atoms, Avogadro's number, present in one mole of any element. To calculate the number of moles in 1.2×10^6 atoms of copper, divide the number of atoms by the number of atoms in one mole.

$$\frac{1.2 \times 10^6 \text{ atoms Cu}}{6 \times 10^{23} \text{ atoms/mole}} = 0.2 \times 10^{-17} = 2.0 \times 10^{-18} \text{ mole}$$

51. **(C)** When an amine reacts with an acid halide, a nucleophilic acyl substitution reaction occurs in which the amine substitutes for the halogen of the acid halide, producing an amide. It may help to see what functional groups are involved by first drawing out each line bond structure.

52. **(B)** A neutralization reaction is one in which an acid and a base react to produce a salt and water. In equation B, the acid, HCl, reacts with the base, $CaCO_3$, to produce the salt, $CaCl_2$ and initially H_2CO_3, carbonic acid.

$$2HCl + CaCO_3 \rightarrow CaCl_2 + H_2CO_3$$

However, carbonic acid is unstable and decomposes to carbon dioxide, CO_2, and water, H_2O.

$$H_2CO_3 \rightarrow CO_2 + H_2O$$

Equation A is a single displacement reaction, displacement of the H in HCl by Mg.

$$Mg + 2HCl \rightarrow MgCl_2 + H_2$$

Equation C is a double displacement reaction, in which the positive and negative ions change partners. The Ba replaces the Na and the Na replaces the Ba.

$$BaCl_2 + Na_2SO_4 \rightarrow BaSO_4 + 2NaCl$$

Equation D is a decomposition reaction, in which $KClO_3$ decomposes to KCl and O_2.

$$2KClO_3 \rightarrow 2KCl + 3O_2$$

53. **(D)** In order to determine the oxidation number of an element in a formula, it is necessary to assign oxidation numbers to all the other elements in the formula. For example, in PO_4^{-3}, oxygen has an oxidation number of –2. There are four atoms of oxygen in the formula, so the total oxidation value of oxygen is $4(-2) = -8$. Since the ion has a charge of –3, the oxidation number of phosphorus should be such that when it is combined with –8, a charge of –3 remains. Therefore, the oxidation number of phosphorus is $-3 = -8 + ?$. The value of $+5 = ?$. Oxygen is assigned an oxidation number of –2, except when it is present in a peroxide, eg. H_2O_2, when the oxidation number is –1.

54. **(B)** Denaturation involves the disruption of noncovalent intermolecular forces (in particular, hydrogen bonding, dipole-dipole interactions). Peptide bonds are covalent, and digestion involves the cleavage of these.

55. **(B)** Molarity is defined as moles of solute divided by liters of solution.

$$M = \frac{\text{moles solute}}{\text{liters solution}} = \frac{\text{grams/molar mass}}{\text{liters solution}}$$

Substituting the given values for sodium hydroxide, NaOH, (molar mass = 40 grams/mole) into the above formula gives

$$2.0\ M = \frac{x/40\ \text{gm per mole}}{0.8\ \text{liter}}$$

Solving for x gives a value of 64 grams.

56. **(B)** Since volume is constant in an autoclave, the equation

$$\frac{P_1V_1}{T_1} = \frac{P_2V_2}{T_2} \text{ reduces to } \frac{P_1}{T_1} = \frac{P_2}{T_2}$$

Temperature in the gas equations is always in Kelvin. Substituting the values given in the problem into the above equation gives

$$\frac{1\ \text{atm}}{27 + 273} = \frac{5.0\ \text{atm}}{x} \qquad x = 1500\ K$$

$$1500 - 273 = 1227°C$$

57. **(D)** The major biomolecular classes are carbohydrates (have multiple alcohol groups), nucleic acids (have phosphates, carbohydrates, and aromatic heterocycles), proteins (have amide/peptide bonds), and lipids (have long carbon chains).

58. **(A)** The correct electron configuration for magnesium, Mg, is $1s^2 2s^2 2p^6 3s^2$. Magnesium is the 12th element in counting the elements from left to right across each row. Therefore, the atomic number, the number of protons, is 12 and the number of electrons is 12 for the neutral atom. The letters s, p, d, and f indicate the type of orbital. The number in front of the symbols, as in 1s, indicates the number of the orbital, in this case 1. The superscript, as in $1s^2$, indicates the number of electrons present in the orbital, in this case 2. The electron configuration of Mg, $1s^2 2s^2 2p^6 3s^2$, shows the 12 electrons in the neutral atom.

59. **(B)** When an alkyl halide is converted to an alkene, a base is used. If the halide is primary or secondary, a strong base is required to accomplish an E2 elimination. NH_3 is a weak base but potassium t-butoxide is a strong base.

60. **(C)** $NaBH_4$ is a hydride-reducing agent that reduces aldehydes and ketones to alcohols.

61. **(D)** Copper (II) sulfide is an ionic compound because it is composed of a metal and a nonmetal. The Roman numeral II indicates that it is in the +2 oxidation state (i.e., +2 charge), thus its formula will be CuS. According to the solubility rules, sulfides are generally insoluble in water.

62. **(D)** ^1H NMR gives information about the hydrogens in a molecule. Since there are three signals, there are three kinds of hydrogen in the molecule. Choice (A) can be excluded since the molecule has only four kinds of hydrogen, and choice (C) can be excluded since the molecule has five kinds of hydrogen. After comparing the number of signals in the spectrum to the number of different kinds of hydrogen in the molecule, look at the splitting pattern and integration information. Simple splitting patterns follow the n + 1 rule, meaning that the splitting pattern for a group of hydrogens will be equal to the number of neighboring hydrogens (those on an adjacent carbon) plus one. A doublet indicates that the hydrogens represented by that signal have one neighboring hydrogen, a singlet indicates that the hydrogens represented by that signal have no neighboring hydrogens, and a septet indicates that the hydrogens represented by that signal have six neighboring hydrogens. Both remaining choices (B) and (D) are consistent with the observed splitting pattern. The next level of comparison should be the chemical shifts of the signals. Since the septet is farthest downfield, the hydrogen represented by the signal must be the most deshielded in the molecule. In choice (B), the signal for the methyl hydrogens (represented by the singlet since there are no neighboring hydrogens) would be farthest downfield (due to the adjacent oxygen)—the singlet is not the signal farthest downfield so (B) can be excluded. That leaves (D) as the correct answer, and indeed the hydrogen represented by the septet (since it has six neighboring hydrogens) is expected to be the signal farthest downfield.

63. **(A)** Resonance structures do not have atoms in different places, only pi and unshared electrons. The only structure for which this is true is choice (A).

64. **(B)** The polarity of covalent bonds is a function of the difference between the electronegativities of the bonded elements. Recall that the most electronegative element is fluorine and the closer an element is to fluorine in the periodic table, the more electronegative it is. The bond with the greatest electronegative difference and thus the most polar is answer B.

65. **(C)** Hydrogen bonding, the strongest intermolecular force, is the attraction between a partial negative atom of one molecule and a *very* partial positive hydrogen of another molecule. In order for the hydrogen to be of sufficient partial positive charge to be termed hydrogen bonding, the hydrogen must be covalently bound to N, O, or halogen. It is only when hydrogen is covalently bonded to one of these atoms that the hydrogen will be partial positive enough to participate in hydrogen bonding.

66. **(A)** The solution is 12 M, which means 12 moles of solute per liter of solution. Molality is the number of moles of solute per kilogram of solvent. The density of the solution is 1.2 g/mL, which means that 1 L of solution would have a mass of 1,200 g. Since the solution is 12 M, there would be 12 moles of solute (total mass of solute is 12 moles $\times$ 33 g/mol = 406 g) in 1 L or 1,200 g of solution. That means there is about 800 g of solvent. Molality would be 12 moles solute/0.800 kg of solvent.

67. **(C)** Cell membranes contain phospholipids, steroid hormones are lipids, and triglycerides in adipose tissue are lipids that store carbon chains for later oxidation through beta oxidation.

68. **(D)** A 1.5 M NaBr solution would contain 1.5 moles of NaBr per liter of solution. Since 100 mL is 0.100 L, then 0.15 moles of NaBr are needed (0.100 L $\times$ 1.5 moles/1 L). The formula weight of NaBr is 103 g/mol so 0.15 moles would have a mass of 15.45 g or 15.5 g. To make 100 mL of solution, water would be added to reach a total volume of 100 mL (adding 100 mL of water may result in less than 100 mL of solution because solutes can result in a contraction of volume).

69. **(C)** Phospholipids are esters of glycerol with one or more fatty acids (long-chain carboxylic acids) and a phosphate (at physiological pH, phosphate groups are negatively charged and therefore polar). The phospholipids contain a hydrophilic region (the phosphate groups) and a hydrophobic region (the long-chain fatty acids) and, when in an aqueous environment, will form a bilayer in which their hydrophobic regions are facing each other with their hydrophilic regions along the edges of the bilayer.

70. **(C)** The conformation of a protein is driven by its amino acid sequence that determines the kinds of amino acid side chains present. The hydrophilic side chains will be oriented toward the exterior of the conformation (where the polar water molecules are) and the hydrophobic side chains oriented toward the interior of the conformation (where water is excluded).

71. **(C)** Boiling point is based on molecular weight (the heavier the molecule, the higher the boiling point) and strength of intermolecular attractions. For the options available, choices (A) and (C) have the lowest molecular weight. For those two, the only intermolecular force possible is van der Waal's force (also known as London force). The more extended molecule in (A) would have more available sites for this type of force, but the more compact molecule in (C) would have fewer available sites (less surface area) so the intermolecular forces among molecules of (C) would be less extensive and it would boil at a lower temperature.

72. **(A)** The citric acid cycle oxidizes acetyl groups (produced from the pyruvate product of glycolysis) to yield substrate level ATP/GTP, as well as the reduced cofactors $FADH_2$ and NADH. The reduced cofactors are oxidized in oxidative phosphorylation with a concomitant production of ATP. Beta-oxidation is the oxidation of fatty acids to yield acetyl groups.

73. **(B)** When the Lewis structure for ammonia is examined, there are four sets of electrons around the nitrogen (a set for the bonds to each of the three hydrogens and a lone pair of electrons). These four sets of electrons will assume a tetrahedral geometry but the molecule's geometry is named from the arrangement of the *atoms* in the molecule. So if one of the tetrahedral positions is occupied by a lone pair of electrons on nitrogen, the three hydrogens will be at the other three positions creating a pyramid with nitrogen at the top and the three hydrogens at the corners of the triangular base. This molecular geometry is called trigonal pyramidal.

74. **(B)** To hydrate an alkene, there are two major options: oxymercuration-demercuration (the reagents in (A)) and hydroboration-oxidation (the reagents in (B)). Oxymercuration-demercuration yields the Markovnikov alcohol (the new H goes on the least highly substituted carbon of the alkene and the OH goes on the more highly substituted carbon of the alkene) and hydroboration-oxidation yields the anti-Markovnikov alcohol (the reverse orientation).

75. **(B)** Each carbon atom in $H_2C = CH_2$ is bonded to three other atoms, bonded by two single bonds to two hydrogen atoms and bonded by a double bond to the other carbon atom. To determine the shape of the molecule, the double bond is considered to be one set of electrons. Therefore, each carbon is assumed to have three electron sets around itself and the shape of the molecule around each carbon atom is trigonal planar with a 120° bond angle. The hybridization of the trigonal planar carbon atom is sp^2.

76. **(A)** The value of the pH measures the acidity or basicity of a solution and is defined as $pH = -\log[H^{+1}]$. Substituting $[H^{+1}] = 1 \times 10^{-5}$ into the pH equation gives a $pH = 5$.

77. **(C)** The reason why there are "gas laws" or equations that describe the behavior of gases in general is because gases behave similarly. One of the gas laws is Boyle's law which states that as the volume of a gas is increased, its pressure will decrease (or $P_1V_1 = P_2V_2$). The Kinetic Molecular Theory of

gases (the theory that summarizes our understanding of gases as a result of the observations of the gas laws) states that the kinetic energy of gas particles increases with increased Kelvin temperature (i.e., they are directly proportional).

78. **(B)** The acetate ion, CH_3COO^{-1} or Ac^{-1}, reacts with water to produce hydroxide ion and consequently the solution is basic.

$$Ac^{-1} + H_2O \rightarrow HAc + OH^{-1}$$

79. **(B)** A buffer solution is one in which the pH remains constant even when small amounts of acid or base are added to the solution. A buffer solution consists of a weak acid and its salt, or a weak base and its salt. Acetic acid, CH_3COOH, is the only weak acid present, along with its salt sodium acetate, CH_3COONa. The other acids, HCl, HNO_3, H_2SO_4, are all strong acids.

80. **(C)** The sigma bond between the two carbons is the end-to-end overlap of sp^2 hybrid orbitals (one from each of the two carbons). The pi bond is the side-to-side overlap of p orbitals. The sigma bond electron density resides between the two carbon nuclei, whereas the pi bond electron density is in two parts—one part above the sigma bond and one part below the sigma bond (kind of like a hot dog bun has two parts—a top and a bottom). The pi bond is weaker than the sigma bond and is therefore more reactive.

81. **(B)** According to the Kinetic Molecular Theory of Matter, the molecules in a solid are close together, the molecules of a liquid are farther apart, and the molecules of a gas are farthest apart. The farther apart molecules are, the more freely they can move.

82. **(D)** Grignard reagents attack carbonyl carbons. The reaction of ethyl Grignard with the ketone in choice (A) would give ethyl cyclopentanol whereas its reaction with choice (C) would give 3-ethyl-3-pentanol. Reaction of ethyl Grignard with the aldehyde in choice (D) gives 3-pentanol.

83. **(A)** To name esters, name the alkyl group attached to the oxygen first (in this case, methyl) and then name the rest of the molecule as if its a carboxylate. Choice (B) is not even an ester (it would be named 2,3-dimethylbutanoate), choice (C) is named 2-methylbutyl ethanoate, and choice (D) is also not an ester (and named 2,2-dimethylbutanoate).

84. **(D)** RNA polymerase is used to synthesize RNA.

85. **(B)** The change in free energy, ΔG, represents the energy which can be used to do work in a reaction. The change in free energy may be used to determine whether a reaction will take place as written or not.

If $\Delta G < 0$, the reaction occurs spontaneously in the direction written.

If $\Delta G > 0$, the reaction does not occur spontaneously in the direction written, but does occur spontaneously in the opposite direction.

If $\Delta G = 0$, the reaction is at equilibrium and no change occurs.

86. **(A)** Entropy is a measure of the amount of disorder in a reaction system. More freedom of movement, or disorder, of molecules is possible in a gas than in a liquid than in a solid. In equation A, a solid is converted to a solid and a gas. More disorder can be present in the reaction system in the products, where a gas is produced, than in the reactants, where a solid is used. Disorder increases. In equation B, a gas is converted to a liquid. Disorder decreases. In equation C, two different gases are converted to a liquid. Disorder decreases. In equation D, a liquid and a gas are converted to a solid. Disorder decreases.

87. **(A)** Only a change in temperature can cause a change in the equilibrium constant of a reaction. An increase in temperature causes the reaction to shift toward the direction that absorbs heat, i.e., the endothermic reaction. A decrease in temperature causes the reaction to shift toward the direction that evolves heat, i.e., the exothermic reaction. Changes in either the volume, answer B, or concentration, answer C, of one of the components in the reaction system will cause a corresponding change in the volume or concentration of another component in the system to maintain a constant equilibrium constant. A catalyst, answer D, will cause a change in the mechanism and the activation energy of a reaction but has no effect upon the equilibrium constant.

88. **(A)** Delta decay is nonsense. Neutralization is the reaction between an acid and a base. Nuclear resonance is what some nuclei do when subjected to radio waves when placed in a magnetic field (what is going on in NMR or MRI). Beta decay is the loss of a nuclear electron (beta particle) resulting in the conversion of a neutron to a proton.

89. **(A)** Meiosis is a special process in cell division comprising two nuclear divisions in rapid succession that result in four gametocytes, each containing half the number of chromosomes found in somatic cells. When the two gametes unite in fertilization, the fusion reconstitutes the diploid number of chromosomes.

90. **(A)** 0% will have white hair color.

	B	B
b	Bb	Bb
b	Bb	Bb

91. **(D)** No explanation needed.

92. **(B)** Malignant cancer (A) includes tumors that spread to neighboring tissue but have broken off and traveled though the bloodstream. Benign (C) is a tumor that is noncancerous. Sarcomic (D) refers to cancer or tumors found in bone or connective tissues.

93. **(B)** RNA polymerase I transcribes genes encoding ribosomal RNA, RNA polymerase II transcribes protein-coding genes into messenger RNAs and RNA polymerase III transcribes genes that encode transfer RNA.

94. **(B)** No explanation needed.

95. **(A)** The proper sequencing is prophase, metaphase, anaphase, and telophase. During prophase, the chromosomes condense, the nuclear membrane deteriorates, and the spindle microtubules attach to the chromosomes. During metaphase, the chromosomes move to the center of the cell. During anaphase, each kinetochore divides and the chromosomes separate. During telophase, the nuclear membrane reforms around each new daughter cell's nucleus.

96. **(D)** Exergonic, or catabolic, reactions release energy by breaking molecules down. Anabolic (A) reactions are energy requiring as they build new molecules.

97. **(D)** An endocrine gland has no ducts. It secretes directly into the blood and relies on the circulatory system to transport the secreted hormone to its target tissue.

98. **(B)** Oxytocin is responsible for producing milk. It is also the "bonding" hormone between mother and child.

99. **(D)** Each cell contains a complete set of genes. The differentiation status of a cell is determined by the subset of the gene expressed in that cell.

100. **(C)** Calcitonin causes blood calcium levels to decrease. It is produced by the parafollicular cells of the thyroid gland, and it increases in response to increased blood calcium level. Low blood calcium may result in weak bones and tetany.

101. **(A)** No explanation needed.

102. **(C)** No explanation needed.

103. **(D)** No explanation needed.

104. **(B)** The Tricuspid valve is the valve closing the orifice between the right atrium and the right ventricle of the heart. The Bicuspid valve is the valve closing the orifice between the left atrium and left ventricle of the heart. Choices C and D are not heart valves.

105. **(B)** The red blood cell would enter the right atrium through the inferior vena cava and pass into the right ventricle. The red blood cell would exit the right ventricle through the pulmonary trunk, pass through the lungs, and return to the left atrium through the pulmonary vein. From the left atrium, the red blood cell would enter the left ventricle and leave the heart through the aorta.

106. **(D)** About 97% of the oxygen transported in blood is bound to the heme portion of hemoglobin inside erythrocytes. About 3% is transported dissolved in plasma.

107. **(C)** The nuclear lamina is made of a type of cytoskeletal element called intermediate filaments. They support the nuclear envelope in animal cells.

108. **(A)** Vitamins function as coenzymes, parts of coenzymes, or parts of enzymes. Most vitamins cannot be synthesized by the body, and they are not broken down before use. Vitamins A, D, E, and K are fat-soluble vitamins.

109. **(B)** Obsessive compulsive disorder (OCD) refers to mental disorders. Trichotillomania refers to the compulsive urge to pull out one's own hair, and hoarding is the extreme attachment to personal belongings.

110. **(C)** A reaction in which the enzyme is the catalyst may be written as follows:

Enzyme + Substrate – Enzyme-Substrate complex – Enzyme + Product

The substrate binds to a specific site on the surface of the enzyme, known as the active site, after which product and enzyme are released. The enzyme is then available to bind another substrate. At low substrate concentration, the reaction rate increases sharply with increasing substrate concentration because there are abundant free enzyme molecules available to bind to an added substrate. At high substrate concentration, the reaction rate reaches a plateau as the enzyme active sites become saturated with substrate. The enzyme-substrate complex and no free enzymes are available to bind the added substrate.

111. **(C)** In a heterozygous cross-height, for example, when T represents the dominant, tall, trait and t represents the recessive, short, trait. Tt represents both parents. A cross between Tt × Tt would produce an occurrence of the dominant trait 75 percent of the time.

	T	t
T	TT	Tt
t	Tt	tt

Tall: 3 (75%)   Short: 1 (25%)

112. **(B)** The villi are specialized, finger-shaped structures in the lower intestine that are designed for absorption of digested nutrients. The alveoli are structures that allow the passage of carbon dioxide and oxygen into the lungs. Nephrons are the functional unit of the kidney. Bowman's capsule is where the filtration of the blood occurs in the nephrons of the kidney.

113. **(D)** The probability is that crossing over increases for genes far apart in a chromosome.

114. **(A)** Skin develops from the ectoderm.

115. **(B)** Vitamins A and D are fat-soluble. As fat was burned, these vitamins could have been released. Answer A is incorrect because the groups were told to keep their diet the same.

116. **(A)** One-fourth of their offspring, on average, will have silver fur. Choices C and D are not a possibility because none of the parents have silver fur.

	B	b
B	BB	Bb
b	Bb	bb

117. **(C)** The T-helper cells (T_4) cells are the most infected.

118. **(A)** Digestion begins in the mouth and salivary amylase breaks down starches.

119. **(B)** No explanation needed.

120. **(D)** Disordered eating patterns occur when concerns about dieting, food restriction, fear of becoming overweight, and dissatisfaction with body image interfere with normal daily life. Bulimia nervosa is an eating disorder in which a person eats a great deal of food and then vomits or uses other purging methods. Individuals with binge-eating disorder eat large amounts of food frequently and repeatedly. Choice (C) is a nonsense answer.

121. **(B)** A major function of white blood cells (WBC) is to fight infections.

122. **(A)** Because mitochondria use oxygen to produce ATP, the greater oxygen consumption indicates that tissue A has either a greater number of mitochondria, larger mitochondria, or more enzymatic activity then tissue B.

Figure 1.

123. **(D)** A large sodium (Na^+) influx into the cell results in the resting potential becoming more positive. An action potential is produced when the charge difference across the plasma membrane reverses and then returns to the resting

condition which requires the movement of sodium (Na⁺) ions into the cell. There is generally a higher concentration of potassium (K⁺) ions inside the cell than outside, and conversely a higher concentration of sodium (Na⁺) ions outside the cell than inside. Following the action potential, the sodium-potassium exchange pump restores ion concentrations by moving sodium (Na⁺) ions out of the cell and potassium (K⁺) ions into the cell.

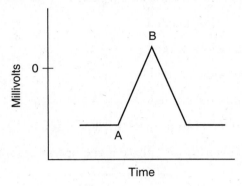

Figure 2.

124. **(C)** The pancreas produces insulin and glucagon. The adrenal glands produce adrenaline and noradrenaline. The pineal gland produces melatonin and serotonin.

125. **(B)** Hormones are secreted in the blood from a specific gland and are distributed by the blood to a specific target site. Blood (answer B) plays a role in the general distribution of hormones.

126. **(A)** In general, the smaller the animal, the farther to the right its curve will be. Therefore, small animals with high metabolic rates and correspondingly high oxygen requirements tend to have hemoglobin that unloads more readily.

Figure 3.

127. **(A)** Vesicles (answer A) deliver cargo proteins such as penicillin to the cell plasma membrane during exocytosis. Answer B is incorrect because the condensing of DNA during prophase by condensin occurs during the cell cycle and would not lead to reduced protein secretion. Answer C is incorrect because there is no indication that the mutant strain has issues with this cytoskeletal protein. Answer D is incorrect because transcription and translation are not affected.

128. **(B)** Neurotransmitters act as a ligand to bind and open ligand-gated channels on a postsynaptic neuron. Once these channels are opened, an influx of ions starts a new action potential in the postsynaptic neuron.

129. **(C)** Glycolipids and glycoproteins are found on the extracellular side of the cell plasma membrane. The number and type of sugars form a unique pattern that helps cells recognize other cells.

130. **(D)** No explanation needed.

131. **(D)** No explanation needed.

132. **(B)** No explanation needed.

133. **(A)** No explanation needed.

134. **(B)** Apoptosis refers to programmed cell death.

135. **(D)** The log (logarithmic) phase is the upward growth of bacteria in culture.

Figure 4.

136. **(C)** Since it multiplies by binary fission at a generation time of 30 minutes, the population within 2 hours (12 noon–2:00 P.M.) is 2 at 12:30, 4 at 1 P.M., 8 at 1:30 P.M., and 16 at 2:00 P.M.

Passage 1

A dreaded disease is striking California's coast live oaks with the ferocity of an oak-tree Ebola virus, <u>causing the trees to sprout sores, hemorrhage sap, and become</u> 137
<u>infested with beetles and various fungi.</u> The trees die within a few weeks of their first symptoms.

A pathologist at the University of California, Davis, announced that his team had found the cause of the disease dubbed "Sudden Oak Death". <u>The tree-slayer is a new</u>
<u>member of the genus Phytophthora,</u> whose name means "plant destroyer". Its kin 139
include pathogens responsible for the Irish potato famine and die-offs in Australian eucalyptus forests and European oak groves. "We don't know if the new species was just recently introduced, or if it has always been here and something else has changed that has allowed it to go crazy," one pathologist says.

<u>The first trees to succumb to the plague 5 years ago were tan oaks, which often</u> 138; 140
<u>grow in the understory of redwood forests. Last year the disease began hitting large</u> 142; 144
<u>numbers of coast live oaks, the signature species in scenic coastal woodlands.</u>
<u>Alarmingly, the pathogen has begun to blight another species, the black oak.</u>

Knowing the culprit doesn't make the outlook much brighter. <u>"Fungicides can</u> 143
<u>save individual oaks," says one pathologist, "but we can't go to Mount Tamalpais</u>
<u>and spray 10,000 trees."</u> And prevention is largely limited to warning people not to carry oak firewood to uninfected areas. The Sierra Nevada hosts black oaks, and
<u>pathologists fear deadly spores could strike groves in beloved Yosemite Valley.</u> 141

Reprinted with permission from *Science*, Vol 289, August 2000. Page 859.

137. **(B)** No explanation needed.

138. **(A)** No explanation needed.

139. **(C)** No explanation needed.

140. **(A)** No explanation needed.

141. **(B)** No explanation needed.

142. **(A)** No explanation needed.

143. **(B)** No explanation needed.

144. **(D)** No explanation needed.

Passage 2

<u>Non-adherence to medication therapy results in numerous adverse effects such as</u> 150
<u>increased hospitalizations and even death. Additionally, it costs the U.S. healthcare</u>
<u>system billions of dollars</u> each year. It is important to assess patients' adherence to medications.

Improper medication adherence encompasses an assortment of behaviors. <u>These</u>
<u>include not having a prescription filled, forgetting or intentionally not taking a</u> 147
<u>medication, consuming an incorrect amount of a medication, taking a medication</u>

at the wrong time, ceasing therapy too soon, or continuing therapy after advised to discontinue. All forms of improper medication-taking behavior may jeopardize health outcomes.

145   Measuring medication-taking behavior is often difficult. The ideal method of measurement should be simultaneously unobtrusive (to avoid patient sensitization and maximize cooperation), objective (to produce discrete and reproducible data

146   for each subject), and practical (to maximize portability and minimize cost). Refill records, pill counts, electronic medication dispensers/caps, patient surveys (interviews), blood-drug level monitoring, and urine assay for drug metabolites can be used as clues to identify improper medication use.

148   Before altering therapy based on the assumption that a patient is taking a medication as prescribed, practitioners should ascertain patient's medication-taking behavior. This becomes especially important when modifying dosages of medications. Due to the advantages and disadvantages of each measurement, it is important for practitioners to use a combination of methods to assess a patient's medication-usage behavior and relate these findings to the patient's clinical presentation.

145.   **(C)** The passage specifically states that the ideal method of measurement should be simultaneously unobtrusive (to avoid patient sensitization and maximize cooperation), objective (to produce discrete and reproducible data for each subject), and practical (to maximize portability and minimize cost).

146.   **(D)** According to the passage, half-life tables, nucleic acid levels, and patient examinations are not techniques for assessing patient's medication usage. Answer D lists techniques used to assess medication usage.

147.   **(A)** According to the passage, improper medication adherence includes those items listed in answer A. Answers B, C, and D are not true.

148.   **(A)** No explanation needed.

149.   **(D)** As the content of the passage primarily discusses the behaviors that encompass medication nonadherence, as well as methods used to measure medication-taking behaviors, answer D represents the most appropriate proposed title. The passage does not address other factors impacting U.S. health care costs, nor does it discuss prevention of or interventions to treat medication nonadherence.

150.   **(B)** Medications may still work even if the patient does not take it as advised, therefore ruling out A. C is not the answer because the passage specifically stated billions and not trillions, and no mention of lawsuits was made. Also, no mention of suicides was made. The first sentence of the passage discussed that nonadherence to medication therapy results in numerous adverse effects such as increased hospitalizations and even death. Therefore, the answer is B.

Passage 3

As many as 50 million Americans have high blood pressure, defined as a systolic blood pressure ≥140 mm Hg and a diastolic blood pressure ≥90 mm Hg. Although blood pressure generally increases with age, the onset of hypertension most often occurs in the third, fourth, or fifth decade of life. The prevalence of hypertension in the elderly population (age ≥ 65 years) is approximately 63% in whites and 76% in blacks. In younger generations (35 to 45 years of age), the prevalence is markedly different with 44% among black men, 37% among black women, 26% among white men, and 17% among white women.　158 151 152

A specific cause of sustained hypertension cannot be found in the vast majority of individuals with high blood pressure. Genetic factors have been suggested to play a role in essential hypertension due to the fact that high blood pressure may be hereditary. Evidence that a single gene may account for specific subtypes of hypertension has also been suggested. Genetic traits include high angiotensin levels, increased aldosterone and other adrenal steroids, and high sodium-lithium countertransport. More direct approaches for preventing or treating hypertension could be achieved by identifying individuals with these traits. Factors such as sodium excretion and transport rates, blood pressure response to plasma volume expansion, electrolyte homeostasis, and glomerular filtration rate help explain the predisposition for a person to develop hypertension.　155 154

Anti-hypertensive drug therapy should be individualized according to various patient characteristics and fundamental pathophysiologic circumstances. Dietary intake has been shown to be similar in all races but blacks ingest less potassium and calcium than whites. Supplemental potassium and calcium has shown to cause a modest reduction in blood pressure in some studies. Therefore, it would seem reasonable to ascertain the affects of increasing the amount of potassium and calcium in the diet as part of the non-pharmacologic regulation of hypertension. The initial treatment for hypertension is life-style unless target-organ damage is present. These changes include sodium reduction, weight reduction, increased physical activity, and ethanol reduction or abstinence. In terms of target-organ damage, diuretics and beta-blockers are first-line therapy. Control of blood pressure and prevention of cardiovascular morbidity and mortality are the goals of antihypertensive therapy. By maintaining arterial blood pressure below 140 mm Hg systolic and 90 mm Hg diastolic and by controlling other risk factors such as smoking, hyperlipidemia, and diabetes, morbidity and mortality may be averted.　156 153 157

151. **(B)** No explanation needed.

152. **(C)** The passage states that, in both younger and elderly generations respectively, the prevalence of hypertension in black individuals is greater than in white individuals.

153. **(B)** Although all choices may represent life-style changes, according to the passage life-style changes that are suggested to lower blood pressure include sodium restriction, weight reduction, increased physical activity, and ethanol reduction or abstinence. Weight gain and increased stress may increase blood pressure.

154. **(B)** No explanation needed.

155. **(D)** No explanation needed.

156. **(A)** No explanation needed.

157. **(D)** The passage states that by maintaining arterial blood pressure below 140 mm Hg systolic and 90 mm Hg diastolic and by controlling other risk factors, morbidity and mortality may be averted.

158. **(C)** No explanation needed.

Passage 4

We humans sense old age through feeling those creaky joints or observing those graying hairs but, according to Apfeld and Kenyon reporting in a recent issue of
161   Nature, the nematode worm senses its age by smelling and tasting the environment. These investigators show that worms with defective olfactory organs (that would normally detect odor molecules in the environment) live longer than their comrades with a keener sense of smell. By comparing these worms with other mutant nematodes that live an unusually long time, the researchers found clues to how a reduced ability to "smell the roses" might lengthen lifespan.

162   The worm's olfactory sense organs—amphids on the head and plasmids on the tail—are composed of a cluster of nerve cells, the ends of which are modified into cilia. The cilia are encircled by a sheath and a socket cell that form a pore in the worm's skin through which the tips of the cilia protrude. Odor molecules and soluble compounds bind to G protein-coupled receptors (similar to the olfactory and taste receptors of mammals) located at the tip of each cilium. Worms with a poor sense of smell—because their olfactory organs have defective or absent cilia, blocked pores, or damaged sheaths—live much longer, yet are otherwise normal (for exam-
160   ple, their feeding and reproductive behaviors are unchanged). Mutations in TAX-4—a channel regulated by cyclic GMP that sits under the G-protein-coupled receptor and transduces the sensory signals into electrical impulses—also imbue the worm with a longer life.

      But mutations in the worms olfactory machinery are not the only defects that
163   extend its lifespan. In an earlier study, Kenyon's group found that defects in the
164   reproductive system could prolong life by decreasing the activity of DAF-2 (a receptor for an insulin-like molecule) and increasing the activity of DAF-16 (a transcrip-
165   tion factor). By looking at worms defective in both sensory perception and reproduction, Apfeld and Kenyon worked out a putative pathway through which smell might influence a worm's longevity.

      An environmental signal, perhaps produced by bacteria (the worm's favorite food), binds to G protein-coupled olfactory receptors on sensory cilia activating
166   TAX-4, which then incites electrical activity in the sensory neurons. This activity triggers secretory vesicles in the neurons to release insulin-like molecules, which bind to DAF-2 and activate the insulin-like signaling pathway. This then switches
159   on genes that will ensure the worm dies at the usual age of 2 weeks. A reduced abil-

ity to sense olfactory cues would result in a decrease in DAF-2 activation and an   168
increase in life-span.

This chain of events is not proven, but insulin-like molecules that might bind to
DAF-2 have been identified in the nematode. Such a pathway would also make
physiological sense. After all, if food is scarce it may behoove the worm to live
longer to ensure that it has the chance to produce its full quota of offspring. A
scarcity of food also promotes longevity in rodents and primates). But so far it seems   167
that in these more complicated creatures a poor sense of smell is not a harbinger of
a ripe old age.

_____

Reprinted with permission from *Science*, Vol 287, January 2000. Page 54.

159. **(D)** No explanation needed.

160. **(A)** No explanation needed.

161. **(D)** No explanation needed.

162. **(C)** No explanation needed.

163. **(D)** No explanation needed.

164. **(A)** No explanation needed.

165. **(B)** No explanation needed.

166. **(A)** No explanation needed.

167. **(D)** No explanation needed.

168. **(B)** No explanation needed.

Passage 5

Presents of the United States are not like you and me. A personality assessment
presented at the American Psychological Association conference in Washington,   169
D.C., shows that, compared to the public they serve, presidents are more likely
to be extroverted, assertive, and disagreeable. They're also less modest and straight-   176
forward.

Says who? Historians who have written book-length biographies of Oval Office   170
occupants. Psychologist Steve Rubenzer of the Mental Health and Mental   171
Retardation Authority of Harris County in Houston, Texas, and colleagues asked the
biographers to fill out three standard personality inventories on their subjects, basing   172
answers on the presidents' behavior during the 5 years preceding their reigns. The
researchers compared the presidents' scores to population norms and compared the
profiles of successful commanders-in-chief with those history hasn't smiled upon.

"Great" presidents, such as Jefferson and Lincoln, they find, "are attentive to their   173
emotions, willing to question traditional values ... imaginative, and more interested
in art and beauty than less successful Chief Executives." They're also more assertive,
stubborn, and "tender-minded," which is a measure of concern for the less fortu-   174

nate. Rubenzer hasn't analyzed the current presidential contenders yet—<u>he prefers</u>
175 <u>to have at least three "unbiased" historians fill out the forms for each president or</u>
<u>presidential wanna-be.</u>

_____

Reprinted with permission from *Science*, Vol 289, August 2000. Page 859.

169. **(C)** No explanation needed.

170. **(A)** No explanation needed.

171. **(B)** No explanation needed.

172. **(D)** No explanation needed.

173. **(B)** No explanation needed.

174. **(B)** No explanation needed.

175. **(A)** No explanation needed.

176. **(A)** No explanation needed.

Passage 6

178 <u>Drug interactions, a common type of drug-related problem, are categorized as phar-</u>
<u>macokinetic, pharmacodynamic, or a combination of both. Pharmacokinetic drug</u>
180 <u>interactions include changes in absorption, distribution, excretion, and metabolism;</u>
whereas, pharmacodynamic drug interactions may lead to antagonistic or synergistic effects. Not all drug interactions are undesirable, in fact, many drug interactions
are used to produce desirable effects. Patients who take drugs with narrow therapeutic indices and drugs that interfere with the pharmacokinetic properties of other
181 drugs are at increased risk of experiencing a drug interaction. <u>Also, patients who</u>
<u>take multiple medications per day or take multiple doses of medications per day are</u>
<u>at increased risk.</u> Because renal transplant patients take immunosuppressive agents
that have narrow therapeutic indices and are subjected to multiple medications per
day, they are vulnerable to experiencing adverse drug events. <u>To prevent adverse</u>
183 <u>drug interactions, an alternative therapy should be considered when possible or the</u>
<u>dose or schedule of the drugs should be adjusted to reduce the occurrence of an</u>
<u>adverse experience.</u> Additionally, adequate monitoring to prevent and detect adverse
effects is an essential part of patient care.

A common pharmacokinetic interaction involves drugs that interfere with the
182 absorption of other medications. <u>Drugs that bind and decrease the gastrointestinal</u>
<u>absorption of another drug, such as cholestyramine decreasing the absorption of</u>
<u>tacrolimus,</u> typically can be prevented by administering the agents two to three hours
177 apart from each other. <u>Prokinetic agents interfere with the rate of absorption. Since</u>
179 <u>many transplant patients take prokinetic agents, such as metochlopromide, this may</u>
<u>increase the bioavailability of other medications. This is of significant importance</u>
<u>since immunosuppressive agents have narrow therapeutic indices and toxicity may</u>

result from this interaction. If the prokinetic agent cannot be avoided, careful mon- 184
itoring (e.g., serum drug levels, clinical presentation of patient) and adjustments
should be made to prevent immunosuppressant toxicity.

177. **(C)** No explanation needed.

178. **(B)** The passage states that drug interactions are characterized as (1) pharmacokinetic, (2) pharmacodynamic, or (3) a combination of both.

179. **(C)** No explanation needed.

180. **(B)** No explanation needed.

181. **(A)** No explanation needed.

182. **(D)** No explanation needed.

183. **(B)** No explanation needed.

184. **(C)** No explanation needed.

185. **(D)** We use the Fundamental Theorem of Calculus for integrals.

$$\int_2^3 \left(10x^4\right) dx = \frac{10x^5}{5}\bigg|_2^3 = 2x^5\bigg|_2^3 = \left(2\cdot(3)^5\right) - \left(2\cdot(2)^5\right) = 486 - 64 = 422$$

186. **(C)** We list the nine values in increasing order: 3, 5, 6, 8, 9, 11, 16, 24, 42.
The median value occurs at the middle position in the list, that is the fifth
entry in the list. So the median is 9.

187. **(A)** Use the conversion formula

Celsius Temp = $\frac{5}{9}$ · (Fahrenheit Temp − 32) = $\frac{5}{9}$ · (86 − 32) = $\frac{5}{9}$ · (54) = 30.

188. **(A)** We use the Quotient Rule for logarithms.

$$\ln\left(\frac{a}{b}\right) = \ln(a) - \ln(b) = 12 - 3 = 9$$

189. **(B)** 12 ounces times 30 mL per ounce = 360 mL total volume

15 mL (x) 3 doses per day = 45 mL per day; 360 mL divided by 45 mL =
8 days

An alternative solution: Since 30 mL = one ounce and 15 mL = one dose,
then each ounce has two doses. Twelve ounces times two doses per ounce =
24 doses; divide by 3 doses per day to obtain 8 days.

190. **(A)** We compute $\dfrac{4+5+11+18+20+22+34+35+38}{9} = \dfrac{187}{9} \approx 20.77$.

191. **(B)** We use the Quotient Rule for derivatives.

$$\frac{d}{dx}\left(\frac{f(x)}{g(x)}\right) = \frac{g(x) \cdot f'(x) - g'(x) \cdot f(x)}{\left(g(x)\right)^2} = \frac{(4+x)\left(3x^2\right) - \left(x^3\right)(1)}{(4+x)^2}$$

$$= \frac{12x^2 + 3x^3 - x^3}{(4+x)^2} = \frac{12x^2 + 2x^3}{(4+x)^2}$$

192. **(A)** A square has the same dimensions on all four sides. Area is calculated by multiplying two sides together. Thus, 210 feet · 210 feet = 44,100 square feet.

Two other lessons should be learned from this question. (1) Since 210 · 210 means the one digit will be a zero, any answer without a zero in the one's place cannot be a correct answer. (2) Estimation can be a means of identifying possible answers. In this case, one can multiply 200 · 200 to get 40,000. Since 210 is greater than 200, the answer must be greater than 40,000. Any number smaller than that cannot be the correct answer.

193. **(B)** Use the Quotient Rule for derivatives.

$$\frac{d}{dx}\left(\frac{f(x)}{g(x)}\right) = \frac{g(x) \cdot f'(x) - g'(x) \cdot f(x)}{(g(x))^2} = \frac{(x^2+3)(1) - (2x)(x)}{(x^2+3)^2}$$

$$= \frac{x^2 + 3 - 2x^2}{(x^2+3)^2} = \frac{3 - x^2}{(x^2+3)^2}$$

194. **(C)** Calculate each number separately such that $10^2 = 100$ and $9^2 = 81$. Added together they equal 181. 181 can also be expressed as 1.81×10^2.

195. **(C)** We calculate the distance using the formula

$$\sqrt{(x_2 - x_1)^2 + (y_2 - y_1)^2} = \sqrt{(-2-6)^2 + (5-8)^2} = \sqrt{64+9} = \sqrt{73}.$$

196. **(D)** Let x = the number of dimes, and $2x$ = the number of quarters. This yields the equation $10 \cdot x + 25 \cdot 2x$ = total money in cents. So, we solve the equation

$$10 \cdot x + 25 \cdot 2x = 660$$

$$60x = 660 \Rightarrow x = \frac{660}{60} = 11$$

Thus, John has 11 dimes, so $11 \cdot 2 = 22$, which means he has 22 quarters.

197. **(B)** We add the expressions by finding a common denominator.

198. **(B)** Given the function $f(x) = 3x - 1$, we solve for y in the equation $x = 3y - 1$.

$$x = 3y - 1$$

$$x + 1 = 3y \Rightarrow y = \frac{x+1}{3}$$

199. **(D)** As x approaches 2 from the right-hand side, the values of $f(x)$ approach 0.

200. **(A)** As x approaches 2 from the left-hand side, the values of $f(x)$ approach -4.

201. **(B)** The left-hand and right-hand limits are not equal.

202. **(B)** The *Product Rule* for logarithms states that

$$\log(M) + \log(N) = \log(M \cdot N)$$

203. **(C)** From 12 Noon to 6 P.M. is 6 hours. At a speed of 100 kilometers (km) per hour, the truck will travel 600 kilometers. Several conversions can be used to change kilometers to miles. One mile = 1.6 kilometers; one kilometer = 0.62 miles

For this problem 600 km (x) 0.62 miles per km = 372 miles.

204. **(A)** We compute $(0.32) \cdot (800) = 256$.

205. **(A)** We use the integration rule.

$$\int_{e}^{e^2} \left(\frac{6}{x} \right) dx = 6\ln(x) \Big]_{e}^{e^2} = 6\ln(e^2) - 6\ln(e) = 6 \cdot 2 - 6 \cdot 1 = 6.$$

206. **(B)** We use the Product Rule for derivatives

$$\frac{d}{dx}\big(f(x) \cdot g(x)\big) = f'(x) \cdot g(x) + f(x) \cdot g'(x)$$

and the fact that $\dfrac{d}{dx} e^{2x} = 2e^{2x}$ and $\dfrac{d}{dx} \sin(x) = \cos(x)$.

207. **(D)** Since x approaches positive infinity, the numerator and denominator are each dominated by their highest-powered terms, that is,

$$\lim_{x \to \infty} \left(\frac{8x^6 + 4x^2 - 10x + 5}{7x^6 + 12x^3} \right) \to \frac{8x^6}{7x^6} = \frac{8}{7}$$

208. **(A)** When a coin is tossed only two outcomes are possible, heads or tails. No matter how many times a coin has been tossed, the probability on any one toss is 50 : 50 or 1 chance out of 2 for either heads or tails. Thus, there is a 50% chance for heads (or tails) on this toss.

209. **(D)** The projectile hits the ground when the height equals zero. So we solve the equation $-0.006x^2 + 12x$.

$$-0.006x^2 + 12x = 0$$

$$x(-0.006x^2 + 12) = 0$$

$$x = 0, \; -0.006x + 12 = 0 \Rightarrow x = \frac{-12}{-0.006} = 2{,}000$$

210. **(C)** Let x = the original price in dollars. The sale price is given by the original price minus the percent discount. Thus, we have the equation

$$210 = x - 0.30x \Rightarrow 210 = 0.7x \Rightarrow x = \frac{210}{0.7} = 300.$$

211. **(A)** The probability event A does not occur is given by the formula:

Probability that A does not occur = 1 – probability of A = $1 - \dfrac{5}{9} = \dfrac{4}{9}$.

212. **(D)** The expression $4x = \dfrac{1}{2}$ can be solved by dividing both sides of the

equation by four to provide the new equation $x = \dfrac{1}{2} \div 4$.

The four can become $\dfrac{4}{1}$. Now the equation is $x = \dfrac{1}{2} \div \dfrac{4}{1}$.

This rearranges for the purpose of division to become $x = \dfrac{1}{2} \times \dfrac{1}{4}$.

Solving yields $x = \dfrac{1}{8}$.

213. **(C)** There were 730 + 185 = 915 patients who had Drug A or Drug B. There were 1,500 total patients.

Thus, probability $\dfrac{915}{1{,}500} = 0.61 = 61\% \approx 60\%$.

214. **(A)** The percentage of patients prescribed Drug D was

$$\frac{466}{1{,}500} \approx 0.31 = 31\%.$$

Thus, the percentage of patients who did NOT have a prescription for Drug D was 1 – 0.31 = 0.69 = 69%.

215. **(C)** 1 milligram (mg) = 1000 micrograms (mcg). You must convert either the concentration of the Digoxin Injection (500 mcg/2 mL = 0.5 mg/2 mL) or the dose desired (0.25 mg = 250 mcg) so that you are working with numbers that have the same dimension.

$$\frac{2 \text{ mL}}{500 \text{ mcg}} \cdot \frac{1{,}000 \text{ mcg}}{1 \text{ mg}} = \frac{4 \text{ mL}}{1 \text{ mg}}$$

So we have the ratio $\dfrac{4 \text{ mL}}{1 \text{ mg}} \cdot \dfrac{0.25}{0.25} = \dfrac{1 \text{ mL}}{0.25 \text{ mg}}$

216. **(A)** We calculate the slope using the formula $\dfrac{\Delta y}{\Delta x} = \dfrac{-6-3}{4-10} = \dfrac{-9}{-6} = \dfrac{3}{2}$.

217. **(B)** Given the function $y = f(x)$, if k is a positive number, then $y = f(x - k)$ shifts the graph of f to the right by k units. Thus, $y = f(x - 3)$ shifts the original graph 3 units to the right.

218. **(B)** We plug into the given formula

$$\text{CrCl} = \left(\frac{(140 - 58)}{(72 \cdot 2.6)}\right) \cdot (76) = \left(\frac{82}{187}\right) \cdot (76) \approx 33.$$

219. **(A)** Since f^{-1} represents the inverse function for f, the domain of f^{-1} corresponds to the range of f.

220. **(A)** The derivative of f is positive when the graph of f has a positive slope. Of the possible choices, the only valid interval is $x > 11.5$.

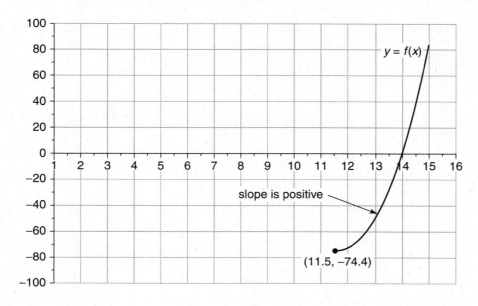

221. **(B)** The graph is concave down when $-\infty < x < 9$.

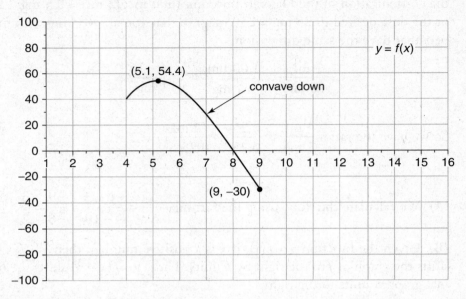

222. **(A)** A relative maximum corresponds to a "peak" on the graph.

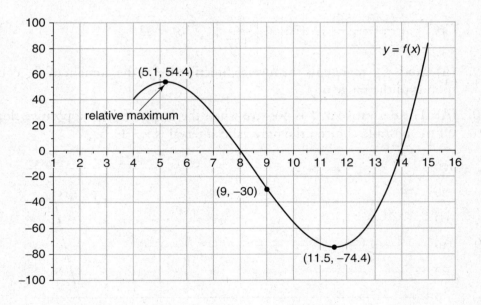

223. **(C)** Note that $\lim\limits_{x\to 8}\left(\dfrac{f(x)-f(8)}{x-8}\right)=f'(8)=$ the slope of the graph when

$x=8$.

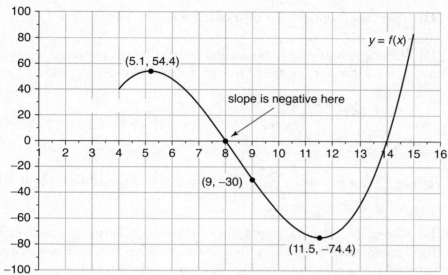

224. **(A)** We compute $\dfrac{f(4)-f(2)}{4-2}=\dfrac{64-8}{2}=28$.

225. **(D)**
$$\sqrt{45}=\sqrt{9\cdot 5}=3\sqrt{5}$$
$$\sqrt{80}=\sqrt{16\cdot 5}=4\sqrt{5}$$
$$3\sqrt{5}+4\sqrt{5}=7\sqrt{5}$$

226. **(A)** The formula for slope (m) of a line is $m=\dfrac{y_2-y_1}{x_2-x_1}$.

Substituting the values into the formula yields $m=\dfrac{5-1}{5-1}=1$.

227. **(C)** Arrange the values in order from least to highest: 8, 9, 9, 9, 10, 10, 10, 11, 12, 12. Because there are an even number of values, you will need to find the average of the two values that fall in the middle of the list (10 and 10 as underlined). Add 10 + 10 = 20. Then, divide 20 by 2, 20 ÷ 2 = 10. The median value is 10.

228. **(D)** There are 5 options for each of the 3 letters. Total = 5^3 = 125.

229. **(D)** If the graph of f has a horizontal tangent line at the point where $x = a$, then $f'(a) = 0$. Applying the Quotient Rule for derivatives yields

$$f'(x) = \frac{(x+2)(1)-(x)(1)}{(x+2)^2} = \frac{x+2-x}{(x+2)^2} = \frac{2}{(x+2)^2} \; .$$

Setting $f'(x) = 0$ yields $\dfrac{2}{(x+2)^2} = 0 \Rightarrow 2 = 0$. Thus, the graph of f never has a horizontal tangent line.

230. **(D)** Choice (A) demonstrates a linear relationship between x and y. Choice (B) demonstrates a quadratic relationship between x and y. Choice (C) demonstrates a cubic relationship between x and y.

231. **(C)** With the understanding that the symbol $\cup$ means the set of elements either in A or B or in both, and the symbol $\cap$ means the set that contains all those elements that A and B have in common, we use the formula

$P(A \cup B) = P(A) + P(B) - P(A \cap B) = 0.35 + 0.22 - 0.09 = 0.48.$

232. **(C)** The exact area of the shaded region is given by the definite integral $\displaystyle\int_{1}^{\sqrt{e}} \frac{3}{x} \, dx$.

Using the Fundamental Theorem of Calculus yields

$$\int_{1}^{\sqrt{e}} \frac{3}{x} \, dx = 3\ln|x|\Big]_{1}^{\sqrt{e}} = \left(3\ln\left(\sqrt{e}\right) - 3\ln(1)\right) = 3 \cdot \left(\frac{1}{2}\right) - 0 = 1.5.$$

Appendix: Weights, Measures, and Conversions

LENGTH

1 inch (in.)		= 2.54 cm
1 foot (ft.)	= 12 in.	= 0.3048 m
1 yard (yd.)	= 3 ft.	= 0.9144 m
1 mile (mi.)	= 1,760 yd.	= 1.6093 km
1 millimeter (mm)		= 0.0394 in.
1 centimeter (cm)	= 10 mm	= 0.3937 in.
1 meter (m)	= 1,000 mm	= 1.0936 yd.
1 kilometer (km)	= 1,000 m	= 0.6214 mi.

AREA

1 square inch (in^2)		= 6.4516 cm^2
1 square foot (ft^2)	= 144 in^2	= 0.093 m^2
1 square yard (yd^2)	= 9 ft^2	= 0.8361 m^2
1 acre	= 4840 yd^2	= 4046.86 m^2
1 square mile (mi^2)	= 640 acres	= 2.59 km^2
1 square centimeter (cm^2)	= 100 mm^2	= 0.155 in^2
1 square meter (m^2)	= 10,000 cm^2	= 1.196 yd^2
1 hectare (ha)	= 10,000 m^2	= 2.4711 acres
1 square kilometer (km^2)	= 100 ha	= 0.3861 mi^2

WEIGHT

1 ounce (oz.)	= 437.5 grains	= 28.35 g
1 pound (lb.)	= 16 oz.	= 0.4536 kg
1 kilogram (kg)	= 1,000 g	= 2.2 lb.
1 short ton	= 2,000 lb.	= 0.9072 metric ton
1 long ton	= 2,240 lb.	= 1.0161 metric ton
1 milligram (mg)		= 0.0154 grain
1 gram (g)	= 1,000 mg	= 0.0353 oz.
1 tonne	= 1,000 kg	= 1.1023 short tons
1 tonne		= 0.9842 long ton

VOLUME

1 cubic inch (in^3)		= 16.387 cm^3
1 cubic foot (ft^3)	= 1,728 $in.^3$	= 0.028 m^3
1 cubic yard (yd^3)	= 27 $ft.^3$	= 0.7646 m^3
1 cubic centimeter (cm^3)		= 0.061 in^3
1 cubic decimeter (dm^3)	= 1,000 cm^3	= 0.0353 ft^3
1 cubic meter (m^3)	= 1,000 dm^3	= 1.3079 yd^3
1 liter (L)	= 1 dm^3	= 0.2642 gal.
1 hectoliter (hL)	= 100 L	= 2.8378 bushel (bu.)
1 fluid ounce (fl. oz.)		= 29.573 mL
1 liquid pint (pt.)	= 16 fl. oz.	= 0.4732 L
1 liquid quart (qt.)	= 2 pt.	= 0.946 L
1 gallon (gal.)	= 4 qt.	= 3.7853 L

TEMPERATURE

$$Celsius° = \frac{5}{9}(F° - 32°)$$

$$Fahrenheit° = \frac{9}{5}(C°) + 32$$

$$Kelvin = 273.15 + C°$$

Index